# Lumbar Spine Access Surgery

AF400166

Joseph R. O'Brien • JeffreyJeffrey B. Weinreb
Joseph C. Babrowicz

Editors

# Lumbar Spine Access Surgery

A Comprehensive Guide to Anterior
and Lateral Approaches

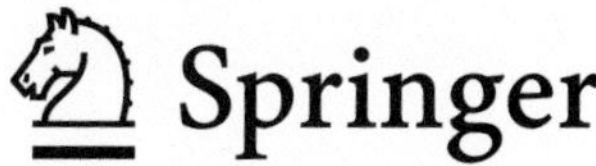
Springer

*Editors*
Joseph R. O'Brien
Aligned Orthopaedics
Bethesda, MD, USA

Joseph C. Babrowicz
Vascular Surgery
Inova Health System
Falls Church, VA, USA

Jeffrey B. Weinreb
Department of Orthopedic Surgery
The George Washington University
Washington, DC, USA

ISBN 978-3-031-48036-2     ISBN 978-3-031-48034-8   (eBook)
https://doi.org/10.1007/978-3-031-48034-8

© The Editor(s) (if applicable) and The Author(s), under exclusive license to Springer Nature Switzerland AG 2023

This work is subject to copyright. All rights are solely and exclusively licensed by the Publisher, whether the whole or part of the material is concerned, specifically the rights of translation, reprinting, reuse of illustrations, recitation, broadcasting, reproduction on microfilms or in any other physical way, and transmission or information storage and retrieval, electronic adaptation, computer software, or by similar or dissimilar methodology now known or hereafter developed.

The use of general descriptive names, registered names, trademarks, service marks, etc. in this publication does not imply, even in the absence of a specific statement, that such names are exempt from the relevant protective laws and regulations and therefore free for general use.

The publisher, the authors, and the editors are safe to assume that the advice and information in this book are believed to be true and accurate at the date of publication. Neither the publisher nor the authors or the editors give a warranty, expressed or implied, with respect to the material contained herein or for any errors or omissions that may have been made. The publisher remains neutral with regard to jurisdictional claims in published maps and institutional affiliations.

This Springer imprint is published by the registered company Springer Nature Switzerland AG
The registered company address is: Gewerbestrasse 11, 6330 Cham, Switzerland

Printed on acid-free paper

Paper in this product is recyclable

# Acknowledgements

I would like to acknowledge Claire van Ekdom and Gabrielle Heller for their thoughtful and diligent work on this textbook. I have no doubt that they will make incredible surgeons one day. I am grateful to my fellow editors: Joe Babrowicz, who has been my co-captain in many operating rooms, and Jeff Weinreb, who is growing into a leader in our field. I am grateful to all the authors of this textbook. Through our collaboration, we have strengthened the bridge between surgical specialties and made these surgical techniques more accessible to patients. My greatest appreciation is for my wife, Janet, and my sons, Brad and Alex.

—Joseph R. O'Brien

To my wife Jessie, thank you for supporting me throughout training and for your indispensable advice.

To my sons Seth and Elias, thank you for making every day exciting and reminding me of the important things in life.

To my family, friends, and mentors, thank you for everything.

—Jeff B. Weinreb

Thank you to my many spine surgery colleagues for the professional relationships and friendships we have developed over the years. Also, thank you to the many patients we have had the privilege to care for together. Finally, and most importantly, thank you to my beautiful supportive wife and amazing, brilliant children. Surgery as a profession is not easy on the surgeon or those around them. It is by the unending support of family that we can do this to our best ability.

—Joseph C. Babrowicz

# Contents

**Part VII   Additional Considerations for Lumbar Spine
Access Surgery**

# Part I
# History and Rationale of Lumbar Spine Access Surgery

# Chapter 1
# Overview of Anterior Lumbar Spine Access Surgery

Emile-Victor Kuyl, Thomas Hong, Tyler Pease, and Jeffrey B. Weinreb

## Introduction

In appropriately selected patients, modern lumbar fusion surgery is considered the gold standard for treatment of multiple spinal pathologies and can result in a significant improvement in pain and disability scores [1–4]. An armamentarium of techniques, approaches, and instrumentation exists to help contemporary surgeons treat patients effectively and safely. Interbody fusion is a technique that allows direct and indirect decompression, a favorable biologic fusion environment, and the ability to correct deformity. Interbody fusions are often classified by the approach taken to place an interbody device and include anterior lumbar interbody fusion (ALIF), posterior lumbar interbody fusion, oblique lumbar interbody fusion, transforaminal lumbar interbody fusion, and lateral lumbar interbody fusion (LLIF) [5]. However, long before various anatomical approaches to lumbar surgery were extensively studied, physicians and scientists were puzzled over how to treat diseases of the spine when conservative or nonsurgical management failed.

E.-V. Kuyl · T. Hong
School of Medicine and Health Sciences,
The George Washington University, Washington, DC, USA

T. Pease (✉)
Department of Orthopedic Surgery, University of Maryland School of Medicine,
Baltimore, MD, USA

J. B. Weinreb
Department of Orthopedic Surgery, University of Maryland School of Medicine,
Baltimore, MD, USA

Department of Orthopedic Surgery, The George Washington University, Washington, DC, USA

© The Author(s), under exclusive license to Springer Nature Switzerland AG 2023
J. R. O'Brien et al. (eds.), *Lumbar Spine Access Surgery*,
https://doi.org/10.1007/978-3-031-48034-8_1

# A History of the Anterior Approach to the Lumbar Spine

In 1779, a surgeon by the name of Percivall Pott described a complication of *Mycobacterium tuberculosis* infection as spastic paralysis of the lower limbs associated with abnormal curvature and deformity of the spine (later to be termed Pott disease) [6, 7]. Failing to resolve with conservative treatment or medical therapy, he recommended draining paraspinal tuberculous abscesses via a surgical incision to drain pus and decompress the spinal canal [7]. When direct surgery of the spine could finally be considered in 1828 after the completion of the first successful laminectomy, only posterior approaches existed, but Pott disease abscesses were largely located on the anterior surface of the spine. In 1906, Müller performed the first successful anterior approach to the lumbar spine but failed to achieve good outcomes—resulting in the abandonment of the procedure altogether [8]. A definitive ventral approach would finally be described by the Japanese orthopedic surgeon Hiromu Ito in 1934 [9]. By accessing the abscess cavity with an extraperitoneal approach, Ito was able to perform a fusion to stabilize the spine after the abscess was resected [9]. As antituberculosis drugs became more efficient in treating Pott disease, the indication for anterior/lateral lumbar surgery became less prevalent for this infectious disease [6].

From 1930 to 1960, surgeons continued to adapt and perfect the anterior approach for various pathologies of the lumbar spine including spondylolisthesis and discectomy [6, 10–13]. As posterior approaches began to be utilized for fusion of spondylolisthesis, Norman Capener described a theoretical anterior operation in 1932 where bilateral grafts were placed in the anterior-posterior direction into L5 and S1 to fuse spondylolisthesis. Notably, Capener advised against his own approach given the theoretical risks [14]. In 1933, Burns developed and performed an anterior L5–S1 fusion using bone drilling and grafting on a 14-year-old boy with traumatic spondylolisthesis, not unlike a modern-day reverse-Bohlman technique [10]. A few years later in 1936, Mercer would perform and modify the Burns technique to include transperitoneal discectomy, graft, and screw placement that closely approximates a modern ALIF technique (Fig. 1.1) [11]. Due to difficulties with posterior visualization of lumbar disc herniations, Lane and Moore described a transperitoneal multilevel ALIF for disc herniations with good results [12]. In 1957, Southwick and Robinson described a retroperitoneal anterolateral approach that was a modification of the general surgery approach generally used for sympathectomy but was also noted to provide excellent exposure of L4 and L5 [13]. Their modification required a 12th rib resection for visualization of L1–L5 and was noted to provide excellent access for psoas abscess debridement and bone grafting [13]. A few years later in 1960, Harmon described his experience with an anterior extraperitoneal lumbar approach for disc herniation with fusion using autologous, allogeneic, and xenogenic bone grafting with a 98% fusion rate with autologous grafting [15]. From the 1960s onwards, improvements in ALIF involved newer instrumentation and techniques that made the procedure less traumatic and more minimally invasive including Fraser's muscle-splitting approaches in 1992 (which limited disruption of

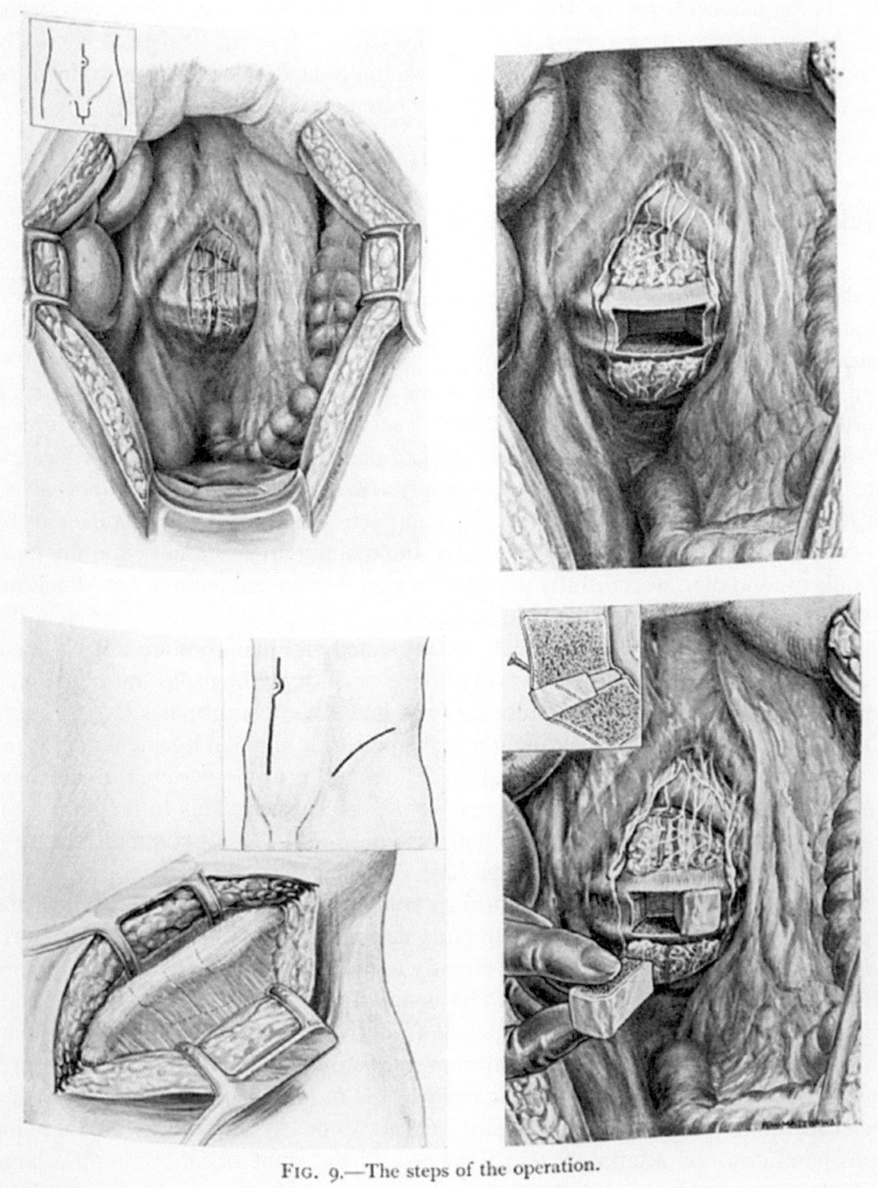



**Fig. 1.1** The original description of the Mercer technique for transperitoneal discectomy and bone grafting (open domain under CC BY 4.0) [11]

the abdominal wall) [6, 16–19]. The mini-open approach (a modified version of Fraser's muscle splitting approach) was proposed by Mayer in 1997 and eventually outperformed laparoscopic approaches—eventually leading to the development of lateral extraperitoneal approaches which are often utilized today [20, 21].

## Relevant Anatomy of the Lateral and Anterior Lumbar Spine

A detailed understanding of the relevant osseous, vascular, urological, and neural anatomy for anterior or lateral spine surgery is essential for optimal outcomes and intraoperative patient safety. The lumbar spine consists of five vertebrae (L1–L5) situated caudal to the thoracic vertebrae and cranial to the sacrum. Between each vertebral body lies an intervertebral disc that serves to mitigate compression forces. Posterior elements of each vertebra consist of pedicles, lamina, spinous processes, and facet joints—all of which are not typically visualized during anterior approaches to the spine. Depending on the specific approach, the entire lumbar spine can be visualized anteriorly, while the location of the diaphragm proximally and the lumbar plexus and iliac crest distally may limit a lateral approach without modifications like rib resection or a transthoracic component. During the anterior approach, the muscle layers of the abdominal wall are separated and therefore are not violated. Lateral approaches require passing anterior to or through the psoas muscle, which originates from the transverse processes and lateral vertebral bodies (L1–L5) and inserts into the femur after passing under the posterior inguinal ligament [22].

The aorta and inferior vena cava (IVC) lie anterior to the vertebral bodies and split into the common iliac arteries and veins, respectively. This bifurcation typically happens at the L4 level. When patients lay supine, the left common iliac vessels can be at increased risk of damage [23]. Placing patients in the lateral decubitus position instead can cause the abdominal contents and vessels to shift out of the operative field due to gravity and help mitigate some of the risks [24–26]. The aorta tends to lie ventrally to the IVC and slightly to the left. For approaches that require dissection at L4–L5, surgeons should be aware of one or more branches of the iliolumbar vein that crosses the psoas muscle from the IVC. Lumbar arteries originating from the aorta run below the inferior endplate of each superior intervertebral disc space. Segmental and spinal branches pass around each vertebral body and enter the dura near the dorsal root ganglia. The venous system of the lumbar spine runs parallel to the arterial system. Drainage of the spine occurs through a large valveless venous plexus (Batson's). Intradural venous drainage passes from radiculomedullary veins into anterior and posterior spinal veins [22].

During lateral and anterior approaches to the lumbar spine, careful attention must be paid to the kidneys and ureters, which lie close to the spine in the retroperitoneal space. The left kidney aligns itself slightly more caudal from T11–12 to L2–L3, whereas the right kidney typically rests between T12–L1 and L3–L4. From the right kidney, the right ureter travels anteromedially along the right aspect of the

IVC and crosses the external iliac artery before entering the pelvis. The left kidney ureter crosses instead over the common iliac artery [22].

The spinal cord terminates as the conus medullaris at the L1 or L2 level and continues as the lumbar and sacral nerve roots, known as the cauda equina. In the lumbar spine, nerve roots exit below their corresponding pedicle and form the lumbar plexus. From L1, the ilioinguinal and iliohypogastric nerves pass laterally and anteriorly into the abdomen. From L1 and L2, the genitofemoral nerve exits the ventral psoas and divides into the femoral and genital branches, lateral to the common and iliac arteries. The obturator and femoral nerves arise from L2–L3 and L4–L5, respectively, and comprise the largest branches of the lumbar plexus. Since the obturator nerve lies medially to the psoas, it is not considered to be at much risk compared to the femoral nerve during lateral transpsoas approaches [22].

## Common Pathologies

Intervertebral discs are composed of an outer annulus fibrosus and an inner nucleus pulposus [27]. The annulus fibrosus is made up of type 1 collagen fibers that pass obliquely between vertebral bodies, while the nucleus pulposus is a gel-like substance made of proteoglycan, water, type II collagen, and elastin fibers [28]. Degeneration of intervertebral discs in the lumbar spine can be a causative factor for lower back pain and contribute to motion segment instability, and compression of the neural elements.

Degenerative disc disease (DDD) is a common condition that increases with age and is most commonly seen in the lower lumbar spine [29]. The main cause of disc degeneration is thought to be excessive mechanical loading [30], which can disrupt the structure of the disc and trigger a series of irreversible cell-mediated responses that cause further damage [31]. Injured discs show increased levels of catabolic cytokines and matrix metalloproteinases (MMPs), which lead to scar formation and renewed matrix turnover [32]. With aging, the overall proteoglycan and water content of the disc decrease, leading to a relative increase in collagen content [33]. Genetics also play a major role in the development of DDD, accounting for 74% of the variability in twin studies [34], and several individual genes have been associated with disc degeneration, including those for type IX collagen, aggrecan, vitamin D receptor, MMP3, and cartilage intermediate layer protein [28, 35–39]. Isolated disc resorption is a subtype of DDD that is characterized by the breakdown of the nucleus pulposus. This can cause the disc to lose its height and ability to absorb shock, leading to pain and other symptoms [40, 41]. Spondylosis refers to the degeneration of spinal structures, including the intervertebral discs, facet joints, and ligaments. It can result in the development of osteophytes and a reduction in the disc's height, which can put pressure on the spinal nerves and cause pain, numbness, and weakness [42, 43].

Motion segment instability, or lumbar instability, is abnormal mobility in the lumbar motion segment, a reference to two adjacent vertebrae in the lumbar spine connected by three joints—the left and right zygapophyseal (facet) joints and the intervertebral discs [44, 45]. Motion segments in the spinal column are made stable by the interactions between the spinal column and its ligaments, the central nervous system, and the various muscles supporting the spine, including the multifidus, transverse abdominis, erector spinae, and quadratus lumborum muscles [46–48]. Motion segment instability can involve conditions such as spondylolisthesis, where one vertebra slips forward or backward in relation to the adjacent vertebra, and scoliosis, a multidimensional spinal curvature [49–51].

## Indications

Indications for an anterior approach to the lumbar spine include DDD, deformity, trauma, infection, tumor, pseudarthrosis, and motion segment instability [52–54]. The decision may depend on patient characteristics such as age, comorbidities, and spinal pathology.

Placement of an interbody device can help restore disc height, decompress nerve roots, and stabilize the affected segment, making it a safe and effective surgical option for DDD [5]. ALIF can also be an effective treatment for motion segment instability and patients with spondylolisthesis have demonstrated good outcomes with ALIF [55–58].

Regarding other pathologies, ALIF can also be a viable option for patients with adjacent segment disease, which is the development of symptoms at levels adjacent to a previous spinal fusion [59, 60]. Pseudarthrosis, which is the failure of a previous fusion, may also be treated with ALIF [61–63]. Recurrent lumbar disc herniation and post-discectomy collapse can be treated with ALIF but may also require additional surgical intervention [52, 64]. Instability after laminectomy or posterior decompression, spinal osteotomy, and kyphosis may also be addressed with ALIF [52, 65, 66].

Contraindications for ALIF may include osteoporosis, infection, and unfavorable anatomy [52]. Osteoporosis can increase the risk of implant failure and may make it difficult to obtain adequate fixation. Infection can lead to implant failure, and existing posterior instrumentation may need to be removed or revised to accommodate the procedure to allow for anterior mobilization. Consultation with the vascular or general surgery team is critical in the context of relative contraindications including previous abdominal surgery with adhesions, unfavorable vascular anatomy, and severe peripheral vascular disease [67]. It is also essential to evaluate other spinal areas to determine if they require surgical intervention and if an anterior approach is the best option.

## Risks of Anterior and Lateral Lumbar Surgery

During an anterior approach there is limited direct visualization of the neural elements and the risk of dural laceration is minimal [68, 69]. However, major concerns remain for serious complications such as vascular injury and retrograde ejaculation [70–78]. Other complications include infection, wound dehiscence, hernia, seroma, ileus, bleeding, thrombosis/embolism, and injury to the bowel, nervous, and genitourinary structures [79–81].

Vascular complications are a potentially devastating risk of the anterior approach. Although in some cases the spine surgeon may feel comfortable addressing vascular injuries, these complications often require the assistance of a vascular approach surgeon and consideration must be paid to the local medicolegal environment [74, 79, 82]. The rate of vascular injury has been reported as greater than 10% in some studies and is a major risk factor for deep vein thrombosis [80, 83, 84]. Intraoperative vascular injury greatly increases procedure time, length of stay (LOS), and readmission rate, placing patients at risk of additional complications and longer recovery time [84, 85].

Retrograde ejaculation (RE) in the context of an anterior approach is poorly described in the literature, making it difficult for approach surgeons to counsel their male patients [86–88]. As surgeons have shifted towards retroperitoneal approaches and away from a transperitoneal approach, damage to intraperitoneal structures has decreased, but injury to major vasculature and the hypogastric plexus remains a major risk [89, 90]. RE typically occurs secondary to damage of the hypogastric plexus which crosses the prevertebral space near L5–S1. The consequent decrease in sympathetic function permits relaxation of the internal bladder sphincter during ejaculation, allowing retrograde flow of ejaculate into the bladder [86]. Some studies have also implicated the use of bone morphogenetic protein 2 (BMP2) during ALIF with the development of RE [72, 82, 86, 87, 91]. Surgeons should be prepared to discuss this potential complication with their male patients, including preoperative sperm banking, as well as the potential for possible self-resolution.

## Contemporary Utilization of Anterior Approach and Future Directions

The anterior approach to lumbar spine surgery has undergone significant changes in utilization over the last few decades. Over the past 10–15 years, there has been a significant increase in ALIF/LLIF utilization in older patients with more comorbidities and higher American Society of Anesthesiologists classifications [92]. Within the same time frame, the utilization of ALIF/LLIF in the smoking population has dropped [92]. Despite the increased use of the approach in higher-risk patients, morbidity has significantly decreased [92, 93]. This may be due to a rise in the use of tranexamic acid, granting spine surgeons greater degrees of hemostatic control

[94–96]. The decrease in LOS over the past decade is likely greatly influenced by new applications of enhanced recovery pathways, multimodal anesthesia, and opioid-sparing/regional analgesic techniques [97–101]. Additionally, there has been increased adoption of BMP to enhance osseointegration and improve fusion rates in ALIF since its approval in 2002 by the U.S. Food and Drug Association [102].

The anterior approach has also evolved to offer a range of surgical techniques, including more traditional retroperitoneal or transperitoneal approaches and newer oblique and lateral approaches. In the anterior retroperitoneal or transperitoneal approaches, an incision is made on either the right or left side between the rectus abdominis muscle and the peritoneum while the patient lies supine [103]. The oblique and lateral approaches place the patient in a lateral decubitus or prone position, and the spine is accessed retroperitoneally. It is possible that an anterolateral approach is preferred for surgeons as it may avoid mandatory involvement of access surgeons [24, 67, 103]. In recent times, LLIF in the prone position has gained popularity because it allows for simultaneous posterior instrumentation, decompression procedures, and corrective osteotomies in a more familiar position [104].

## Conclusion

Anterior access via an anterior or lateral approach is commonly utilized in modern spine surgery. Initially described for treating Pott disease, anterior approaches have since been adapted for the treatment of spondylolisthesis, lumbar disc herniations, malignancy, degenerative conditions, trauma, and deformity. Safe and effective surgery through anterior exposure requires a multidisciplinary team of providers who should be aware of the unique anatomy, pathophysiology, indications, and associated risks. With the further development of variant approaches, enhanced recovery pathways, biologics, and instrumentation technologies, the anterior approach may continue to reshape surgical treatment for spinal pathologies.

## References


1. Reid PC, Morr S, Kaiser MG. State of the union: a review of lumbar fusion indications and techniques for degenerative spine disease. J Neurosurg Spine. 2019;31:1–14.
2. Makanji H, Schoenfeld AJ, Bhalla A, et al. Critical analysis of trends in lumbar fusion for degenerative disorders revisited: influence of technique on fusion rate and clinical outcomes. Eur Spine J. 2018;27:1868–76.
3. Brox JI, Sørensen R, Friis A, et al. Randomized clinical trial of lumbar instrumented fusion and cognitive intervention and exercises in patients with chronic low back pain and disc degeneration. Spine (Phila Pa 1976). 2003;28:1913–21.
4. Fritzell P, Hägg O, Wessberg P, et al. 2001 Volvo Award Winner in Clinical Studies: lumbar fusion versus nonsurgical treatment for chronic low back pain: a multicenter randomized controlled trial from the Swedish Lumbar Spine Study Group. Spine (Phila Pa 1976). 2001;26:2521–32; discussion 2532–4.

5. Teng I, Han J, Phan K, et al. A meta-analysis comparing ALIF, PLIF, TLIF and LLIF. J Clin Neurosci. 2017;44:11–7.
6. Matur AV, Mejia-Munne JC, Plummer ZJ, et al. The history of anterior and lateral approaches to the lumbar spine. World Neurosurg. 2020;144:213–21.
7. Pott P. Farther remarks on the useless state of the lower limbs, in consequence of a curvature of the spine: being a supplement to a former treatise on that subject. 1782. Clin Orthop Relat Res. 2007;460:4–9.
8. Muller W. Transperitoneale freilegung der wirbelsaule bei tuberkuloser spondylitis. Dtsch Z Chir. 1906;85:128–35.
9. Ito H, Tsuchiya J, Asami G. A new radical operation for Pott's disease: report of ten cases. JBJS. 1934;16:499.
10. Burns BH. An operation for spondylolisthesis. Lancet. 1933;221:1233.
11. Mercer W. Spondylolisthesis: with a description of a new method of operative treatment and notes of ten cases. Edinb Med J. 1936;43:545–72.
12. Lane JD, Moore ES. Transperitoneal approach to the intervertebral disc in the lumbar area. Ann Surg. 1948;127:537–51.
13. Southwick WO, Robinson RA. Surgical approaches to the vertebral bodies in the cervical and lumbar regions. JBJS. 1957;39:631–44.
14. Capener N. Spondylolisthesis. Br J Surg. 1932;19:374–86.
15. Harmon PH. Anterior extraperitoneal lumbar disk excision and vertebral body fusion. Clin Orthop Relat Res. 1960;18:169–98.
16. Obenchain TG. Laparoscopic lumbar discectomy: case report. J Laparoendosc Surg. 1991;1:145–9.
17. Fraser RD, Gogan WJ. A modified muscle-splitting approach to the lumbosacral spine. Spine (Phila Pa 1976). 1992;17:943–8.
18. Regan JJ, Aronoff RJ, Ohnmeiss DD, et al. Laparoscopic approach to L4–L5 for interbody fusion using BAK cages: experience in the first 58 cases. Spine (Phila Pa 1976). 1999;24:2171–4.
19. Bassani R, Gregori F, Peretti G. Evolution of the anterior approach in lumbar spine fusion. World Neurosurg. 2019;131:391–8.
20. Mayer HM. A new microsurgical technique for minimally invasive anterior lumbar interbody fusion. Spine (Phila Pa 1976). 1997;22:691–9; discussion 700.
21. Brau SA. Mini-open approach to the spine for anterior lumbar interbody fusion. Spine J. 2002;2:216–23.
22. Richardon AM, Manzano G, Levi AD. Relevant surgical anatomy of the lateral and anterior lumbar spine. In: Lumbar interbody fusions. London: Elsevier; 2019. p. 27–35.
23. Bečulić H, Sladojević I, Jusić A, et al. Morphometric study of the anatomic relationship between large retroperitoneal blood vessels and intervertebral discs of the distal segment of the lumbar spine: a clinical significance. Med Glas (Zenica). 2019;16:260–4. https://doi.org/10.17392/1011-19.
24. Malham GM, Wagner TP, Claydon MH. Anterior lumbar interbody fusion in a lateral decubitus position: technique and outcomes in obese patients. J Spine Surg. 2019;5:433–42.
25. Jin C, Jaiswal MS, Jeun S-S, et al. Outcomes of oblique lateral interbody fusion for degenerative lumbar disease in patients under or over 65 years of age. J Orthop Surg Res. 2018;13:38.
26. Xi Z, Burch S, Mummaneni PV, et al. Supine anterior lumbar interbody fusion versus lateral position oblique lumbar interbody fusion at L5–S1: a comparison of two approaches to the lumbosacral junction. J Clin Neurosci. 2020;82:134–40.
27. Humzah MD, Soames RW. Human intervertebral disc: structure and function. Anat Rec. 1988;220:337–56.
28. Adams MA, Roughley PJ. What is intervertebral disc degeneration, and what causes it? Spine. 2006;31:2151–61.

29. Videman T, Battié MC, Gill K, et al. Magnetic resonance imaging findings and their relationships in the thoracic and lumbar spine. Insights into the etiopathogenesis of spinal degeneration. Spine (Phila Pa 1976). 1995;20:928–35.
30. Adams MA. Biomechanics of back pain. Acupunct Med. 2004;22:178–88.
31. Riley GP, Curry V, DeGroot J, et al. Matrix metalloproteinase activities and their relationship with collagen remodelling in tendon pathology. Matrix Biol. 2002;21:185–95.
32. Kang JD, Georgescu HI, McIntyre-Larkin L, et al. Herniated lumbar intervertebral discs spontaneously produce matrix metalloproteinases, nitric oxide, interleukin-6, and prostaglandin E2. Spine (Phila Pa 1976). 1996;21:271–7.
33. Roberts S, Evans H, Trivedi J, et al. Histology and pathology of the human intervertebral disc. J Bone Joint Surg Am. 2006;88(Suppl 2):10–4.
34. Sambrook PN, MacGregor AJ, Spector TD. Genetic influences on cervical and lumbar disc degeneration: a magnetic resonance imaging study in twins. Arthritis Rheum. 1999;42:366–72.
35. Paassilta P, Lohiniva J, Göring HH, et al. Identification of a novel common genetic risk factor for lumbar disk disease. JAMA. 2001;285:1843–9.
36. Kawaguchi Y, Osada R, Kanamori M, et al. Association between an aggrecan gene polymorphism and lumbar disc degeneration. Spine (Phila Pa 1976). 1999;24:2456–60.
37. Seki S, Kawaguchi Y, Chiba K, et al. A functional SNP in CILP, encoding cartilage intermediate layer protein, is associated with susceptibility to lumbar disc disease. Nat Genet. 2005;37:607–12.
38. Videman T, Gibbons LE, Battié MC, et al. The relative roles of intragenic polymorphisms of the vitamin d receptor gene in lumbar spine degeneration and bone density. Spine (Phila Pa 1976). 2001;26:E7–12.
39. Takahashi M, Haro H, Wakabayashi Y, et al. The association of degeneration of the intervertebral disc with 5a/6a polymorphism in the promoter of the human matrix metalloproteinase-3 gene. J Bone Joint Surg Br. 2001;83:491–5.
40. Venner RM, Crock HV. Clinical studies of isolated disc resorption in the lumbar spine. J Bone Joint Surg Br. 1981;63B:491–4.
41. Jaffray D, O'Brien JP. Isolated intervertebral disc resorption. A source of mechanical and inflammatory back pain? Spine (Phila Pa 1976). 1986;11:397–401.
42. Garfin SR, Eismont FJ, Bell GR, et al., editors. Rothman-Simeone and Herkowitz's the spine. 7th ed. Philadelphia: Elsevier; 2018.
43. Seichi A. [Lumbar spondylosis]. Nihon Rinsho 2014;72:1750–4.
44. Dupuis PR, Yong-Hing K, Cassidy JD, et al. Radiologic diagnosis of degenerative lumbar spinal instability. Spine (Phila Pa 1976). 1985;10:262–76.
45. Bogduk N, Bogduk N. Clinical and radiological anatomy of the lumbar spine. 5th ed. New York: Churchill Livingstone; 2012.
46. Panjabi MM. The stabilizing system of the spine. Part I. Function, dysfunction, adaptation, and enhancement. J Spinal Disord. 1992;5:383–9; discussion 397.
47. Phillips S, Mercer S, Bogduk N. Anatomy and biomechanics of quadratus lumborum. Proc Inst Mech Eng H. 2008;222:151–9.
48. Russo M, Deckers K, Eldabe S, et al. Muscle control and non-specific chronic low back pain. Neuromodulation. 2018;21:1–9.
49. Fujiwara A, Lim TH, An HS, et al. The effect of disc degeneration and facet joint osteoarthritis on the segmental flexibility of the lumbar spine. Spine (Phila Pa 1976). 2000;25:3036–44.
50. Hasegewa K, Kitahara K, Hara T, et al. Biomechanical evaluation of segmental instability in degenerative lumbar spondylolisthesis. Eur Spine J. 2009;18:465–70.
51. Aebi M. The adult scoliosis. Eur Spine J. 2005;14:925–48.
52. Mobbs RJ, Loganathan A, Yeung V, et al. Indications for anterior lumbar interbody fusion. Orthop Surg. 2013;5:153–63.
53. Wang JC, Mummaneni PV, Haid RW. Current treatment strategies for the painful lumbar motion segment: posterolateral fusion versus interbody fusion. Spine (Phila Pa 1976). 2005;30:S33–43.

54. Burkus JK, Schuler TC, Gornet MF, et al. Anterior lumbar interbody fusion for the management of chronic lower back pain: current strategies and concepts. Orthop Clin North Am. 2004;35:25–32.
55. Takahashi K, Kitahara H, Yamagata M, et al. Long-term results of anterior interbody fusion for treatment of degenerative spondylolisthesis. Spine (Phila Pa 1976). 1990;15:1211–5.
56. Ishihara H, Osada R, Kanamori M, et al. Minimum 10-year follow-up study of anterior lumbar interbody fusion for isthmic spondylolisthesis. J Spinal Disord. 2001;14:91–9.
57. Johnson LP, Nasca RJ, Dunham WK. Surgical management of isthmic spondylolisthesis. Spine (Phila Pa 1976). 1988;13:93–7.
58. Hsieh PC, Koski TR, O'Shaughnessy BA, et al. Anterior lumbar interbody fusion in comparison with transforaminal lumbar interbody fusion: implications for the restoration of foraminal height, local disc angle, lumbar lordosis, and sagittal balance. J Neurosurg Spine. 2007;7:379–86.
59. Gumbs AA, Hanan S, Yue JJ, et al. Revision open anterior approaches for spine procedures. Spine J. 2007;7:280–5.
60. Fisher CG, Vaccaro AR, Whang PG, et al. Evidence-based recommendations for spine surgery. Spine (Phila Pa 1976). 2013;38:E30–7.
61. Gertzbein SD, Hollopeter MR, Hall S. Pseudarthrosis of the lumbar spine. Outcome after circumferential fusion. Spine (Phila Pa 1976). 1998;23:2352–6; discussion 2356–7.
62. Etminan M, Girardi FP, Khan SN, et al. Revision strategies for lumbar pseudarthrosis. Orthop Clin North Am. 2002;33:381–92.
63. Barrick WT, Schofferman JA, Reynolds JB, et al. Anterior lumbar fusion improves discogenic pain at levels of prior posterolateral fusion. Spine (Phila Pa 1976). 2000;25:853–7.
64. Hlubek RJ, Mundis GM. Treatment for recurrent lumbar disc herniation. Curr Rev Musculoskelet Med. 2017;10:517–20.
65. Mayer HM. The ALIF concept. Eur Spine J. 2000;9(Suppl 1):S35–43.
66. Mummaneni PV, Haid RW, Rodts GE. Lumbar interbody fusion: state-of-the-art technical advances. Invited submission from the Joint Section Meeting on Disorders of the Spine and Peripheral Nerves, March 2004. J Neurosurg Spine. 2004;1:24–30.
67. Mobbs RJ, Phan K, Malham G, et al. Lumbar interbody fusion: techniques, indications and comparison of interbody fusion options including PLIF, TLIF, MI-TLIF, OLIF/ATP, LLIF and ALIF. J Spine Surg. 2015;1:2–18.
68. Phan K, Thayaparan GK, Mobbs RJ. Anterior lumbar interbody fusion versus transforaminal lumbar interbody fusion--systematic review and meta-analysis. Br J Neurosurg. 2015;29:705–11.
69. Gennari A, Yuh S-J, Le Petit L, et al. Anterior Longitudinal Ligament Flap technique: description of anterior longitudinal ligament opening during anterior lumbar spine surgery and review of vascular complications in 189 patients. World Neurosurg. 2022;165:e743–9.
70. Bassani R, Morselli C, Baschiera R, et al. New trends in spinal surgery: less invasive anatomical approach to the spine. The advantages of the anterior approach in lumbar spinal fusion. Turk Neurosurg. 2021;31:484–92.
71. Brau SA, Delamarter RB, Schiffman ML, et al. Vascular injury during anterior lumbar surgery. Spine J. 2004;4:409–12.
72. Burkus JK, Dryer RF, Peloza JH. Retrograde ejaculation following single-level anterior lumbar surgery with or without recombinant human bone morphogenetic protein-2 in 5 randomized controlled trials: clinical article. J Neurosurg Spine. 2013;18:112–21.
73. Phan K, Xu J, Scherman DB, et al. Anterior lumbar interbody fusion with and without an "access surgeon": a systematic review and meta-analysis. Spine (Phila Pa 1976). 2017;42:E592–601.
74. Quraishi NA, Konig M, Booker SJ, et al. Access related complications in anterior lumbar surgery performed by spinal surgeons. Eur Spine J. 2013;22(Suppl 1):S16–20.
75. Zahradnik V, Lubelski D, Abdullah KG, et al. Vascular injuries during anterior exposure of the thoracolumbar spine. Ann Vasc Surg. 2013;27:306–13.

76. Wood KB, Devine J, Fischer D, et al. Vascular injury in elective anterior lumbosacral surgery. Spine (Phila Pa 1976). 2010;35:S66–75.

77. Rao PJ, Loganathan A, Yeung V, et al. Outcomes of anterior lumbar interbody fusion surgery based on indication: a prospective study. Neurosurgery. 2015;76:7–23; discussion 23–4.

78. Garg J, Woo K, Hirsch J, et al. Vascular complications of exposure for anterior lumbar interbody fusion. J Vasc Surg. 2010;51:946–50; discussion 950.

79. Mobbs RJ, Phan K, Daly D, et al. Approach-related complications of anterior lumbar interbody fusion: results of a combined spine and vascular surgical team. Global Spine J. 2016;6:147–54.

80. Wert WG, Sellers W, Mariner D, et al. Identifying risk factors for complications during exposure for anterior lumbar interbody fusion. Cureus. 2021;13:e16792.

81. Fantini GA, Pawar AY. Access related complications during anterior exposure of the lumbar spine. World J Orthop. 2013;4:19–23.

82. Bateman DK, Millhouse PW, Shahi N, et al. Anterior lumbar spine surgery: a systematic review and meta-analysis of associated complications. Spine J. 2015;15:1118–32.

83. Nourian AA, Cunningham CM, Bagheri A, et al. Effect of anatomic variability and level of approach on perioperative vascular complications with anterior lumbar interbody fusion. Spine (Phila Pa 1976). 2016;41:E73–7.

84. Ho VT, Martinez-Singh K, Colvard B, et al. Increased vertebral exposure in anterior lumbar interbody fusion associated with venous injury and deep venous thrombosis. J Vasc Surg Venous Lymphat Disord. 2021;9:423–7.

85. Elia CJ, Arvind V, Brazdzionis J, et al. 90-day readmission rates for single level anterior lumbosacral interbody fusion: a nationwide readmissions database analysis. Spine (Phila Pa 1976). 2020;45:E864–70.

86. Body AM, Plummer ZJ, Krueger BM, et al. Retrograde ejaculation following anterior lumbar surgery: a systematic review and pooled analysis. J Neurosurg Spine. 2021;35:427–36.

87. Comer GC, Smith MW, Hurwitz EL, et al. Retrograde ejaculation after anterior lumbar interbody fusion with and without bone morphogenetic protein-2 augmentation: a 10-year cohort controlled study. Spine J. 2012;12:881–90.

88. Brickman B, Tanios M, Patel D, et al. Clinical presentation and surgical anatomy of sympathetic nerve injury during lumbar spine surgery: a narrative review. J Spine Surg. 2022;8:276–87.

89. Gornet MF, Burkus JK, Dryer RF, et al. Lumbar disc arthroplasty with Maverick disc versus stand-alone interbody fusion: a prospective, randomized, controlled, multicenter investigational device exemption trial. Spine (Phila Pa 1976). 2011;36:E1600–11.

90. Lindley EM, McBeth ZL, Henry SE, et al. Retrograde ejaculation after anterior lumbar spine surgery. Spine (Phila Pa 1976). 2012;37:1785–9.

91. Singh K, Ahmadinia K, Park DK, et al. Complications of spinal fusion with utilization of bone morphogenetic protein: a systematic review of the literature. Spine (Phila Pa 1976). 2014;39:91–101.

92. Oezel L, Okano I, Hughes AP, et al. Longitudinal trends of patient demographics and morbidity of different approaches in lumbar interbody fusion: an analysis using the American College of Surgeons National Surgical Quality Improvement Program Database. World Neurosurg. 2022;164:e183–93.

93. Katz AD, Mancini N, Karukonda T, et al. Approach-based comparative and predictor analysis of 30-day readmission, reoperation, and morbidity in patients undergoing lumbar interbody fusion using the ACS-NSQIP Dataset. Spine. 2019;44:432–41.

94. Franchini M, Mannucci PM. The never ending success story of tranexamic acid in acquired bleeding. Haematologica. 2020;105:1201–5.

95. Yoo JS, Ahn J, Karmarkar SS, et al. The use of tranexamic acid in spine surgery. Ann Transl Med. 2019;2019:S172.

96. Cheriyan T, Maier SP, Bianco K, et al. Efficacy of tranexamic acid on surgical bleeding in spine surgery: a meta-analysis. Spine J. 2015;15:752–61.

97. Soffin EM, Beckman JD, Tseng A, et al. Enhanced recovery after lumbar spine fusion. Anesthesiology. 2020;133:350–63.
98. Soffin EM, Okano I, Oezel L, et al. Impact of ultrasound-guided erector spinae plane block on outcomes after lumbar spinal fusion: a retrospective propensity score matched study of 242 patients. Reg Anesth Pain Med. 2022;47:79.
99. Owen RJ, Quinlan N, Poduska A, et al. Preoperative fluoroscopically guided regional erector spinae plane blocks reduce opioid use, increase mobilization, and reduce length of stay following lumbar spine fusion. Global Spine J. 2023;13(4):954–60.
100. Gabriel RA, Swisher MW, Sztain JF, et al. State of the art opioid-sparing strategies for postoperative pain in adult surgical patients. Expert Opin Pharmacother. 2019;20:949–61.
101. Reisener M-J, Hughes AP, Okano I, et al. The association of transversus abdominis plane block with length of stay, pain and opioid consumption after anterior or lateral lumbar fusion: a retrospective study. Eur Spine J. 2021;30:3738–45.
102. Katsuura Y, Wright-Chisem J, Wright-Chisem A, et al. The importance of surface technology in spinal fusion. HSS J. 2020;16:113–6.
103. Allain J, Dufour T. Anterior lumbar fusion techniques: ALIF, OLIF, DLIF, LLIF, IXLIF. Orthop Traumatol Surg Res. 2020;106:S149–57.
104. Barkay G, Wellington I, Mallozzi S, et al. The prone lateral approach for lumbar fusion-a review of the literature and case series. Medicina (Kaunas). 2023;59:251.

# Chapter 2
# History and Evolution of Anterior Lumbar Spine Access Surgery

Neil Kelly, Francis C. Lovecchio, and Sheeraz A. Qureshi

## Introduction

From the earliest reports of nonoperative management of spine disorders in the Edwin Smith papyrus to the first successful spine surgery performed in 1829 by Alban Smith, there has long been a culture of forward thinking in spine care [1, 2]. Spine surgery has advanced tremendously in a relatively short period of time and has revolutionized the care for a myriad of spine conditions. This revolution in care is due in part to expanding modes of access to the spine. Over time, the field has evolved to include anterior, lateral, and oblique approaches to surgical treatments of the spine. With each approach now recognized for distinct advantages and indications, the purpose of this chapter is to highlight the history and evolution from posterior to anterolateral surgical approaches of the spine (Fig. 2.1).

N. Kelly · F. C. Lovecchio
Weill Cornell Medical College, New York, NY, USA

S. A. Qureshi (✉)
Weill Cornell Medical College, New York, NY, USA

Department of Orthopaedic Surgery, Hospital for Special Surgery, New York, NY, USA

© The Author(s), under exclusive license to Springer Nature Switzerland AG 2023
J. R. O'Brien et al. (eds.), *Lumbar Spine Access Surgery*,
https://doi.org/10.1007/978-3-031-48034-8_2

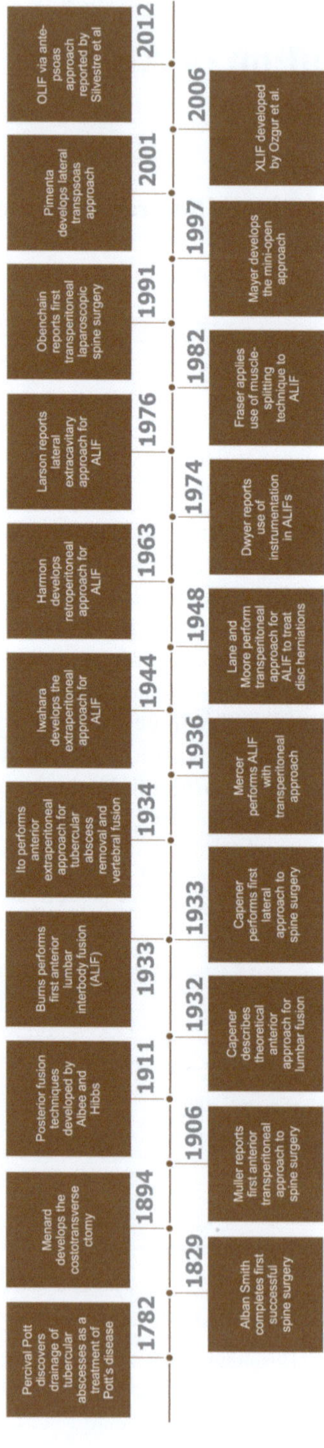


**Fig. 2.1** Timeline of significant events in the history of anterolateral lumbar spine access

## History of Anterior Lumbar Spine Access

Spine surgery has been performed for nearly two centuries, the first third of which was spent exclusively using a posterior surgical approach. The first alternatives to a posterior approach were developed in the early twentieth century to improve the treatment of Pott's disease. In the following decades, the use of anterior lumbar spine access would continue to expand to include new indications, instrumentation, and minimally invasive techniques. Now, modern anterior approach techniques are recognized for advantages which include direct access and wide exposure to the anterior spinal column, ease of insertion of large implants, avoidance of paraspinal muscle dissection and denervation, enhanced indirect decompression of intervertebral neural foramen, and improved fusion rates and sagittal profile [3]. Additionally, rates of complications associated with the anterior approach, such as vascular injury, ileus, and retrograde ejaculation, are relatively low when performed by experienced surgeons [4].

## *A Need for Anterior Access to the Lumbar Spine*

Although the posterior approach has been the mainstay since the inception of spine surgery, it has several key limitations which spurred initial interest in an alternative anatomical access route. For example, posterior lumbar dissection leads to damage, detachment, and denervation of the paraspinal musculature, while access to the disc space is limited by the retraction of the neural elements [5]. Pott's disease was the original impetus for finding a new approach to the spine.

First referenced in ancient medical texts between 3200 and 1800 BCE and later formally described by Percival Pott in 1779 CE, Pott's disease (i.e., tuberculous spondylitis) is osteomyelitis of the spine which develops from a *Mycobacterium tuberculosis* infection [6]. Infection spread also commonly affects the nearby paraspinal and psoas muscles, resulting in tubercular abscesses. In fact, Pott's observation that drainage of superficial paraspinal abscesses led to neurologic improvement spurred interest in developing a strategy to drain deeper, anterior abscesses, which were difficult to access surgically via a posterior approach [7]. Among the first alternatives to a posterior approach was costotransversectomy reported in 1894 by Menard and the anterior transperitoneal approach reported in 1906 by Müller [8, 9]. Shortly thereafter, posterior fusion techniques to prevent postinfectious kyphosis were developed independently by Albee and Hibbs in 1911 [10, 11]. In 1934, Ito combined and expanded the work of Müller, Albee, and Hibbs [12]. By performing an anterior extraperitoneal approach through which deep and anterior abscesses could be removed and fusion of the affected segments could be performed, Ito developed the first definitive anterior surgical treatment for Pott's disease [12]. Surgical improvements and alternative approaches to treat Pott's disease were pursued through 1960 when Hodgson et al. employed the use of anterior, lateral, and several other approaches along the length of the spine [13]. With the eventual development of antitubercular medications, however, medical treatment supplanted surgical treatment in the management of Pott's disease.

While anterior approaches were being developed for the treatment of Pott's disease, they were simultaneously being considered for the treatment of spondylolisthesis. In 1932, Capener first described a theoretical anterior approach for lumbar fusion and shortly thereafter, in 1933, Burns successfully performed the first anterior lumbar interbody fusion (ALIF) to treat a case of traumatic L5–S1 spondylolisthesis [14, 15]. Whereas Capener's proposed technique involved the use of bilateral anteroposterior grafts to fuse L5 and S1, Burns used autologous bone graft to fill a hole drilled through the center of the L5 and S1 vertebral bodies [14, 15]. After learning Burns' ALIF technique, Mercer then modified it in 1936 by utilizing a transperitoneal approach to remove and replace the intervertebral disc with bone graft [16]. The success of Mercer's ALIF technique spurred further applications of the anterior lumbar approach to include lumbar discectomy for degenerative conditions in addition to spondylolisthesis. In 1948, Lane and Moore described transperitoneal ALIF for the treatment of disc herniations at L3–S1 [17]. Extraperitoneal ALIF approaches were subsequently proposed and developed by Iwahara in 1944, Southwick and Robinson in 1957, and Harmon in 1960 [18–21].

## Evolution of the Anterior Approach

The technical development of ALIF continued through the 1960s as Harmon developed a retroperitoneal approach to perform discectomies and fusions and Dwyer began the use of instrumentation in ALIF [22, 23]. Despite continued and exciting ALIF developments, the technique remained controversial throughout the 1960s and 1970s. This was, in part, due to conflicting reports about surgical outcomes. Whereas Hodgson and Wong reported that more than 80% of patients undergoing ALIF showed complete fusion and more than 99% showed symptomatic improvement, Stauffer and Coventry found a fusion rate of 56%, with only 36% of patients reporting a good clinical result [24, 25]. Several other investigators reported similarly disparate results [26–28]. However, during the 1980s, anterior approaches reemerged as case series describing high union rates and clinical improvement were published [29–31]. In conjunction with increasing ALIF support and popularity, the 1980s also saw Fraser apply his muscle-splitting technique to the ALIF to minimize operative damage to the abdominal wall [32]. Further advancements in the following decades similarly focused on minimizing surgical morbidity and enhancing recovery by applying minimally invasive techniques to the ALIF.

Accordingly, the next step toward minimally invasive anterior lumbar access came in 1991 when Obenchain et al. reported the first transperitoneal laparoscopic lumbar discectomy [33]. Reports of transperitoneal laparoscopic ALIF followed shortly thereafter, the first of which was published by Mathews et al. in 1995 [34]. In the early 2000s, advancements in the field of laparoscopic ALIF focused on transitioning from the transperitoneal approach, which was hampered by the drawbacks of carbon dioxide insufflation (i.e., limited ability to use suction instruments or remove tissue), to a gasless extraperitoneal approach known as the balloon-assisted endoscopic retroperitoneal gasless technique [35]. Despite excellent outcomes when performed by experienced surgeons, the extra training required to become proficient in laparoscopic spine surgery limited its popularity. Moreover, laparoscopic techniques were largely limited to the L5–S1 level. This was in contrast with a separate, less technically challenging, minimally invasive technique known as the mini-open approach which could access the L2–S1 levels. With the mini-open approach in development at the same time as the laparoscopic approach and a lack of superiority data for laparoscopy, the mini-open ultimately became the favored approach within the field [36].

The mini-open approach was developed by Mayer and first published in 1997 [37]. Building on Fraser's muscle-splitting technique for ALIF, Mayer included a self-retaining spreader frame for retraction and employed microsurgical techniques which allowed lumbar access through a 4-cm incision [32, 37, 38]. Mayer's mini-open approach provided single- and two-level access to L2–L3, L3–L4, and L4–L5 via a retroperitoneal approach and to L5–S1 via a transperitoneal approach. Mayer's original mini-open approach continues to be optimized for single- and multilevel lumbar access [39–41].

## History of Lateral and Oblique Lumbar Spine Access

### First Descriptions of Lateral Lumbar Spine Surgery

The first lateral approach to the spine was performed by Capener in 1933 for a thoracolumbar decompression [42, 43]. The origins of Capener's lateral approach (termed the "lateral rhachotomy") are traced back to Menard's costotransversectomy [8]. Much as Capener modified Menard's approach, Capener's approach was later modified by Larson who developed the lateral extracavitary approach [44]. Initially developed for the treatment of Pott's disease in the 1950s, Larson's lateral extracavitary approach was applied to fractures and disc herniations of the thoracic and lumbar spine in the 1970s and 1980s [44–46]. The contributions of Menard, Capener, and Larson form the foundation of lateral spine access.

### Development of the Transpsoas Approach

The contemporary lateral transpsoas approach was first described by Pimenta in 2001 [47]. Today, indications for lateral lumbar interbody fusion (LLIF) include spondylolisthesis, disc herniation, degenerative disc disease (DDD), post-laminectomy kyphosis, adjacent segment disease, and degenerative scoliosis [48]. Use of the LLIF confers advantages such as not requiring a general surgeon for access, avoidance of the peritoneum and great vessels, the use of small incisions, direct visualization, and early postoperative mobilization [49, 50]. The LLIF, however, is limited in that the L5–S1 (and sometimes even the L4–L5) disc space can be obscured by the iliac crest. Furthermore, the anatomy of the lumbar plexus can increase neurologic morbidity of lateral access to L4–L5 [49]. Some authors have described relative contraindications to LLIF, including a lumbarized sacrum, high-grade spondylolisthesis, and severe canal stenosis [49, 51].

## *Development of the Ante-Psoas or Anterior-to-Psoas Approach*

Investigators have attempted to circumvent limitations of the transpsoas approach with use of an ante-psoas (or anterior-to-psoas) approach. The ante-psoas approach is performed with the patient in the lateral position but allows for reliable access to the L5–S1 and L4–L5 disc spaces. The ante-psoas approach was first performed by Mayer during his development of the mini-open anterior approach in 1997 [37]. Mayer's technique would eventually evolve into the oblique lumbar interbody fusion (OLIF) as reported by Silvestre et al. in 2012 [52]. Although the ante-psoas technique improves L5–S1 access and avoids the lumbar plexus, it is still relatively contraindicated in cases of high-grade spondylolisthesis and severe canal stenosis, much like the transpsoas approach [49]. When compared, the LLIF carries a higher risk of nerve and muscle injury and infection while the OLIF carries a higher risk of vascular injury [53].

## Current State of Anterolateral Lumbar Spine Surgery

Anterolateral lumbar spine surgery is currently performed for numerous indications, including infection, fracture, correction of deformity, spondylolisthesis, DDD, and increasing the fusion area for arthrodesis. Currently, one of the most hotly debated indications is whether the indirect decompression induced by disc space distraction is sufficient to relieve symptoms of central and lateral recess spinal stenosis [54]. The need for posterior instrumentation (especially after LLIF) is an additional topic of debate (Fig. 2.2). While most series show high fusion rates after stand-alone LLIF, a recent systematic review demonstrated that high-grade subsidence occurs in 11.1% of stand-alone LLIF [55]. As surgeons gain more experience and longer follow-up, the indications for stand-alone procedures will likely become more nuanced.

The advantages and disadvantages of various approaches are secondary to inherent anatomical constraints [56]. Surgeons debate the advantage of one approach over another when either could be used. For example, OLIF and LLIF may be

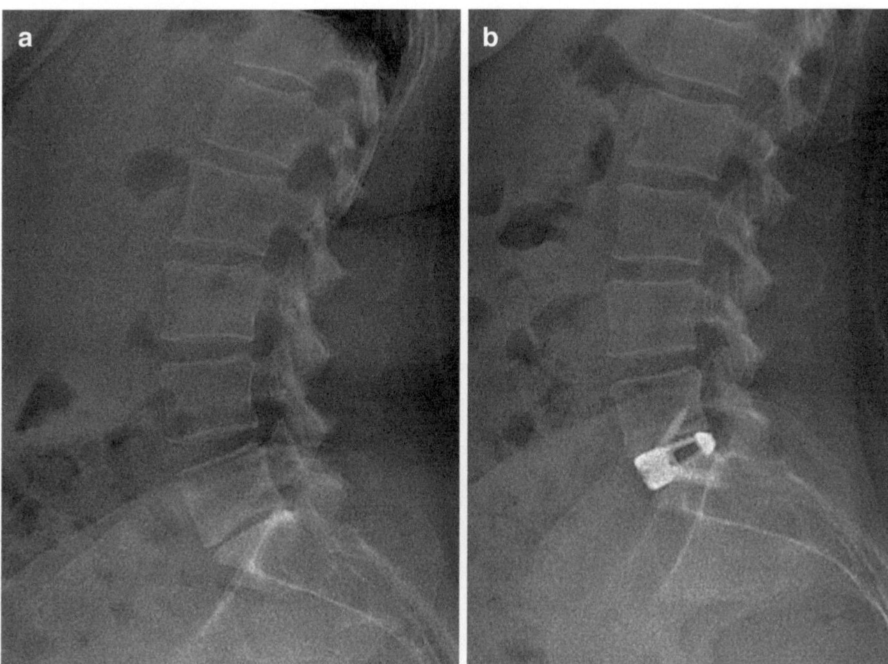

**Fig. 2.2** Example of a standalone interbody fusion performed in a young healthy male for single-level DDD

utilized to access the same levels, both with the patient in the same position. Walker et al. compiled the outcomes from 59 studies to examine whether complication rates were higher in OLIF or LLIF [53]. Notably, the results were consistent with the anatomical dangers of each approach—the OLIF group had a higher rate of sympathetic nerve injury and vascular injury, while the LLIF group had a higher rate of transient hip flexor weakness and sensory symptoms [53]. Given the fusion rates were similar between the cohorts, it can be concluded that each surgeon should use whichever approach is safest in their hands and for each patient's individual anatomy. As with most matters in surgical training, surgeons should do their best to avail themselves of all possible knowledge and experience with every type of anterolateral approach to the lumbar spine.

Finally, new technologies allow for anterolateral approaches to be performed more precisely and with fewer adverse effects to the patient and surgical team. Urakawa et al. demonstrated that three-dimensional (3D) intraoperative navigation could be safely and accurately used for LLIF, with a potential decrease in radiation dose during the procedure [56]. Technology has also been utilized to develop "single-position" anterolateral and posterior surgery. While initial series described navigated posterior instrumentation with the patient in the lateral position, more recent series describe a navigated lateral approach with the patient in the prone position (i.e., "prone lateral fusion") (Fig. 2.3) [57–60].

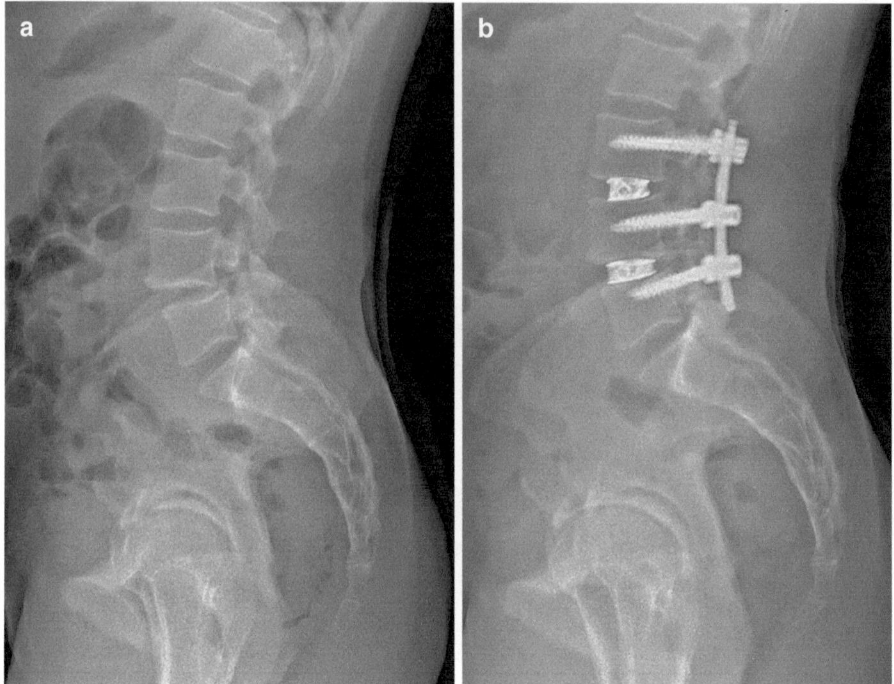

**Fig. 2.3** Example of a robotic-assisted "prone-lateral" two-level interbody fusion with posterior instrumentation

## Conclusion

As with many matters in medicine, anterolateral approaches to the spine were developed to manage a previously untreatable condition. The indications for the anterolateral approach have continued to grow over the last few decades. Outcomes also continue to improve as surgeons become more familiar with techniques and implant technology improves. Today, it is not uncommon for anterior, lateral, and oblique approaches to be performed in the same surgical setting. New developments in 3D navigation, robotics, and data science will allow surgeons to continue to innovate to improve patient safety and clinical outcomes.

## References


1. van Middendorp JJ, Sanchez GM, Burridge AL. The Edwin Smith papyrus: a clinical reappraisal of the oldest known document on spinal injuries. Eur Spine J. 2010;19(11):1815–23.
2. Smith AG. Account of a case in which portions of three dorsal vertebrae were removed for the relief of paralysis from fracture, with partial success. N Am Med Surg J. 1829;8(15):94.

3. Bassani R, Gregori F, Peretti G. Evolution of the anterior approach in lumbar spine fusion. World Neurosurg. 2019;131:391–8.
4. Phan K, Xu J, Scherman DB, Rao PJ, Mobbs RJ. Anterior lumbar interbody fusion with and without an "access surgeon": a systematic review and meta-analysis. Spine (Phila Pa 1976). 2017;42(10):E592–601.
5. Talia AJ, Wong ML, Lau HC, Kaye AH. Comparison of the different surgical approaches for lumbar interbody fusion. J Clin Neurosci. 2015;22(2):243–51.
6. Matur AV, Mejia-Munne JC, Plummer ZJ, Cheng JS, Prestigiacomo CJ. The history of anterior and lateral approaches to the lumbar spine. World Neurosurg. 2020;144:213–21.
7. Pott P. Farther remarks on the useless state of the lower limbs, in consequence of a curvature of the spine: being a supplement to a former treatise on that subject. 1782. Clin Orthop Relat Res. 2007;460:4–9.
8. Menard V. Causes de la paraplegia dans le mal de Pott. Son traitement chirurgical par l'ouverture direct du foyer tuberculeux des vertebras [Causes of paraplegia in Pott's disease. Its surgical treatment by directly opening the tuberculous focus of the vertebras]. Rev Orthop. 1894;5:47–64.
9. Muller W. Transperitoneale freilegung der wirbelsaule bei tuberkuloser spondylitis [Transperitoneal exposure of the spine in tuberculosis spondylitis]. Dtsch Ztschr Chir. 1906;85:128.
10. Albee FH. Transplantation of a portion of the tibia into the spine for Pott's disease. J Am Med Assoc. 1911;57:885–6.
11. Hibbs RA. An operation for progressive spinal deformities: a preliminary report of three cases from the service of the orthopaedic hospital. 1911. Clin Orthop Relat Res. 2007;460:17–20.
12. Ito H, Tsuchiya J, Asami G. A new radical operation for Pott's disease. J Bone Jt Surg. 1934;16(3):499–515.
13. Hodgson AR, Stock FE, Fang HS, Ong GB. Anterior spinal fusion. The operative approach and pathological findings in 412 patients with Pott's disease of the spine. Br J Surg. 1960;48:172–8.
14. Capener N. Spondylolisthesis. Br J Surg. 1932;19(75):374–86.
15. Burns BH. An operation for spondylolisthesis. Lancet. 1933;221:1233.
16. Mercer W. Spondylolisthesis: with a description of a new method of operative treatment and notes of ten cases. Edinb Med J. 1936;43(9):545–72.
17. Lane JD Jr, Moore ES Jr. Transperitoneal approach to the intervertebral disc in the lumbar area. Ann Surg. 1948;127(3):537–51.
18. Iwahara T. A new method of vertebral body fusion. Surgery. 1944;8:271–87.
19. Iwahara T, Ikeda K, Hirabayashi K. Results of anterior spine fusion by extraperitoneal approach for spondylolysis and spondylolisthesis. Nihon Seikeigeka Gakkai Zasshi. 1963;36:1049–67.
20. Southwick WO, Robinson RA. Surgical approaches to the vertebral bodies in the cervical and lumbar regions. J Bone Joint Surg Am. 1957;39-A(3):631–44.
21. Harmon PH. Anterior extraperitoneal lumbar disk excision and vertebral body fusion. Clin Orthop Relat Res. 1960;18:169–98.
22. Harmon PH. Anterior excision and vertebral body fusion operation for intervertebral disk syndromes of the lower lumbar spine: three-to five-year results in 244 cases. Clin Orthop Relat Res. 1963;26:107–27.
23. Dwyer AF, Newton NC, Sherwood AA. An anterior approach to scoliosis. A preliminary report. Clin Orthop Relat Res. 1969;62:192–202.
24. Hodgson AR, Wong SK. A description of a technic and evaluation of results in anterior spinal fusion for deranged intervertebral disk and spondylolisthesis. Clin Orthop Relat Res. 1968;56:133–62.
25. Stauffer RN, Coventry MB. Anterior interbody lumbar spine fusion. Analysis of Mayo Clinic series. J Bone Joint Surg Am. 1972;54(4):756–68.
26. Goldner JL, Urbaniak JR, McCollum DE. Anterior disc excision and interbody spinal fusion for chronic low back pain. Orthop Clin North Am. 1971;2(2):543–68.

27. Flynn JC, Hoque MA. Anterior fusion of the lumbar spine. End-result study with long-term follow-up. J Bone Joint Surg Am. 1979;61(8):1143–50.
28. Sacks S. Anterior interbody fusion of the lumbar spine. Indications and results in 200 cases. Clin Orthop Relat Res. 1966;44:163–70.
29. Chow SP, Leong JC, Ma A, Yau AC. Anterior spinal fusion or deranged lumbar intervertebral disc. Spine (Phila Pa 1976). 1980;5(5):452–8.
30. Crock HV. Anterior lumbar interbody fusion: indications for its use and notes on surgical technique. Clin Orthop Relat Res. 1982;165:157–63.
31. Inoue S, Watanabe T, Hirose A, et al. Anterior discectomy and interbody fusion for lumbar disc herniation. A review of 350 cases. Clin Orthop Relat Res. 1984;183:22–31.
32. Fraser RD. A wide muscle-splitting approach to the lumbosacral spine. J Bone Joint Surg Br. 1982;64(1):44–6.
33. Obenchain TG. Laparoscopic lumbar discectomy: case report. J Laparoendosc Surg. 1991;1(3):145–9.
34. Mathews HH, Evans MT, Molligan HJ, Long BH. Laparoscopic discectomy with anterior lumbar interbody fusion. A preliminary review. Spine (Phila Pa 1976). 1995;20(16):1797–802.
35. Vazquez RM, Gireesan GT. Balloon-assisted endoscopic retroperitoneal gasless (BERG) technique for anterior lumbar interbody fusion (ALIF). Surg Endosc. 2003;17(2):268–72.
36. Inamasu J, Guiot BH. Laparoscopic anterior lumbar interbody fusion: a review of outcome studies. Minim Invasive Neurosurg. 2005;48(6):340–7.
37. Mayer HM. A new microsurgical technique for minimally invasive anterior lumbar interbody fusion. Spine (Phila Pa 1976). 1997;22(6):691–9; discussion 700.
38. Fraser RD, Gogan WJ. A modified muscle-splitting approach to the lumbosacral spine. Spine (Phila Pa 1976). 1992;17(8):943–8.
39. Tay BB, Berven S. Indications, techniques, and complications of lumbar interbody fusion. Semin Neurol. 2002;22(2):221–30.
40. Brau SA. Mini-open approach to the spine for anterior lumbar interbody fusion: description of the procedure, results and complications. Spine J. 2002;2(3):216–23.
41. Bassani R, Querenghi AM, Cecchinato R, et al. A new "keyhole" approach for multilevel anterior lumbar interbody fusion: the perinavel approach-technical note and literature review. Eur Spine J. 2018;27(8):1956–63.
42. Seddon HJ. Pott's paraplegia: prognosis and treatment. Br J Surg. 1935;22:769–99.
43. Capener N. The evolution of lateral rhachotomy. J Bone Joint Surg Br. 1954;36-B(2):173–9.
44. Larson SJ, Holst RA, Hemmy DC, Sances A Jr. Lateral extracavitary approach to traumatic lesions of the thoracic and lumbar spine. J Neurosurg. 1976;45(6):628–37.
45. Lifshutz J, Lidar Z, Maiman D. Evolution of the lateral extracavitary approach to the spine. Neurosurg Focus. 2004;16(1):E12.
46. Maiman DJ, Larson SJ, Luck E, El-Ghatit A. Lateral extracavitary approach to the spine for thoracic disc herniation: report of 23 cases. Neurosurgery. 1984;14(2):178–82.
47. Pimenta L. Lateral endoscopic transpsoas retroperitoneal approach for lumbar spine surgery. Presented at: The VIII Brazilian Spine Society Meeting; 2001; Belo Horizonte, Minas Gerais, Brazil.
48. Arnold PM, Anderson KK, McGuire RA Jr. The lateral transpsoas approach to the lumbar and thoracic spine: a review. Surg Neurol Int. 2012;3(Suppl 3):S198–215.
49. Mobbs RJ, Phan K, Malham G, Seex K, Rao PJ. Lumbar interbody fusion: techniques, indications and comparison of interbody fusion options including PLIF, TLIF, MI-TLIF, OLIF/ATP, LLIF and ALIF. J Spine Surg. 2015;1(1):2–18.
50. Ozgur BM, Aryan HE, Pimenta L, Taylor WR. Extreme Lateral interbody Fusion (XLIF): a novel surgical technique for anterior lumbar interbody fusion. Spine J. 2006;6(4):435–43.
51. Smith WD, Youssef JA, Christian G, Serrano S, Hyde JA. Lumbarized sacrum as a relative contraindication for lateral transpsoas interbody fusion at L5-6. J Spinal Disord Tech. 2012;25(5):285–91.

52. Silvestre C, Mac-Thiong JM, Hilmi R, Roussouly P. Complications and morbidities of mini-open anterior retroperitoneal lumbar interbody fusion: oblique lumbar interbody fusion in 179 patients. Asian Spine J. 2012;6(2):89–97.
53. Walker CT, Farber SH, Cole TS, et al. Complications for minimally invasive lateral interbody arthrodesis: a systematic review and meta-analysis comparing prepsoas and transpsoas approaches. J Neurosurg Spine. 2019:1–15. https://doi.org/10.3171/2018.9.SPINE18800.
54. Manzur MK, Samuel AM, Morse KW, et al. Indirect lumbar decompression combined with or without additional direct posterior decompression: a systematic review. Global Spine J. 2022;12(5):980–9.
55. Manzur MK, Steinhaus ME, Virk SS, et al. Fusion rate for stand-alone lateral lumbar interbody fusion: a systematic review. Spine J. 2020;20(11):1816–25.
56. Urakawa H, Sivaganesan A, Vaishnav AS, Sheha E, Qureshi SA. The feasibility of 3D intraoperative navigation in lateral lumbar interbody fusion: perioperative outcomes, accuracy of cage placement and radiation exposure. Global Spine J. 2021;13(3):737–44.
57. Buckland AJ, Ashayeri K, Leon C, et al. Single position circumferential fusion improves operative efficiency, reduces complications and length of stay compared with traditional circumferential fusion. Spine J. 2021;21(5):810–20.
58. Guiroy A, Carazzo C, Camino-Willhuber G, et al. Single-position surgery versus lateral-then-prone-position circumferential lumbar interbody fusion: a systematic literature review. World Neurosurg. 2021;151:e379–86.
59. North RY, Strong MJ, Yee TJ, Kashlan ON, Oppenlander ME, Park P. Navigation and robotic-assisted single-position prone lateral lumbar interbody fusion: technique, feasibility, safety, and case series. World Neurosurg. 2021;152:221–30. e221
60. Godzik J, Ohiorhenuan IE, Xu DS, et al. Single-position prone lateral approach: cadaveric feasibility study and early clinical experience. Neurosurg Focus. 2020;49(3):E15.

# Chapter 3
# Rationale for Anterior Lumbar Spine Surgery

Lauren E. Matteini

## Introduction

Indicating patients for surgery is a skill requiring time and expertise. The spine surgeon has multiple options when deciding how to accomplish their goals based on the individual patient and underlying pathology. Anterior spine surgery has become a popular option to treat numerous conditions in the thoracolumbar and lumbosacral spine. This approach was first described by Capener in 1932 in the treatment of spondylolisthesis and since then has become more sophisticated and diverse in its applications [1].

## Rationale for Anterior Lumbar Spine Surgery

Due to advancements in techniques, improvements in retractors and implants, and a favorable risk profile, anterior lumbar interbody fusion (ALIF) has become an increasingly attractive option for spine surgeons, particularly those treating degenerative conditions necessitating fusion [2, 3]. The most commonly affected levels are L4–L5 and L5–S1, which are easily accessed via an anterior approach. Individual surgeons' comfort performing anterior surgery varies, and many spine surgeons combine their efforts with a highly skilled general or vascular surgeon to perform the approach.

An ALIF restores biomechanical and structural integrity, restores lumbar lordosis, reduces spondylolisthesis, and can help achieve coronal and sagittal balance [3–5]. A large interbody implant increases the neuroforaminal height which indirectly decompresses the nerve root and may obviate the need for posterior surgery

L. E. Matteini (✉)
Fox Valley Orthopedics, Geneva, IL, USA

© The Author(s), under exclusive license to Springer Nature Switzerland AG 2023
J. R. O'Brien et al. (eds.), *Lumbar Spine Access Surgery*,
https://doi.org/10.1007/978-3-031-48034-8_3

[6, 7]. Thus, ALIF can safely be performed for conditions such as degenerative disc disease, degenerative and isthmic spondylolisthesis, degenerative lumbar scoliosis, failed back surgery, and pseudoarthrosis.

The ALIF is a surgical option in the patient who has recurrent disc herniations in the setting of previous posterior decompression with scar formation [6, 7]. After prior posterior microdiscectomies, a repeat posterior approach for discectomy and fusion may entail an increased complication risk profile due to scar tissue formation. An anterior approach, however, avoids altered posterior anatomy and allows for discectomy, implant placement with distraction, and height restoration and fusion.

Other advantages of the anterior approach to the lumbar spine are apparent with comparison to posterior techniques. Posterior structures are spared when the spine is accessed anteriorly. The surgeon avoids paraspinal muscle stripping and associated postoperative pain. The posterior bony and ligamentous elements are spared, leaving the posterior tension band intact [3, 8]. As the ALIF technique may achieve indirect decompression, a direct posterior decompression may not be necessary, which can decrease the risk of neurologic injury or durotomy [5, 9].

Direct access to the anterior column via the anterior approach provides visualization of the entire disc space and adjacent vertebral bodies. This affords the opportunity for complete discectomy as well as corpectomy, which may be indicated in trauma, deformity correction, or tumor resection [10]. While anterior corpectomy and fusion with cage placement is generally supplemented with posterior instrumentation, it allows for significant anterior vertebral column height and sagittal profile restoration without some of the risks of neural or vascular injury associated with large posterior corrective osteotomies such as vertebral column resection or pedicle subtraction osteotomy. The anterior approach may also be utilized in the context of infection, including osteodiscitis, if surgery is indicated. Loose hardware, including interbody devices placed from a posterior approach, can be removed from an anterior approach, and revision may be accomplished in the context of infection or pseudoarthrosis [11].

Advancements in the anterior approach have also reduced its complication profile. Reports of operative times under 90 minutes have been published in the literature which are associated with reduced blood loss and transfusion rates [3, 4, 8, 12]. These characteristics make the anterior approach attractive, especially considering the general trend towards less invasive surgery, which some surgeons consider performing in an outpatient setting.

However, the anterior approach does carry its own unique risk profile. Complications specific to the anterior anatomy, including major vessel injury (common iliac vein, inferior vena cava, and ascending iliolumbar vein); direct injury to the viscera, including ureteral injury, peritoneal tears and bowel injury; and approach-related neural injury, including presacral superior hypogastric plexus injury leading to retrograde ejaculation or sympathetic trunk injury leading to sympathetic dysfunction have been described [13, 14]. Postoperative complications including deep venous thrombosis, arterial thrombosis, and ileus may also occur as a result of the anterior approach and should be considered and discussed with the patient prior to surgery [13].

## Conclusion

The anterior approach to the lumbar spine is safe and effective when performed with care and attention to detail. Through one incision, multiple levels of the anterior lumbar spine can be visualized and accessed, allowing complete discectomy and application of a large footprint implant for height restoration, indirect decompression, anterior column support, and lordosis correction. The anterior approach may preclude the need for direct exposure or retraction of the dura and neural elements from a posterior approach. Indications for an anterior approach vary and may include spondylosis, radiculopathy, claudication, or deformity correction. The risk profile is generally favorable but does entail some unique risks including large vessel injury, visceral injury, or approach-related neural injury. Generally, the anterior approach to the lumbar spine represents a safe and effective approach to treat multiple lumbar pathologies.

## References


1. Capener N. Spondylolisthesis. Br J Surg. 1932;19:374–86.
2. Mobbs RJ, Phan K, Malham G, Seex K, Rao PJ. Lumbar interbody fusion: techniques, indications and comparison of interbody fusion options including PLIF, TLIF, MI-TLIF, OLIF/ATP, LLIF and ALIF. J Spine Surg. 2015 Dec;1(1):2–18.
3. Mobbs RJ, Loganathan A, Yeung V, Rao PJ. Indications for anterior lumbar interbody fusion. Orthop Surg. 2013;5(3):153–63.
4. Burke PJ. Anterior lumbar interbody fusion. Radiol Technol. 2001;72:423–30.
5. Pradhan BB, Nassar JA, Delamarter RB, Wang JC. Single-level lumbar spine fusion: a comparison of anterior and posterior approaches. J Spinal Disord Tech. 2002;15:355–61.
6. Chen D, Fay LA, Lok J, Yuan P, Edwards WT, Yuan HA. Increasing neuroforaminal volume by anterior interbody distraction in degenerative lumbar spine. Spine. 1995;20:74–9.
7. Duggal N, Mendiondo I, Pares HR, et al. Anterior lumbar interbody fusion for treatment of failed back surgery syndrome: an outcome analysis. Neurosurgery. 2004;54:636–43.
8. Mummaneni PV, Haid RW, Rodts GE. Lumbar interbody fusion: state-of-the-art technical advances. J Neurosurg Spine. 2004;1:24–30.
9. Shen FH, Samartzis D, Khanna AJ, Anderson DG. Minimally invasive techniques for lumbar interbody fusions. Orthop Clin North Am. 2007;38:373–86.
10. Mühlbauer M, Pfisterer W, Eyb R, Knosp E. Minimally invasive retroperitoneal approach for lumbar corpectomy and anterior reconstruction. J Neurosurg. 2000;93(1):161–7. https://doi.org/10.3171/spi.2000.93.1.0161.
11. Buttermann GR, Glazer PA, Hu SS, Bradford DS. Revision of failed lumbar fusions: a comparison of anterior autograft and allograft. Spine. 1997;22:2748–55.
12. Strube P, Hoff E, Hartwig T, Perka CF, Gross C, Putzier M. Stand-alone anterior versus anteroposterior lumbar interbody single-level fusion after a mean follow-up of 41 months. J Spinal Disord Tech. 2012;25:362–9.

                                                      

13. Czerwein JK, Thakur N, Migliori SJ, Lucas P, Palumbo M. Complications of anterior lumbar surgery. J Am Acad Orthop Surg. 2011;19(5):251–8.
14. Samudrala S, Khoo LT, Rhim SC, Fessler RG. Complications during anterior surgery of the lumbar spine: an anatomically based study and review. Neurosurg Focus. 1999;7(6):e9.

# Part II
# Preoperative Care for Lumbar Spine Access Surgery

# Chapter 4
# Patient Selection for Anterior Lumbar Access Surgery

Rebecca L. Kelso

## Introduction

While patient selection has always been a crucial point in surgical planning, lumbar access surgery exemplifies its importance. The introduction of minimally invasive access surgery with the options of anterior, oblique, lateral, and transforaminal lumbar interbody fusion has changed the landscape of patient evaluation. It is important to know not only the surgical plan and instrumentation capabilities, but also how a patient's unique factors can act in concert to increase surgical complexity and perioperative considerations that can be evaluated to minimize risk. The purpose of this chapter is to review specific considerations when evaluating a patient for anterior lumbar access surgery to help facilitate a safe and effective surgical procedure.

## General Considerations

As spine surgery is often elective, health and function optimization are imperative. Prior to consulting an access surgeon, the spine surgeon has usually already passed judgement on the suitability of a patient for surgery in general. This is done after considering pathology, symptoms, treatment options, and imaging. Additional evaluation takes factors such as comorbidities and surgical history into consideration to confirm the patient's surgical candidacy. The anterior approach for anterior lumbar interbody fusion (ALIF) surgery requires assessment of several specific areas.

R. L. Kelso (✉)
Novant Health Heart and Vascular Institute, Charlotte, NC, USA
e-mail: rlkelso@novanthealth.org

© The Author(s), under exclusive license to Springer Nature Switzerland AG 2023
J. R. O'Brien et al. (eds.), *Lumbar Spine Access Surgery*,
https://doi.org/10.1007/978-3-031-48034-8_4

The patient's medical record can provide a snapshot of their history with the caveat that the documentation may be incomplete. A review of comorbidities with special attention paid to cardiopulmonary diagnoses can provide an overview of the patient's overall health. Medical conditions such as obesity, coronary artery disease, and chronic obstructive pulmonary disease require special attention given their association with anesthesia risk and complications. A medication list may also provide useful information. A blood thinner may suggest an underlying condition such as atrial fibrillation, a history of embolism, thrombosis (venous or arterial), or thrombophilia, which have implications in perioperative management. Antiplatelet therapy may point to atherosclerotic vessel diseases with possible prior interventions such as stent placement.

Preoperatively, anticoagulation medication should be stopped at a predetermined level as agreed upon by the surgical team. In a similar fashion, prophylactic doses should be resumed when medically safe. Patients with a history of deep venous thrombosis (DVT) are at an increased risk during the perioperative period. Those with increased iliac vein manipulation or May-Thurner syndrome (left common iliac vein compression by an overlying right common iliac artery) are at a theoretical increased risk. However, it is difficulty to isolate the exact risk as the rate of DVT after ALIF is approximately 0–5% [1–3]. Patients with a vascular injury during surgery will also require appropriate management with antiplatelets or anticoagulation depending on the situation and reconstruction required.

Vascular disease can also affect the access procedure. Patients with aneurysms or atherosclerosis may have increased surgical complexity. Iliac or hypogastric aneurysms make access to the lower lumbar spine difficult and may be a contraindication for an anterior lumbar approach. There are some anecdotal reports of patients undergoing concomitant aneurysm and spine surgery; however, many surgeons prefer to not combine surgeries due to surgical complexity. Significant atherosclerotic disease can be identified on preoperative imaging as calcification or on physical exam as diminished pulses. Manipulation of heavily calcified vessels can cause plaque disruption leading to leg ischemia and additional procedures. In patients undergoing open surgery, scarring around the vessels can make access through regular techniques more challenging. In addition, endovascular stents within the iliac vessels must be carefully managed or avoided. Stents in general are associated with an inflammatory reaction and vessel scarring. Within the iliac system, stents can be balloon expandable or self-expanding. Balloon expandable stents are more common within the common iliac artery and compression with a retractor can lead to stenosis or occlusion. This requires immediate identification and treatment to minimize ischemia. Self-expanding stents differ by nature of their composition and will re-expand following compression. Knowing the patient's history and thoroughly reviewing imaging can help with decision-making. Patients with May-Thurner's syndrome may have a self-expanding iliac stent. Imaging review shows the location of the stent relative to the disc space (Fig. 4.1). Adjusting the location of the incision, accessing from the left versus the right pelvis, or performing anterior versus oblique or lateral approaches are all considerations for safer surgery. Review of the extent of iliac disease is important especially in exposure of the L4–L5 level as this location

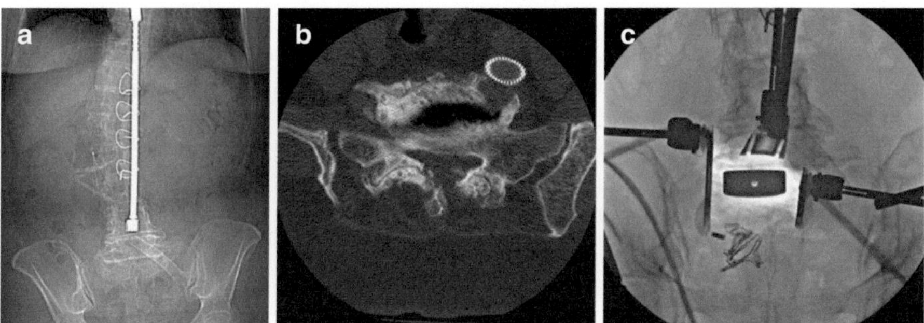

**Fig. 4.1** Vascular stents can affect surgical planning. Example of a self-expanding stent placed for May-Thurner's syndrome. (**a**) Plain film images showing location relative to the L5–S1 disc space. (**b**) Computed tomography at the level of the mid-disc space with stent in the lateral position preserving the access window. (**c**) Intraoperative images with good exposure and a midline trial. Note the stent is not in proximity to the retractor blades and there is no stent deformation

requires the greatest vessel manipulation and is thus the most common level for vascular injuries [2, 3].

In the obese patient, abdominal depth can make spine access surgery challenging. Obesity causes an increase in surgical time and incision size. Some studies suggest there are no differences in technical or intraoperative complication rates after surgery [4]. However, there may be differences in fusion rates, ileus occurrence, and wound complications [4, 5]. Ultimately, the absolute limitation in obese patients is surgical instrument length. All instruments, including forceps, cautery, and retractor systems, have a maximum available length. The longest retractor blades are often 200 or 220 mm. The L5–S1 level is often the deepest in the pelvis due to the natural lordosis of the spine. Weight loss will improve access, decrease infection risk, and improve postoperative recovery. Decreased force on the spine with weight loss may also mitigate some of the patient's symptoms, thus decreasing the need for surgery. In considering anterior lumbar fusion specifically, there has been recognition that lateral positioning can help facilitate access to the retroperitoneum by using gravity to retract the abdominal contents inferiorly, allowing a better window within the lower quadrant, anterior to the iliac crest. These techniques include the oblique lateral interbody fusion, anterior to psoas, or lateral ALIF approaches.

## Specific Considerations

Patient selection is often based on individual anatomy, including considerations of previous surgery. Contraindications to surgery are based on potential pitfalls related primarily to postsurgical scar tissue formation. As more surgeons gain experience and comfort operating in the retroperitoneum, the list of absolute contraindications will naturally shift towards relative contraindications. Careful case selection with gradually increasing complexity is advised when starting to perform access surgery. Most access surgeons favor a retroperitoneal approach rather than a transabdominal approach given the natural planes that provide direct access to the anterior spine. It also eliminates any manipulation or injury to the bowel. It is easiest to consider surgical risk by looking at the two main areas of dissection: the abdominal wall and the retroperitoneum. In addition, some special characteristics regarding previous spine surgery and infection will be discussed.

## Abdominal Wall

The abdominal wall is regarded by many as the guardian of the abdomen and entire chapters have been devoted to its construction and anatomic variation. Any surgery that fuses the natural planes between the posterior rectus sheath or transversalis fascia and the peritoneum bears mentioning (Table 4.1). These include the pre-peritoneal dissection of laparoscopic inguinal hernia repair, open prostate surgery, and abdominal wall reconstruction. The first two usually encompass a more focal area of the lower abdominal wall near the inguinal ligament or the space of Retzius. A clean, unoperated window into the retroperitoneum can often be found more cra-nially or laterally to the previously dissected space. Most hernia repairs use mesh, and its integration can obliterate the retroperitoneal plane, making dissection more difficult. In larger ventral hernia repairs, laparoscopic tacks are used and can be seen on preoperative X-rays, though more recent implants include nonmetallic options. The term "abdominal wall reconstruction" can encompass a broad scope of proce-dures and may include small umbilical hernias or diastasis recti repair to large

**Table 4.1** Anterior abdominal wall risk factors affecting anterior spine access

| Anterior abdominal wall |
| --- |
| Existing ventral hernia |
| Open or laparoscopic hernia repair with mesh |
| Component of parts separation |
| Congenital abdominal wall repair |
|    Gastroschisis, omphalocele |
| Panniculectomy |
| Abdominoplasty |
| Ostomy |
|    Ileostomy, colostomy, urostomy, ileo-conduit |
| Ostomy reversal |
| Open prostate surgery |
| Transverse rectus abdominus muscle flap |
| Deep inferior epigastric perforators flap |
| Previous anterior spine surgery |

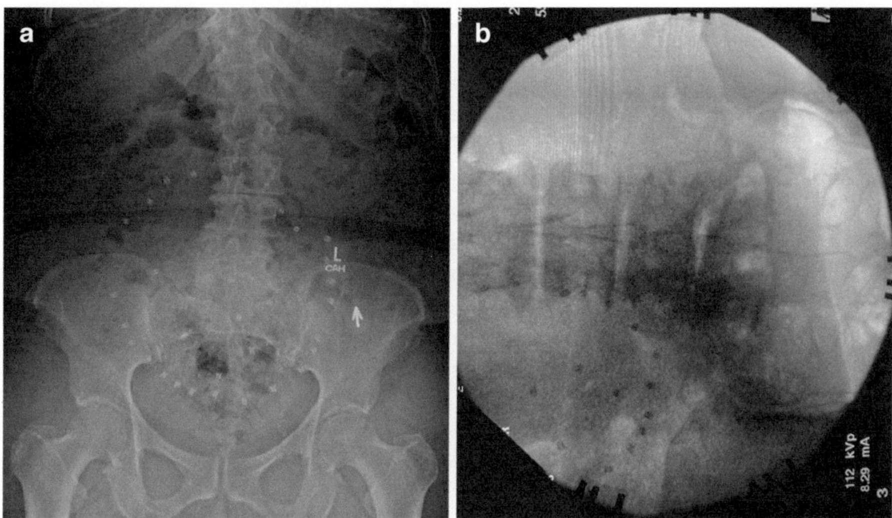

**Fig. 4.2** Alternative positioning for patient with lower abdominal hernia repair. (a) Upright abdominal X-ray showing tacks outlining the mesh edges of a laparoscopic hernia repair. (b) Patient in the lateral decubitus position with gravity-assisted movement of the mesh providing access to the undissected planes of the lower quadrant for lateral or oblique access window

abdominal wall hernias and loss of abdominal domain. These larger constructs require larger repairs with either mesh, component separation (separating layers of the abdominal wall), or a combination of the two. When performed in the lower abdomen, there is complete obliteration of this natural plane with scar tissue and/or mesh. These larger reconstructions often prevent the standard supine ALIF approach; however, depending on the extent of dissection, a lateral or oblique ALIF may be considered (Fig. 4.2). A careful review of the previous operative reports can provide key information of the extent of abdominal wall surgery.

In a similar fashion, plastic surgery can involve the abdominal wall. Cosmetic surgery with an abdominoplasty or panniculectomy, while common, does not violate the rectus sheath or the pre-peritoneal space. Plastic reconstructive surgery, however, utilizes two abdominal wall flaps including the transverse rectus abdominis myocutaneous (TRAM) and the deep inferior epigastric perforator (DIEP) flaps. TRAM flaps include the rectus muscle, leaving behind a large defect which is replaced with mesh. In contrast, DIEP flaps require dissection only around the epigastric vessels while the rectus remains intact, and portions of the pre-peritoneal plane lateral to this dissection are free of scar tissue. DIEP flaps do not tend to pose much difficulty with access surgery. ALIF in patients with unilateral TRAM flaps will be candidates for contralateral retroperitoneal dissection, whereas bilateral TRAM flaps may be a contraindication for ALIF. Transabdominal access is a consideration in these circumstances with the caveat that the construct of the mesh will be violated, and bowel adhesions may be present.

An ostomy creates a defect in the rectus sheath connecting the bowel or ureter to the external skin. Small bowel, colon, ureter, and ileo-conduits make up the most common ostomies and tend to have a standard abdominal wall placement. Reversed ostomies will be associated with a fused pre-peritoneal plane and there may be a hernia isolated to the area of closure. Dissection into the retroperitoneum may be easier by initially avoiding this area. Surgery with patent ostomies requires careful discussion of infection risk and stoma management with the patient and surgical team. Temporary purse-string closure of the ostomy may be required for clean skin prep. Dissection of the abdominal wall can be performed contralateral to the ostomy. If a retroperitoneal structure like the ureter is involved, there may be dissection around both the iliac vessels leading to more significant scar tissue formation. Careful review of the patient's records, imaging, and time since ostomy surgery can prove helpful in decision-making.

## *Retroperitoneum*

The retroperitoneum, in contrast to the abdominal wall, consists of specific structures that are encountered in ALIF surgery (Table 4.2). These structures lead to a higher risk of complications or injuries. Most notable are the iliac vessels, as they are the vessels most prone to injury during surgery. While all vessels are at risk, venous injuries, especially the left iliac vein, tend to be the most common [1]. Previous vascular surgery for an aneurysm or iliac stenting is a risk during ALIF exposure. Other retroperitoneal surgeries include iliac lymph node dissection, open bladder suspension, colon resection, and kidney transplant. Lymph node dissection may accompany surgeries for pelvic or groin cancers, including rectum, ovarian, prostate, or melanoma. They are often identified by surgical clips along the vessels with imaging. Open abdominal bladder suspension is less common today in favor of the more minimally invasive transvaginal versus laparoscopic-assisted approaches. Colon resection on either side will violate the white line of Toldt, making dissection more difficult in this area. It is especially difficult for higher level ALIF surgery along the left side. Kidney transplants will also violate the retroperitoneum making ipsilateral L5–S1 and bilateral L4–L5 exposure difficult; however, contralateral dissection for L5–S1 may still be possible. Primary left kidney surgery (both laparoscopic and open) also involves the retroperitoneum and Gerota's fascia and is a consideration when planning ALIF at higher levels or laterality for lateral surgery.

Diagnoses that obliterate the retroperitoneal planes include pelvic radiation and retroperitoneal fibrosis. Retroperitoneal fibrosis can be extensive and cause excessive scar tissue and even occlude vessels. Surgery in this situation is not recommended due to increased risk of injury and synergism causing increased fibrosis. Anatomic anomalies that can limit access surgery include vascular variations (hypogastric iliolumbar/lumbar anomalies, left-sided/duplicated inferior vena cava) or pelvic space-occupying masses (pelvic/horseshoe kidney, fibroids, and ovarian masses). In these situations, the anatomy may not preclude an anterior approach, but

**Table 4.2** Retroperitoneal risk factors affecting anterior spine access

| Retroperitoneum |
| --- |
| *Existing diagnosis* |
|    Iliac or hypogastric aneurysm |
|    Extensive iliac atherosclerotic disease |
|    Retroperitoneal fibrosis |
|    Large uterine or ovarian mass |
| *History* |
|    Pelvic radiation |
|    Iliac lymph node dissection |
|    Iliac artery or vein stents |
|    Open aortoiliac vascular surgery |
|    Sigmoid colon resection |
|    Kidney transplant |
|    Bladder sling/suspension |
|    Posterior spine surgery |
|    Infection |
|    Spinal osteomyelitis/discitis in location of planned surgery |
|    Upper pelvic abscess |
| *Anatomic anomalies* |
|    Venous variation—hypogastric, iliolumbar veins |
|    Lumbar artery variation |
|    Left sided inferior vena cava |
|    Duplicate inferior vena cava |
|    Pelvic kidney |
|    Horseshoe kidney |
| *Space-occupying pelvic masses* |
|    Ovarian cyst |
|    Fibroid |
|    Cancer of low pelvic structures |

may necessitate additional preoperative discussion and affect laterality. The mass effect from a large lesion may limit the ability to mobilize the lower quadrant contents across the midline and expose the entire vertebral surface.

Previous spine surgery can also cause additional scarring. Clearly differentiating previous posterior from anterior approaches is important, as revision ALIF surgery is more complex following a prior anterior procedure. Previous posterior surgery can lead to inflammation or thickening within the anterior longitudinal ligament (ALL) and adjacent tissues, even if the surgery was at a different level. In revision ALIF surgery, prior surgical laterality should be considered as a contralateral approach may minimize scar tissue encountered.

Infection in the retroperitoneum is often difficult to detect during history taking but can be an important factor in assessing potential scarring around the ALL and iliac veins. Active vertebral osteomyelitis or discitis can be seen as inflammation or phlegmon on imaging. Infection in this space can arise from perforated diverticulitis or appendicitis with a pelvic abscess that overlays the iliac vessels and/or ALL. If a history of any of these infections is identified during patient discussion, a more extensive conversation on intraoperative complications and vein injury is important. Alternative surgical techniques may be utilized to minimize dissection around the vessels and thus decrease risk of injury. Many access surgeons consider an en bloc dissection of all the tissue above the ALL, rather than direct vein dissection to decrease vessel injury. When dissection is carefully performed from a midline to lateral direction, one can minimize dissection to only the window needed for an implant. Careful preoperative review of vessel location is important in this technique.

## Conclusion

A thorough review and assessment of the available history and imaging can provide clues to the status of a patient's unique anatomy. Awareness of a patient's comorbidities and surgical history is essential to proper patient selection and consideration of potential complications will assist in proper preoperative risk discussion. Imaging review is useful in identifying characteristics related to the spine such as the vessel windows, transitional spinal anatomy, and pelvic incidence. Any evidence of vessel disease, previous surgery, and anatomic anomalies are crucial for an access surgeon to recognize and communicate with their spine colleagues. This not only improves preoperative preparation, but is ultimately key to technical success, decreased injury, and improved outcomes.

## References


1. Zahradnik V, Lubelski D, Abdullah KG, Kelso R, Mroz T, Kashyap VS. Vascular injuries during anterior exposure of the thoracolumbar spine. Ann Vasc Surg. 2013;27:306–13.
2. Hamdam AD, Malek JY, Schermerhorn ML, Aulivola B, Blattman SB, Pomposelli FB Jr. Vascular injury during anterior exposure of the spine. J Vasc Surg. 2008;48:650–4.
3. Chririano J, Abou-Zamzam AM Jr, Urayeneza O, Zhang WW, Cheng W. The role of the vascular surgeon in anterior retroperitoneal spine exposure: preservation of open surgical training. J Vasc Surg. 2009;50:148–51.
4. Phan K, Rogers P, Rao PJ, Mobbs RJ. Influence of obesity on complications, clinical outcome, and subsidence after anterior lumbar interbody fusion (ALIF): prospective observational study. World Neurosug. 2017;107:334–41.
5. Katsevaman GA, Daffner SD, Brandmeir NH, Emery SE, France JC, Sedney CL. Complexities of spine surgery in obese patient populations: a narrative review. Spin J. 2020;20(4):501–11.

# Chapter 5
# Imaging Review for Anterior Lumbar Access Surgery

Devin Zarkowsky, Jonathan E. Schoeff, and Aparna Baheti

## Introduction

There are a variety of imaging modalities used to diagnose, plan, and prepare for spine surgery. These include plain radiographs, angiography, computed tomography (CT), and magnetic resonance imaging (MRI). Most surgeons are familiar with interpreting radiographs. Higher-level imaging, including CT and MRI, may offer added value, especially in preoperative planning. Additional techniques, with a particular focus on vascular imaging, may also play a role in preoperative planning and in complex scenarios such as revision spine surgery.

## Radiographs (X-Ray, XR)

"Plain films"—usually including an anteroposterior projection and lateral projections in flexion and extension—are available prior to surgery on most spinal patients. Within the spectrum of imaging requiring ionizing radiation, this is the lowest dose and most cost-effective way to evaluate osseous pathology. Radiographs can offer key insights for spinal access surgeons. First, they provide a sense of the overall size of the patient and the distance from the skin to the spine. Additionally, they depict general spinal anatomy, prior hardware, or fractures. Radiographs also will give

D. Zarkowsky (✉)
Scripps Clinic, La Jolla, CA, USA

J. E. Schoeff
Rocky Mountain Advanced Spine Access, Lone Tree, CO, USA

A. Baheti
Vascular and Interventional Radiologist, Tacoma, WA, USA

© The Author(s), under exclusive license to Springer Nature Switzerland AG 2023
J. R. O'Brien et al. (eds.), *Lumbar Spine Access Surgery*,
https://doi.org/10.1007/978-3-031-48034-8_5

insight into prior abdominal or pelvic surgeries, signified by radiopaque, retained surgical objects in the abdomen or pelvis. Dense vascular calcifications, or evidence of previous endovascular stent intervention, forewarn challenging vascular mobilization. Calculating parameters such as sacral slope relative to the pubic bone can provide insight into accessibility of the lower lumbar spine. When the sacral slope corresponds to a skin intersection caudal to the pubic bone, it may prove difficult to access the L5–S1 level. Although rare, this may obviate the role of an anterior spine procedure in such a patient. Additionally, severe deformity and/or protruding anterior osteophytes should raise concern for inflammation at the affected level(s). Radiographs may also reveal a prior inferior vena cava (IVC) filter, which could complicate anterior access depending on its dwell time and possible erosion into adjacent vertebral bodies. Therefore, it is imperative that radiographs be reviewed preoperatively to aid in planning.

In addition to traditional spinal radiographs which are obtained when the patient is supine, one might note that "standing" or "scoliosis" films that provide basic spinopelvic and global sagittal alignment parameters can be useful for determining spine alignment. Additionally, oblique views may be obtained, which are used to better assess the pars interarticularis.

## Angiography

The gold-standard evaluation of venous pathology remains the diagnostic venogram. This is an invasive procedure performed by a vascular surgeon or other interventional specialist. Patients lay supine on a fluoroscopy table and the femoral or internal jugular vein is accessed percutaneously with a sheath placed to secure vascular access. Digital subtraction angiography is then performed in multiple projections, with sub-selective angiography as necessary. Conventional venography is useful if there is suspicion of preexisting pathology, such as in patients with a prior deep venous thrombosis or trauma. It affords the highest spatial resolution of all the imaging modalities. Venograms can be diagnostic or interventional—the treating physician may embolize vessels predicted to complicate spinal access procedures. Additionally, venous stent placement especially in the setting of venous compressive disorders, such as May-Thurner syndrome, can redirect flow and significantly reduce venous collaterals. Access site complications, including hematoma and arteriovenous fistula, are the main risk associated with angiography, currently 3–4% for arteriography [1, 2] and 3–4% for venography [3, 4].

Enthusiasm for laparoscopy in the late 1990s prompted surgeons in Chicago to evaluate venous and arterial angiography in relationship to the L3–L4, L4–L5, and L5–S1 disc spaces [5]. Angiographic images obtained for indications other than spinal access were reviewed from a total of 43 patients, 22 with arterial images and 21 with venous images. Discs were deemed "accessible" if the target space's central portion and an adjacent 30% was free from overlying vascular structure. Retraction on the aorta was deemed unsafe during laparoscopic exposure; therefore, at L3–L4, only 2 of 21 (9%) of patients were assessed to have an accessible disc, 38% at L4–L5, and 95% at L5–S1. Similarly, the vena cava courses along the right lateral aspect of the disc at L3–L4, rendering 100% of discs accessible at this level in relationship to venous anatomy, 73% at L4–L5, and 60% at L5–S1.

## Computed Tomography (CT)

The main advantage of CT over radiographs is the ability to see a structure in all three planes and thereby better understand the relationships between various structures. CT offers some soft tissue resolution as well, which is often difficult to evaluate with radiographs. CT gives clear evaluation of facet disease, spinal canal narrowing, and osseous anatomy.

Traditional spine CTs, CT myelograms, and CT discograms are usually performed as "noncontrast" exams. When radiologists refer to contrast-enhanced exams, they are referring to intravenous contrast administration, which is not required for standard evaluation of the lumbar spine. Dedicated spine CTs are "coned down" or collimated to only include the spine and do not give information about the entire abdomen/pelvis, just the soft tissues directly adjacent to the spine. Included with the cross-sectional imaging is a "scout scan." This is a very-low-dose radiograph that the CT technologist performs before the CT scan to ensure they are capturing the correct field of view for their cross-sectional images.

Catheter-based angiography has been supplanted by CT imaging over the last decade. Iodinated contrast, which appears hyperdense or "bright" on CT, is injected through a peripheral IV and is used to evaluate the vessels. A CT angiogram is a generic term for a CT scan where the contrast bolus is timed to look at vascular anatomy, typically the arterial phase if not specified by the ordering provider. A CT venogram (CTV) to evaluate the venous vasculature requires a longer delay between injection and scan acquisition as compared with arteriograms. The portal venous CT, generically termed a CT abdomen/pelvis with contrast, is performed at a 70-s delay. In contrast, in the CTV, an arterial phase is performed earlier, with a 30–40-s delay and a venous phase between a 90- and 150-s delay. Most modern imaging systems employ "bolus triggering" to determine the exact timing of the scan.

An advantage of the CT angiogram is the ability to use post-processing to create high-quality multiplanar reconstruction and maximum intensity projection reformats, which is helpful to understand the path of vascular structures relative to the operative field. While CTV can facilitate clearer identification of venous anatomy, it remains somewhat unpredictable in terms of quality and clarity of reconstruction and additionally does not provide critical data regarding the retrovascular fat plane and, consequently, the relative mobility of the vasculature. Advanced applications include bone subtraction, which can be performed manually on traditional CT scanners and can be automated on newer dual-energy CT scanners.

Kleeman et al. evaluated vascular anatomy with MRI and CT preoperative imaging when planning laparoscopic anterior spinal exposures [6]. Patients were classified into categories based on the relationship of the aortic bifurcation and left iliac vein relative to the L4–L5 disc space. These categories guided procedural technique.

## Magnetic Resonance Imaging (MRI)

Compared to CT, MRI offers superior soft tissue resolution to evaluate discs, foramina, facets, and other non-osseous spinal components. Additionally, MRI avoids ionizing radiation risks incurred by XR and CT. A complete MRI of the spine can take anywhere between 30 and 90 min to complete, depending on the sequences requested and a patient's ability to lay still.

MRI is the preferred study when evaluating the overlying vasculature of the spine, providing considerable information, both direct and extrapolative, regarding the absolute location of vessels relative to the spine, general landmarks such as bifurcations and branches, along with critical data regarding the relative adherence and mobility of the venous structures directly in contact with the spine.

As with CT, most spine MRI is performed without contrast. However, if there is concern for a vascular pathology or tumor, contrast can be administered. MRI contrast is a gadolinium-based solution as opposed to the iodinated solution of contrast CTs. Many sequences can be performed after contrast administration to address different points of enhancement in the vascular system (i.e., arterial, portal venous, and venous). MR angiogram (MRA) is usually performed using a 3D gradient echo technique. MRA can detect normal intradural vessels as well as vessels in patients with dural atriovenous fistulas.

Ng et al. defined the "vascular corridor" as the horizontal distance between the rightmost border of the left common iliac vein (LCIV) and the leftmost border of the right common iliac vein (RCIV) which is similar to the "vascular free window" concept [7]. In a retrospective review of 379 patient MRIs, these authors measured the vascular corridor at the L5–S1 level and assessed the fat plane as either present or absent. Of these patients, access to L5–S1 was characterized as "easy" in 37%, "advanced" in 61%, and "difficult" in 2%. Employing MRI to evaluate soft tissue adjacent to vascular structures represents an evolution in preoperative planning, an opportunity not afforded by angiography or CT.

While planning oblique lateral interbody fusion cases, Chung et al. examined both iliac vein juxtaposition with the disc space and mobility afforded by the retrovenous fat pad to classify their patients into three types [8]. Type 1 patients had no requirement for mobilization and the LCIV ran laterally for more than two-thirds of the length of the left side of the L5–S1 disc; type 2 patients had easy mobilization and the LCIV obstructed the L5–S1 disc space, but the perivascular adipose tissue was present under the LCIV; and type 3 patients had potentially difficult mobilization and no perivascular adipose tissue under the LCIV. Interobserver variability statistics demonstrated excellent correlation between attending surgeons, which was of particular importance in the type 3 patients, as this group suffered venous injury with statistically greater frequency than type 1 or type 2 patients (33% vs. 0% vs. 11% respectively, $p < 0.003$). Furthermore, this group demonstrated the necessity to transmit planning information, as there was a progressive decline in interobserver reliability when attending surgeons' classification choices were compared with fellow- and resident-level trainees.

This critical data point informs preoperative discussions around vascular injury during anterior access. Translating 2D static, supine imaging into a spatial understanding of the dynamic, 3D operative space requires consistent practice reviewing T2-weighted series with axial images reformatted to be inline with the disc spaces. This latter tactic—orthogonal reformatting—presents vessel-disc relationships as they will appear intraoperatively. Finally, patient volume status affects venous anatomy's appearance on MRI and we encourage scans to be completed in well-hydrated patients.

## Conclusion

Spinal access surgeons must collaborate closely with their spine surgery colleagues to obtain appropriate preoperative imaging. This information is essential to a multidisciplinary approach in spine patient care. Involving radiology colleagues when developing imaging protocols can inform this process, and we recommend all three specialties communicate during spinal imaging protocol development to achieve the best patient-centered results.

## References


1. Ramirez JL, Zarkowsky DS, Sorrentino TA, et al. Antegrade common femoral artery closure device use is associated with decreased complications. J Vasc Surg. 2020;72:1610–7. e1
2. Siracuse JJ, Farber A, Cheng TW, et al. Common femoral artery antegrade and retrograde approaches have similar access site complications. J Vasc Surg. 2019;69:1160–6. e2
3. Park JY, Ahn JH, Jeon YS, Cho SG, Kim JY, Hong KC. Iliac vein stenting as a durable option for residual stenosis after catheter-directed thrombolysis and angioplasty of iliofemoral deep vein thrombosis secondary to May-Thurner syndrome. Phlebology. 2014;29:461–70.
4. Ishikawa E, Miyazaki S, Mukai M, et al. Femoral vascular complications after catheter ablation in the current era: the utility of computed tomography imaging. J Cardiovasc Electrophysiol. 2020;31:1385–93.
5. Vraney RT, Phillips FM, Wetzel FT, Brustein M. Peridiscal vascular anatomy of the lower lumbar spine. An endoscopic perspective. Spine (Phila Pa 1976). 1999;24:2183–7.
6. Kleeman TJ, Michael Ahn U, Clutterbuck WB, Campbell CJ, Talbot-Kleeman A. Laparoscopic anterior lumbar interbody fusion at L4-L5: an anatomic evaluation and approach classification. Spine (Phila Pa 1976). 2002;27:1390–5.
7. Ng JP, Scott-Young M, Chan DN, Oh JY. The feasibility of anterior spinal access: the vascular corridor at the L5-S1 level for anterior lumbar Interbody fusion. Spine (Phila Pa 1976). 2021;46:983–9.
8. Chung NS, Jeon CH, Lee HD, Kweon HJ. Preoperative evaluation of left common iliac vein in oblique lateral interbody fusion at L5-S1. Eur Spine J. 2017;26:2797–803.

# Chapter 6
# Informed Consent for Anterior Lumbar Access Surgery

Steven E. Raper

## Introduction

Informed consent is a keystone of the surgeon-patient relationship. The consent process is rooted in the ethical principles of autonomy and beneficence. There are numerous stakeholders contributing to informed consent, creating a process in constant evolution. All healthcare institutions have policies regarding how informed consent should be obtained. Within each state and federal government exists some combination of legislation, case law, and regulation that sets out the requirements of consent. Governmental agencies such as the Centers for Medicare and Medicaid Services and the Joint Commission also promulgate conditions healthcare institutions must meet for providing and documenting informed consent. National and international professional societies have also developed principles to which surgeon members are encouraged to adhere.

Informed consent remains an important part of the preoperative process for patients undergoing spine access and spine surgery. Material risks that should be discussed at a minimum have been identified. A recent development is the necessary disclosure to patients that their operation might overlap with that of another patient. Lack of consent comprises a significant proportion of allegations raised in malpractice lawsuits against neurosurgeons and orthopedic surgeons who perform spine surgery. Evolution is facilitated by researchers who are developing novel approaches

---

This chapter is written for educational purposes only and should not be taken as legal advice. Should specific legal questions arise, consult your Office of General Counsel or other attorney licensed in your jurisdiction.

---

S. E. Raper (✉)
Department of Surgery, Perelman School of Medicine, University of Pennsylvania, Philadelphia, PA, USA
e-mail: steven.raper@pennmedicine.upenn.edu

© The Author(s), under exclusive license to Springer Nature Switzerland AG 2023

J. R. O'Brien et al. (eds.), *Lumbar Spine Access Surgery*,
https://doi.org/10.1007/978-3-031-48034-8_6

49

to improving the process of informed consent. As society recognizes that elements of social justice are necessary to ensure all patients can give fully informed consent, so too have these concerns been addressed in spine access and spinal operations.

## Principles of Informed Consent

Two ethical principles—autonomy and beneficence—are considered imperatives in any discussion about informed consent. Respect for autonomy states persons should be free to choose and act without controlling constraints imposed by others. Autonomy is generally the prevailing principle in the twenty-first century. Beneficence is essentially the paternalistic "doctor who knows what is best for the patient" principle and subsumes four elements: do not inflict evil or harm, prevent evil and harm, remove evil and harm, do and promote good [1].

It is unclear if the ancients got consent. However, beneficence was the prevailing ethical principle: Hippocrates wrote "Declare the past, diagnose the present, predict the future. Make a habit of two things: to help or to at least do no harm." A leading medieval physician Henri deMondeville noted "patients should obey their surgeons implicitly in everything appertaining to their cure." During the enlightenment, Benjamin Rush advocated that "The obedience of a patient to the prescriptions of his physician should be prompt, strict, and universal." But Rush did want patients sufficiently educated that they could understand the physician's recommendations as motivation to comply. In 1847, while the westward expansion of *Manifest Destiny* was underway, the American Medical Association (AMA) was founded and published its first code of medical ethics. This code was lifted almost verbatim from a work of Thomas Percival: *The Medical Ethics*. Here again, physician beneficence was the prevailing principle, but did suggest that "to silence a patient with blunt authority may only result in a worsening of the patient's condition." Truth-telling was not a requirement and lies could be told if the physician thought it in the best interests of the patient. Percival's influence persisted in the AMA code up until the 1980s [1].

In 1982, Ronald Reagan established the President's Commission for the Study of Ethical Problems in Medicine and Biomedical and Behavioral Research that released a report, the basic framework for consent that remains to this day [2]. The President's Commission noted that the informed consent doctrine is first and foremost an ethical imperative that nonetheless has substantial foundations in law. Ethically valid consent is a process of shared decision-making based upon mutual respect of physician and patient, not merely ritual rote repetition of the contents of a form that details the risks of particular treatments. Informed consent is rooted in the legal presumption of competency; adults are entitled to accept or reject health-care interventions based on their own personal values and the pursuit of personal goals [2].

## The Law and Informed Consent

Unlike ethics, the law has teeth. The legal system can hold accountable those healthcare providers found negligent in the care of patients. For lack of informed consent, there are two theories of liability under the law: negligence and battery. Negligence requires a plaintiff to demonstrate a duty, breach of the duty, proximate causation, and damages. Medical malpractice—a special type of negligence—is the cause of action in most jurisdictions. Rarely, a jurisdiction exists in which consent is considered a battery or unauthorized touching. Three legal standards evolved for medical malpractice in general and informed consent in specific: the professional standard, the reasonable patient standard, and the subjective standard. The *professional standard* arose from the old beneficence concept in which the physician knew what was best. Basically, the standard required the individual physician to abide by the customary practices of the professional community. A major criticism of the professional standard is that physicians do not have sufficient expertise to know what is in the best interests of the patient. The *reasonable patient standard* focuses on materiality of the risks, alternatives, and consequences a patient would reasonably want to know. This is the prevailing standard in most jurisdictions although materiality of information is ambiguous, and the reasonable patient is not defined. The *subjective standard* requires the physician to disclose the information material to the individual patient. A criticism of this standard is that it allows the patient to make idiosyncratic choices [1].

There are a number of other stakeholders who may adapt the informed consent process. All healthcare organizations have a policy or policies on informed consent. These policies usually are written to comply with various regulatory requirements and may vary widely in scope depending on the state or federal jurisdiction. It is important that surgeons familiarize themselves with *local policy* and procedure. Regulatory bodies such as the Joint Commission look at how closely healthcare organizations adhere to their own policies and procedures.

Often, informed consent policies are shaped by legislatures and the courts. State or federal legislation on informed consent is often enacted and the details can vary widely. Courts, through adjudication of malpractice lawsuits, also have significant impact. The following four landmark cases highlight important legal principles; there are many more. Each state will have a similar case law that is binding in the particular jurisdiction. Consent did not always have to be secured.

In *Schlondorff v. Society of New York Hospital*, the patient agreed to the exam under anesthesia, but no operation. The surgeon removed a giant fibroid tumor without consent and the patient sued. Benjamin Nathan Cardozo, a famous jurist, uttered one of the most famous pronouncements in medicolegal jurisprudence: "Every human being of adult years and sound mind has a right to determine what shall be done with his own body; and a surgeon who performs an operation without his patient's consent commits an assault, for which he is liable in damages" [3]. Consent had to be informed beginning in the 1950s. Salgo suffered lower extremity paralysis after a translumbar aortogram. In response to a claim of inadequate consent, an appeal the court held that "for physicians, in discussing the element of risk, a certain amount of discretion must be employed consistent with the full disclosure of facts necessary to an informed consent" [4]. Natanson alleged negligence after suffering severe radiation burns after mastectomy. In the resulting lawsuit, the court held to a professional standard of practice [5]. But the court further held that even if medical care was flawless, *injury from a known risk undisclosed* to the patient might subject the physician to liability. Canterbury underwent a laminectomy and suffered paralysis after falling out of bed. The court rejected the professional standard and developed the reasonable patient standard "a patient's right of self-determination demands a standard set by law for physicians" [6].

Healthcare facilities that accept Medicare and Medicaid payments must also agree to follow the Centers for Medicare and Medicaid Services (CMS) Hospital Conditions of Participation [7]. The CMS mandated Conditions of Participation and details on how to assess compliance are set out in a State Operations Manual [7]. There are three informed consent sections requiring (1) that the patient or his or her representative (as enacted by state law) has the right to make informed decisions regarding his or her care, (2) that properly executed informed consent forms for procedures and treatments are required and medical staff bylaws must state that physicians must have privileges to perform the procedures for which consent is required, and (3) except in emergencies, properly executed informed consent forms for the operation must be in the patient's chart before surgery [8].

## Informed Consent in Spine Access and Spine Surgery

### *Material Risks*

One concern is what constitutes a *material risk* of either the choice of access or the spine operation itself? One way to determine materiality is to study the complications experienced by patients undergoing spine access procedures [9]. In a study of 660 consecutive patients undergoing anterior lumbar interbody fusion, the rates of intraoperative complications (e.g., vascular injury, ureter injury, retroperitoneal hematoma) and 90-day postoperative complications (e.g., urinary tract infection, scar revision, ileus, deep vein thrombosis, pulmonary embolism, readmission) were reported [10]. In a separate study of 1178 patients, 57 exposure-related complications occurred, including 17 vascular injuries and 3 bowel injuries. Twenty patients sustained venous thromboembolism, and 16 patients developed a retroperitoneal hematoma/seroma. Four patients had a postoperative myocardial infarction, two had a stroke, and two died. Postoperatively, 31 patients developed incisional complications (e.g., surgical site infection, incisional hernia) [11]. In a comparison study of oblique lateral interbody fusion and lateral lumbar interbody fusion spine exposure, vascular injuries were rare with either approach [12].

One strategy to ensure material risks are covered is to standardize the consent process. The "three-legged stool" has been advocated: the first leg is an information booklet, written at a level a reasonable patient understands. The second leg is a patient-surgeon conversation including the risks of the proposed treatment, about which a reasonable patient would want to know. The conversation is best documented in the medical record. The third leg is the actual consent for signed by the patient [13]. Often, the advice is to list frequent complications that lead to lesser injury and rare complications that lead to serious injury. However, it can be hard to determine specific examples of what rare complications should be listed. One review of 100 patient charts showed none mentioned postoperative visual loss, a rare but serious complication of prone positioning for spinal surgery [14]. There is often a discrepancy between what patients and surgeons expect to accomplish with spine surgery. The authors demonstrated wide discrepancies between the patient and the surgeon regarding the expected outcome of surgery, highlighting a need for clearer explanations of the association between the spinal diagnosis and neurological deficits of pain and function after spine surgery [15].

## Overlapping Surgery and Informed Consent (Multiple Rooms)

In April 2016, the American College of Surgeons (ACS) revised its Statements on Principles; a significant change was the articulation of a position on concurrent and overlapping surgery. Concurrent surgery, defined as two operations by the same surgeon in which the key or critical elements are being performed simultaneously, is deemed inappropriate. Overlapping operations may be allowed but subject to conditions. First, when the key or critical elements of an operation are completed without a reasonable expectation that the surgeon will need to return to that operation, a second operation can start in a different operating room while a qualified practitioner finishes the first operation. Second, when the key or critical elements an operation have been completed and the primary attending surgeon is performing key or critical portions of a second operation in another room, the surgeon must assign immediate availability in the first operating room to another attending surgeon. The patient needs to be informed in either of these circumstances [16]. Major neurosurgical societies have issued a similar position statement [17].

The Senate Finance Committee has jurisdiction over the Medicare and Medicaid programs. Committee staff became aware of the practice of overlapping surgery. Committee staff examined the Statement on Principles promulgated by the ACS and other materials and subsequently released a report "Concurrent and Overlapping Surgery: Additional Measures Warranted." The Committee characterized their findings as a patient safety issue. The committee was concerned that lack of evidence was not the same as evidence that such concurrent procedures were safe. Citing the ACS Statements of Principles with favor, the Committee suggested healthcare institutions and oversight bodies strengthen policies regarding concurrent and overlapping surgery. Additionally, healthcare institutions were encouraged to assure patients understand their surgery will overlap with others, develop frequently asked questions, and educate patients far enough in advance to allow full consideration of their options [18].

In one survey of patients undergoing spine surgery, patients had an overall positive attitude toward having residents participate, knew, and were comfortable with the role that residents played in their healthcare [19]. Knowledge about concurrent and overlapping surgery was low in a separate survey of patients and family members. Only 60% of those surveyed felt comfortable with overlapping surgery and essentially all wanted the surgeon to disclose the participation of surgical residents and fellows. Patient comfort rose with those in the fourth and fifth years of surgical training. The authors concluded that a general lack of knowledge about concurrent or overlapping surgery impairs informed consent [20].

## *Medical Malpractice and Lack of Spine Surgery Consent*

Although not the most common source of medical malpractice claims, lack of informed consent issues leads to an appreciable number of lawsuits against spine surgeons [21, 22]. In one study of 978 medical malpractice claims in the United Kingdom, the primary allegation was failure to warn/informed consent in 80 (8.13%) of the cases [23]. A study of a large legal database showed that lack of informed consent was present in 34% of spine surgery lawsuits [24]. In a separate review, there was a perception that informed consent was not adequate in 24% of state and federal malpractice lawsuits [25].

## Novel Approaches to Improve the Informed Consent Process

In spine surgery, as in many other disciplines, efforts are being made to try and improve the informed consent process. A French spinal surgery society developed an Internet-based model information sheet. The prospective study documented improved understanding in patients scheduled for spinal surgery [26]. Preoperatively prepared patient-specific 3D models were used in a small series of patients undergoing posterior lumbar fixation to improve patient understanding and informed consent. The models were shared with neurosurgical trainees who reported better understanding of spine anatomy [27]. Patients were sent a video recording of the counselling and consent discussion—the Oxford Video Informed Consent tool—prior to spinal surgery. The intervention improved satisfaction over traditional consenting methods [28]. To encourage patients to ask more questions and create a more interactive consent process, a question prompt list was developed. Self-reported questionnaires documented high satisfaction [29]. Using validated tests, patient anxiety could be correlated with unfulfilled information needs and pain during the informed consent consultation [30]. One mixed-methods study showed variation in the disclosure of potential harms during informed consent discussions for lumbar spine surgery among Canadian spine surgeons. Patients wanted more information specifically about postoperative care. A proposal to develop guidelines should reduce practice variation making consent discussions more effective [31].

Three randomized clinical trials also attempted to improve informed consent. In one trial, a written sheet of surgical risks given at the informed consent discussion significantly increased recall of surgical risks for elective lumbar spine surgery [32]. Patients were randomized to an intervention consisting of an e-book containing information about their disease process. The use of mobile technology—an electronic booklet—significantly improved patients' knowledge of their surgical procedure [33]. Patients undergoing spine surgery were randomized to receive either an interactive videodisc (with a booklet) or a booklet alone. Those who viewed the videodisc chose surgery less often although the choice did not reach significance due in large part to sample size [34]. Seventy randomized clinical trials designed to test interventions that might improve informed consent were reviewed. The data suggested that validated interventions and assessments of comprehension, patient satisfaction, and minimizing anxiety or depression were more effective than non-validated instruments [35].

## Social Justice and Informed Consent

To adequately describe material risks, issues of language, literacy, learning needs, and cost have not been adequately studied—in any specialty—attempting to improve the informed consent process [35]. A systematic review of spine surgery consent practices noted that understanding the baseline health literacy level, knowledge, and information needs of each patient regarding the treatment will help surgeons tailor their communication to an appropriate level [36]. Patient recall is also a concern. Overall, problems in written consent for elective lumbar spinal surgery were partly reflected in the poor patient recall. Younger age and longer consent-to-surgery time improved patient recall of risks like paralysis and return of symptoms [37]. A multicenter multispecialty observational study of neurosurgeons recorded while providing informed consent for noninstrumented spine surgery was conducted. In approximately half of the video recordings, risks were not explained in words patients were likely to understand [38].

## Conclusion

The process of informed consent is a foundational part of the surgeon-patient relationship. Patients deciding whether to undergo an operation need to understand the procedure under discussion in a form the patient can understand and be free of coercive restraint. Surgeons must be familiar with the fact that many stakeholders have input into the details of consent, local policies, the relevant law, and the regulations put forth by federal agencies like CMS. In addition to the material risks of which the patient is apprised, other aspects of the procedure are necessary as found in professional society statements. Consent discussions, done properly, are an important way to maintain good communication with the patient and are best tailored to the patient's language, literacy, and learning needs. Well-informed patients are better able to participate in their care and often will have better outcomes.

## References


1. Faden RR, Beauchamp TL. Pronouncement and practice in clinical medicine. In: Faden RR, Beauchamp TL, King N, editors. A history and theory of informed consent. New York: Oxford University Press; 1986. p. 53–113.
2. President's Commission for the Study of Ethical Problems in Medicine and Biomedical and Behavioral Research. Vol. 1: report: making health care decisions: the ethical and legal implications of informed consent in the patient-practitioner relationship. ASI 16088--1.1. Washington, DC: US Government Printing Office; 1982.
3. *Schloendorff v Society of New York Hospitals 211 N.Y.125, 105 N.E. 92* (1914).
4. *Salgo v. Leland Stanford Jr. University Board of Trustees, 317 P.2d 170* (1957).
5. *Natanson v. Kline 350 P.2d 1093* (1960).
6. *Canterbury v. Spence 464 F.2d 772 (D.C. Cir. 1972).*
7. Centers for Medicare and Medicaid Services Hospital Conditions of Participation. Quality, safety & oversight – certification & compliance. https://www.cms.gov/Medicare/Provider-Enrollment-and-Certification/CertificationandComplianc/Hospitals. Last accessed 26 Jan 2022.
8. Raper SE, Joseph J. Informed consent for academic surgeons: a curriculum-based update. MedEdPORTAL. 2020;16:10985. https://doi.org/10.15766/mep_2374-8265.10985.
9. Wert WG Jr, Sellers W, Mariner D, Obmann M, Song B, Ryer EJ, Nikam S. Identifying risk factors for complications during exposure for anterior lumbar interbody fusion. Cureus. 2021;13(7):e16792. https://doi.org/10.7759/cureus.16792.
10. Momin AA, Barksdale EM III, Lone Z, Enders JJ, Nowacki AS, Winkelman RD, Krantz M, Hardy DM, Steinmetz MP. Exploring perioperative complications of anterior lumber interbody fusion in patients with a history of prior abdominal surgery: a retrospective cohort study. Spine J. 2020;20:1037–43.
11. Manunga J, Alcala C, Smith J, Mirza A, Titus J, Skeik N, Senthil J, Stephenson E, Alexander J, Sullivan S. Technical approach, outcomes, and exposure-related complications in patients undergoing anterior lumbar interbody fusion. J Vasc Surg. 2021;73:992–8.
12. Aguirre AO, Soliman MAR, Azmy S, Khan A, Jowdy PK, Mullin JP, Pollina J. Incidence of major and minor vascular injuries during lateral access lumbar interbody fusion procedures: a retrospective comparative study and systematic literature review. Neurosurg Rev 2022;45(2):1275-1289 https://doi.org/10.1007/s10143-021-01699-8.

13. Powell JM, Rai A, Foy M, Casey A, Dabke H, Gibson A, Hutton M. The 'three-legged stool': a system for spinal informed consent. Bone Joint J. 2016;98-B:1427–30.
14. Greenway F, Tulloch I, Laban J. Consent for postoperative visual loss in prone spinal surgery: aligning clinical practice with legal standards. Br J Neurosurg. 2018;32(6):604–9. https://doi.org/10.1080/02688697.2018.1519111.
15. Lattig F, Fekete TF, O'Riordan D, Kleinstück FS, Jeszenszky D, Porchet F, Mutter U, Mannion AF. A comparison of patient and surgeon preoperative expectations of spinal surgery. Spine. 2013;38(12):1040–8.
16. American College of Surgeons Statements on Principles. https://www.facs.org/about-acs/statements/stonprin#iid. Last visited 22 Jan 2022.
17. Position statement on intraoperative responsibility of the primary neurosurgeon. https://www.aans.org/-/media/Files/AANS/Advocacy/PDFS/Position-Statements/Neurosurgery-Position-Statement-on-Overlapping-Surgery-FINAL.ashx. Last visited 22 Jan 2022.
18. Senate Finance Committee. Concurrent and overlapping surgeries: additional measures warranted. https://www.finance.senate.gov/imo/media/doc/Concurrent%20Surgeries%20Report%20Final.pdf. Last visited 21 Jan 2022.
19. Fiani B, Cathel A, Arshad M, Hadi H, Khan YR, Quadri SA, Alastra A, Siddiqi J. Patient perspectives on the participation of neurosurgery resident physicians in their care. Cureus. 2020;12(2):e6880. https://doi.org/10.7759/cureus.6880.
20. Kim A, Alluri R, Kang H, Wang J, Hah R. Not without my attending: a survey of patient and family member attitudes and perceptions about concurrent and overlapping surgery. Spine J. 2021;21(6):889–98.
21. Epstein NE. What can spine surgeons do to improve patient care and avoid medical negligence suits? Surg Neurol Int. 2020;11(38):1–5.
22. Jackson KL, Rumley J, Griffith M, Linkous TR, Agochukwu U, DeVine J. Medical malpractice claims and mitigation strategies following spine surgery. Global Spine J. 2021;11(5):782–91.
23. Machin JT, Hardman J, Harrison W, Briggs TWR, Hutton M. Can spinal surgery in England be saved from litigation: a review of 978 clinical negligence claims against the NHS. Eur Spine J. 2018;27:2693–9. https://doi.org/10.1007/s00586-018-5739-1.
24. Makhni MC, Park PJ, Jimenez J, Saifi C, Caldwell JM, Ha A, Figueroa-Santana B, Lehman RA Jr, Weidenbaum M. The medicolegal landscape of spine surgery: how do surgeons fare? Spine J. 2018;18:209–15.
25. Agarwal N, Gupta R, Agarwal P, Matthew P, Wolferz R Jr, Shah A, Adeeb N, Prabhu AV, Kanter AS, Okonkwo DO, Kojo Hamilton D. Descriptive analysis of state and federal spine surgery malpractice litigation in the United States. Spine. 2018;43(14):984–90.
26. Madkouri R, Grelat M, Vidon-Buthion A, Lleu M, Beaurain J, Mourier K-L. Assessment of the effectiveness of SFCR patient information sheets before scheduled spinal surgery. Orthop Traumatol Surg Res. 2016;102:479–83.
27. Liew Y, Beveridge E, Demetriades AK, Hughes MA. 3D printing of patient-specific anatomy: a tool to improve patient consent and enhance imaging interpretation by trainees. Br J Neurosurg. 2015;29(5):712–4. https://doi.org/10.3109/02688697.2015.1026799.
28. Mawhinney G, Thakar C, Williamson V, Rothenfluh DA, Reynolds J. (OxVIC): a pilot study of informed video consent in spinal surgery and preoperative patient satisfaction. BMJ Open. 2019;9:e027712. https://doi.org/10.1136/bmjopen-2018-027712.
29. Renovanz M, Julian Haaf J, Nesbigall R, Gutenberg A, Laubach W, Ringel F, Fischbeck S. Information needs of patients in spine surgery: development of a question prompt list to guide informed consent consultations. Spine J. 2019;19:523–31.
30. Fischbeck S, Petrowski K, Renovanz M, Nesbigall R, Haaf J, Ringel F. Anxiety is associated with unfulfilled information needs and pain at the informed consent consultation of spine surgery patients: a longitudinal study. Eur Spine J. 2021;30:2360–7.
31. Zahrai A, Bhanot K, Mei XY, Crawford E, Tan Z, Yee A, Palda V. Surgeon clinical practice variation and patient preferences during the informed consent discussion: a mixed-methods analysis in lumbar spine surgery. Can J Surg. 2020;63(3):E284–91.

32. Mauffrey C, Prempeh EM, John J, Vasario G. The influence of written information during the consenting process on patients' recall of operative risks. A prospective randomised study. Int Orthop. 2008;32:425–9.
33. Bethune A, Davila-Foyo M, Valli M, da Costa L. e-Consent: approaching surgical consent with mobile technology. Can J Surg. 2018;61(5):339–44.
34. Phelan EA, Deyo RA, Cherkin DC, Weinstein JN, Ciol MA, Kreuter W, Howe JF. Helping patients decide about back surgery: a randomized trial of an interactive video program. Spine. 2001;26(2):206–12.
35. Raper SE, Clapp JT, Fleisher LA. Improving surgical informed consent: unanswered questions. Ann Surg. 2021;2(1):e030–8. https://doi.org/10.1097/AS9.0000000000000030.
36. Nathan A, Shlobin NA, Mark Sheldon M, Sandi LS. Informed consent in neurosurgery: a systematic review. Neurosurg Focus. 2020;49(5):E6.
37. Lo WB, McAuley CP, Gillies MJ, Grover PJ, Pereira EAC. Consent: an event or a memory in lumbar spinal surgery? A multi-centre, multi-specialty prospective study of documentation and patient recall of consent content. Eur Spine J. 2017;26:2789–96. https://doi.org/10.1007/s00586-017-5107-6.
38. Ng ALC, McRobb LS, White SJ, Cartmill JA, Cyna AM, Seex K. Consent for spine surgery: an observational study. ANZ J Surg. 2021;91:1220–5.

# Part III
# Intraoperative Care for Lumbar Spine Access Surgery

# Chapter 7
# Patient Positioning and Marking for Anterior Lumbar Access Surgery

Sashi Kilaru and Brian Kuhn

## Introduction

Proper patient positioning is important in achieving surgical success when planning lumbar fusion surgery. The following book chapter provides details on proper patient and operating room positioning for anterior and lateral approaches to the lumbar spine and how to avoid complications from positioning including nerve and soft tissue injuries.

## Patient Positioning and Marking for Anterior Lumbar Interbody Fusion

When a patient is taken to the operating room for anterior lumbar interbody fusion surgery, they are placed in the neutral supine position with the shoulders abducted at or less than 90° on arm boards to prevent brachial plexus injury. Alternatively, the arms may be folded and secured over the chest. When the arms are on arm boards, the palms should be facing up and fingers should be extended. It is preferred to place foam padding under the elbows and wrists. Hyperabduction of the arms should be avoided at all times. A pillow may be placed under the knees to maintain normal lumbar

S. Kilaru (✉)
Section of Vascular Surgery, The Christ Hospital, Cincinnati, OH, USA

B. Kuhn
Trihealth Heart Institute, Cincinnati, OH, USA

© The Author(s), under exclusive license to Springer Nature Switzerland AG 2023
J. R. O'Brien et al. (eds.), *Lumbar Spine Access Surgery*,
https://doi.org/10.1007/978-3-031-48034-8_7

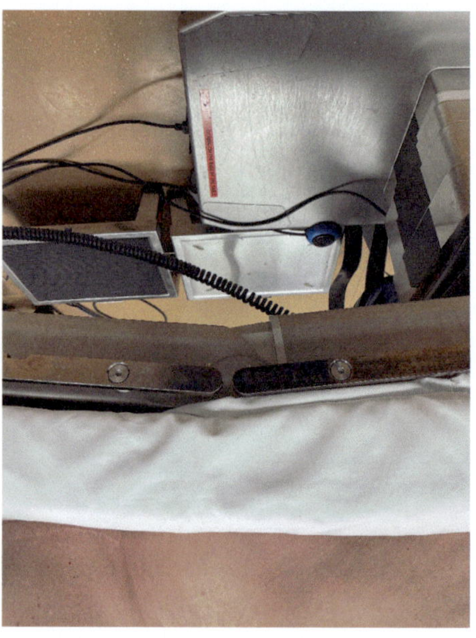

**Fig. 7.1** Patient's lumbar area positioned at the break of the table allows for adjusting lordosis

lordosis and prevent strain on the back and thighs. The legs should be placed parallel and uncrossed to prevent peroneal and tibial nerve injury and avoiding compression of the circulation. Sequential compression devices should be placed on the legs for deep venous thrombosis prophylaxis depending on individual institutional protocols. The supine position should place the patient's cervical, thoracic, and lumbar spine in a straight line. All pressure points should be padded. The safety strap is placed over the mid- to upper thighs and not over a bony prominence to prevent a pressure injury.

It is generally not recommended to place bumps or bolsters under the lumbar spine because hyperlordosis of the lumbar spine will increase the tension on the iliac vessels and may hinder adequate discectomy and distraction of the posterior disc space. It is recommended to place the patient on the operating table such that the break in the table is under the lumbar area so the amount of lordosis can be adjusted as needed (Fig. 7.1).

Once the patient is appropriately positioned, it is important to localize the disc space with fluoroscopy for proper incision placement. This allows for a focused incision that is smaller in length. Fluoroscopy is done in a lateral position with the image intensifier as close to the patient as possible to maximize the view. A long straight metal instrument is placed along the side of the patient and visualized with fluoroscopy (Fig. 7.2). The instrument can then be moved cranially or caudally and

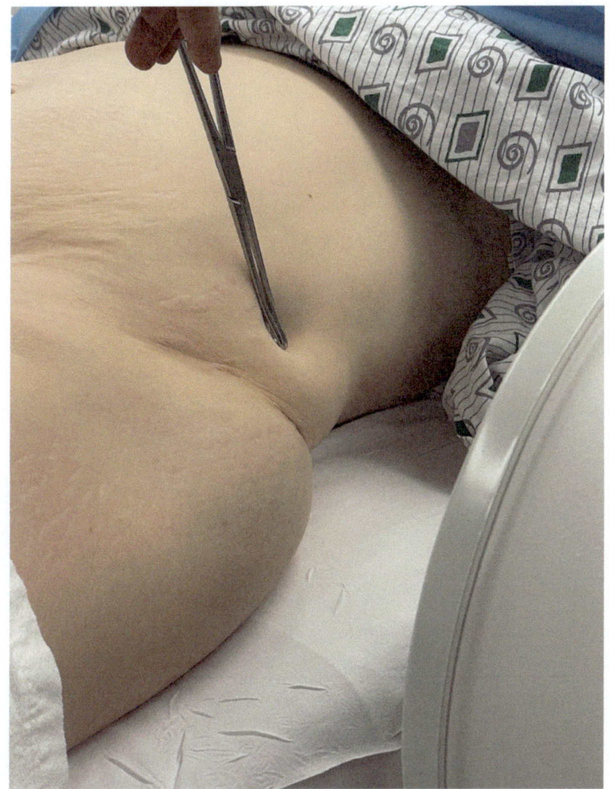

**Fig. 7.2** A long straight metal instrument is placed along the side of the patient so as to visualize it during fluoroscopy

the angle of the instrument can be changed to match the angle of the disc space (Fig. 7.3). A line is then drawn on the abdomen perpendicular to the instrument to finalize the location of the incision. Proper placement of the small incision is crucial. The incisions can be horizontal, oblique, or vertical based on the preference and experience of the surgeon. It is generally preferred to place the incision more caudad than cephalad based on the angle of the disc space to facilitate implant placement.

Another method to localize the disc spaces is using lateral plain films of the lumbar spine. The location of the iliac crest can be used in relation to the location of the L4–L5 disc space. The films can also help one determine the sacral slope and the angle of the L5–S1 disc space. The iliac crest can be palpated and one can determine the proximal and distal extent of the incision based on its relation to the L4–L5 disc space.

**Fig. 7.3** The instrument is positioned to match the angle of the disc space

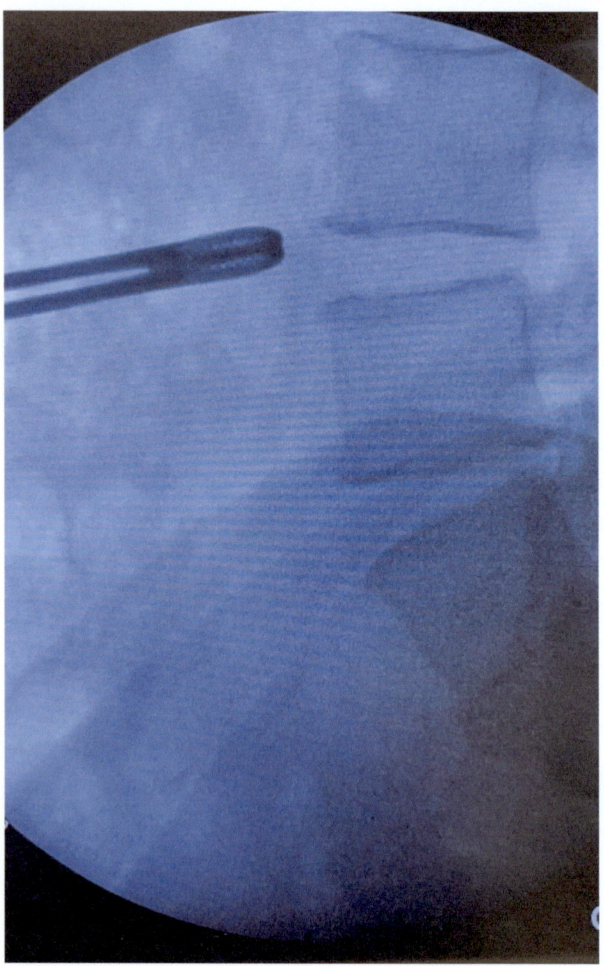

# Patient Positioning and Marking for Lateral Lumbar Interbody Fusion

The standard lateral surgical positioning is right lateral decubitus or left side up as the left-sided vasculature is more robust and less prone to injury. Consideration should be given to ease of access, previous surgeries, surgeon preference, and preoperative imaging when deciding whether to approach from the right or left side. Sagittal and axial images of MRI or CT scans can help localize the arterial and venous bifurcations in relation to the underlying disc spaces and help plan with location of the incision.

The patient is placed in a lateral decubitus position on an adjustable surgical table such that the patient's greater trochanter is directly over the break in the table.

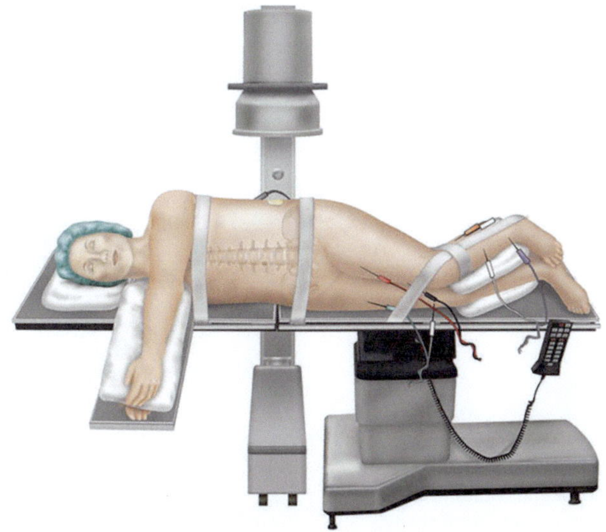

**Fig. 7.4** Care should be taken to make sure that the base of the table is reversed so as to allow for fluoroscopy

Care should be taken to make sure that the base of the table is reversed so as to allow for fluoroscopy (Fig. 7.4). A pillow is placed under the patient's head with the dependent ear assessed after positioning. The patient's arms are supported and secured on parallel arm boards with one arm on each arm board and both arms abducted less than 90°. An axillary roll is placed under the patient's dependent thorax, distal to the axillary fold, at the level of the seventh to the ninth rib to avoid compression of the axillary vessels and the brachial plexus. Bilateral radial pulses are verified after placement of the axillary roll. The patient's dependent leg is flexed at the hip and knee. The patient's upper leg is positioned straight and supported with pillows between the legs. Lateral braces, kidney braces, and beanbag positioners may be used as needed. The patient is then secured to the table with surgical tape in four locations: over the greater trochanter, over the thoracic region beneath the shoulder, over the thigh, and over the calf. The patient is placed in a slight reverse Trendelenburg position and then the head of the table is dropped, therefore allowing better access to the lumbar spine by increasing the distance between the iliac crest and the lower rib as well as widening the disc space to be accessed.

Once the patient has been secured to the table, the table is adjusted so that the true lateral and anterior-posterior (A/P) projections are obtained when the C-arm is set at 90° and 0°, respectively. True A/P orientation is obtained when the spinous process is centered directly equidistant between the pedicles; the pedicles are round and appear as a single line on fluoroscopy (Fig. 7.5). True lateral orientation is noted when the neural foramina align perfectly on fluoroscopy and the endplates appear as a straight line (Fig. 7.6).

The first step in localizing and marking the incision site is done by using two crossed K-wires laid on top of the skin. The anterior and posterior margins of the targeted disc space are marked. In addition, the angle of the disc space, the midpoint

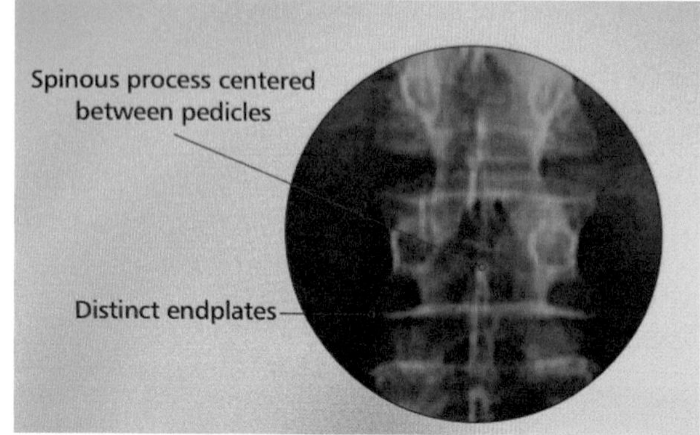



**Fig. 7.5** True A/P orientation is obtained when the spinous process is centered directly equidistant between the pedicles; the pedicles are round and appear as a single line on fluoroscopy

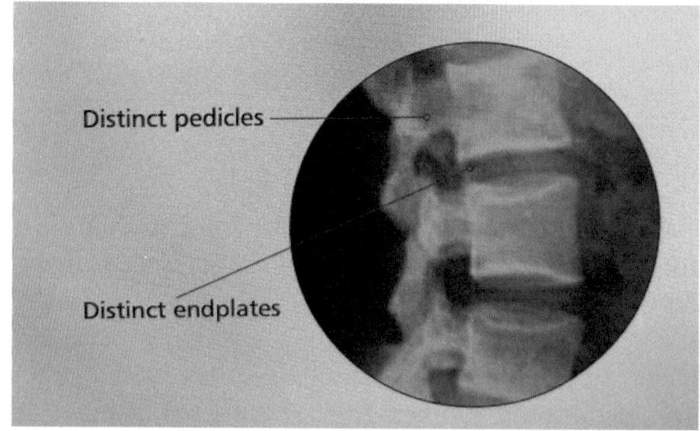



**Fig. 7.6** True lateral orientation is noted when the neural foramina align perfectly on fluoroscopy and the endplates appear as a straight line

of the space, and the anterior superior iliac spine are marked. The incision point for a single level should be in line with the disc of the level to be fused. For two levels, the incision is centered over the vertebral body separating the two discs. The orientation of the incision may be horizontal, oblique, or vertical based on surgeon preference.

## Complications from Improper Positioning

Positioning patients appropriately for spine surgeries is critical for optimal operative site exposure. Patients undergoing spine surgery are often placed in nonphysiological positions that can lead to complications. Although the incidence is relatively low, these complications can result in significant disability, functional loss, and potential for litigation. The incidence of perioperative peripheral nerve injury (PPNI) is 0.03–0.1% [1, 2]. One of the main mechanisms of PPNI is nerve ischemia [3, 4]. Slowing of nerve conduction occurs due to ischemia leading to demyelination [5–7]. Stretch of the peripheral nerve can also lead to injury from disruption of the axons [8]. Diseases affecting the microcirculation such as hypertension and diabetes, tobacco use, and intraoperative conditions such as hypovolemia, dehydration, hypotension, hypoxia, electrolyte disturbances, and induced hypothermia have all been associated with nerve injury [9].

Ulnar neuropathy is the most common site of PPNI [2]. Ulnar neuropathy can lead to significant morbidity and loss of function. Ulnar nerve injury results in the inability to abduct or adduct the fingers and loss of sensation to the fifth finger and the radial half of the fourth finger. Permanent injury will lead to a clawlike hand deformity due to atrophy of the intrinsic muscle of the hand including the third and fourth lumbricals and dorsal and palmar interossei. The ulnar nerve has a superficial path along the medial epicondyle of the humerus within the cubital tunnel [10]. The ulnar collateral artery and vein run in close proximity to the ulnar nerve and may be affected by external pressure leading to reduced perfusion, ischemia, and nerve injury [11]. Compression of the ulnar nerve and its blood supply (the posterior ulnar collateral artery) at the area of the tubercle of the coronoid may lead to ischemia [12]. The ulnar nerve is relatively more sensitive to ischemia compared to the median and radial nerves [13].

The brachial plexus is the second most common site of PPNI, usually secondary to compression and stretch. Shoulder braces, head-down positioning, improper arm positioning, and prolonged neck extension were commonly identified mechanisms for brachial plexus injury [14]. Shoulder abduction greater than 90°, external rotation of the arm, and posterior shoulder displacement can stretch the brachial plexus [9, 15]. Downward tilting of the head and hyperabduction of the independent arm in the lateral position may stretch the brachial plexus and lead to brachial plexus injury [16]. Extension and lateral flexion of the head in the supine position may contribute to stretch of the brachial plexus on the contralateral side [9].

Median and radial nerve injuries are quite rare and are typically due to operative positioning and direct pressure. Extension of the elbow may overstretch the median nerve leading to injury [17]. Prolonged hyperextension of the wrist may lead to slowing of nerve conduction and median nerve injury across the carpal tunnel [18].

## Conclusion

Safe and appropriate patient positioning and adequate fluoroscopic imaging is critically important to achieve successful patient outcomes during lumbar spine fusion surgery. The exposing surgeon should have complete knowledge of all the intricacies related to positioning to ensure excellent outcomes.

## References

1. Welch MB, Brummett CM, Welch TD, Tremper KK, Shanks AM, Guglani P, Mashour GA. Perioperative peripheral nerve injuries: a retrospective study of 380,680 cases during a 10-year period at a single institution. Anesthesiology. 2009;111:490–7.

2. Cassoria L, Lee JW. Patient positioning in anesthesia. In: Miller RD, editor. Miller's anesthesia. 7th ed. Philadelphia: Elsevier; 2009. p. 1151–70.
3. Myers RR, Yamamoto T, Yaksh TL, Powell HC. The role of focal nerve ischemia and Wallerian degeneration in peripheral nerve injury producing hyperesthesia. Anesthesiology. 1993;78:308–16.
4. Bonner SM, Pridie AK. Sciatic nerve palsy following uneventful sciatic nerve block. Anaesthesia. 1997;52:1205–7.
5. Warner MA, Warner ME, Martin JT. Ulnar neuropathy. Incidence, outcome, and risk factors in sedated or anesthetized patients. Anesthesiology. 1994;81:1332–40.
6. Sunderland S. The intraneural topography of the radial, median and ulnar nerves. Brain. 1945;68:243–99.
7. Aguayo A, Nair CP, Midgley R. Experimental progressive compression neuropathy in the rabbit. Histologic and electrophysiologic studies. Arch Neurol. 1971;24:358–64.
8. Winfree CJ, Kline DG. Intraoperative positioning nerve injuries. Surg Neurol. 2005;63:5–18; discussion 18
9. Sawyer RJ, Richmond MN, Hickey JD, Jarrratt JA. Peripheral nerve injuries associated with anaesthesia. Anaesthesia. 2000;55:980–91.
10. Britt BA, Gordon RA. Peripheral nerve injuries associated with anaesthesia. Can Anaesth Soc J. 1964;11:514–36.
11. Prielipp RC, Morell RC, Walker FO, Santos CC, Bennett J, Butterworth J. Ulnar nerve pressure: influence of arm position and relationship to somatosensory evoked potentials. Anesthesiology. 1999;91:345–54.
12. Contreras MG, Warner MA, Charboneau WJ, Cahill DR. Anatomy of the ulnar nerve at the elbow: potential relationship of acute ulnar neuropathy to gender differences. Clin Anat. 1998;11:372–8.
13. Swenson JD, Hutchinson DT, Bromberg M, Pace NL. Rapid onset of ulnar nerve dysfunction during transient occlusion of the brachial artery. Anesth Analg. 1998;87:677–80.
14. Cheney FW, Domino KB, Caplan RA, Posner KL. Nerve injury associated with anesthesia: a closed claims analysis. Anesthesiology. 1999;90:1062–9.
15. Wadsworth TG. The external compression syndrome of the ulnar nerve at the cubital tunnel. Clin Orthop Relat Res. 1977;124:189–204.
16. Ngamprasertwong P, Phupong V, Uerpairojkit K. Brachial plexus injury related to improper positioning during general anesthesia. J Anesth. 2004;18:132–4.
17. American Society of Anesthesiologists Task Force on Prevention of Perioperative Peripheral Neuropathies. Practice advisory for the prevention of perioperative peripheral neuropathies: an updated report by the American Society of Anesthesiologists Task Force on Prevention of Perioperative Peripheral Neuropathies. Anesthesiology. 2011;114:741–54.
18. Chowet AL, Lopez JR, Brock-Utne JG, Jaffe RA. Wrist hyperextension leads to median nerve conduction block: implications for intra-arterial catheter placement. Anesthesiology. 2004;100:287–91.

# Chapter 8
# Adjunctive Measures: Neuromonitoring, Perfusion Monitoring, Foley

**David Y. Zhao and Faheem A. Sandhu**

## Introduction

Intraoperative care begins prior to surgery with a detailed discussion with the anesthesia and neuromonitoring teams. Special attention should be paid to the patient's comorbid medical conditions, and consideration should be made to institute adjunctive measures to optimize patient safety during the case.

Intraoperative multimodality neuromonitoring is employed based upon the structures at risk of injury. During anterior and lateral lumbar surgery, modalities specifically addressing the lumbar and sacral nerve roots as well as the lumbar plexus are most commonly selected. This chapter will highlight the clinical utility and limitations of somatosensory evoked potentials (SSEPs), electromyography (EMG), and motor evoked potentials (MEPs), with specific attention to anterior and lateral lumbar approaches. Cardiovascular perfusion monitoring via an arterial line is helpful for maintenance and augmentation of blood pressure. Evidence from the management of acute spinal cord injury can be applied to intraoperative care when neural structures are at risk or damaged. Foley catheterization is routinely used to monitor fluid balance during lumbar surgery. Consideration should be given to urinary catheterization depending on case type, duration, and patient risk factors for postoperative urinary retention.

D. Y. Zhao
Department of Neurosurgery, MedStar Georgetown University Hospital,
Washington, DC, USA

F. A. Sandhu (✉)
Center for Minimally Invasive Spine Surgery, MedStar Georgetown University Hospital,
Washington, DC, USA

© The Author(s), under exclusive license to Springer Nature
Switzerland AG 2023
J. R. O'Brien et al. (eds.), *Lumbar Spine Access Surgery*,
https://doi.org/10.1007/978-3-031-48034-8_8

# Neuromonitoring

Judicious use of multimodality intraoperative neuromonitoring allows the surgeon to optimally monitor the functional integrity of the spinal cord and spinal nerves during surgery. Robust evidence exists to support its use as a diagnostic adjunct to enhance the safety of spine surgery [1–13], in particular for anterior and lateral approaches to the lumbar spine [14–20].

## *Somatosensory Evoked Potentials*

### Background and Physiology

Somatosensory evoked potentials (SSEPs) provide continuous, direct monitoring of the dorsal column-medial lemniscus ascending pathway that mediates fine touch, two-point discrimination, vibration, and proprioception. In the lower extremity, the posterior tibial and peroneal nerves are typically selected via placement of stimulating needle electrodes, while the median and ulnar nerves in the upper extremity are usually selected for SSEP monitoring.

Upon repetitive electrical stimulation of the distal peripheral sensory and motor fibers, action potentials ascend via neuronal axons, through the dorsal root ganglia, entering the spinal cord and projecting via the gracilis and cuneatus fasciculi. After synapsing and decussating in the lower medulla, these signals travel to the ventral posterior lateral nucleus of the thalamus, synapse, and ultimately project to the somatosensory cortex. Recording electrodes in the dorsal neck and scalp detect the summated electrical signal potentials, and peripheral electrodes at the popliteal fossa or at the level of the brachial plexus provide a positive control determination (Fig. 8.1).

### Clinical Utility and Alarm Criteria

Since its inception in the 1970s, SSEP has become a mainstay intraoperative neuromonitoring modality during spinal instrumentation procedures. Owing to a very high specificity (95–100%) for new postoperative neurological deficits, recent guidelines have demonstrated with Level II evidence the reliability of SSEP as a diagnostic adjunct for spine surgery [7, 8]. Even stronger Level I recommendations exist for multimodality intraoperative neuromonitoring whereby SSEP is combined with MEP as a diagnostic adjunct in the assessment of spinal cord integrity [8].

A decrease in amplitude by greater than 50% from baseline and/or increase in latency by greater than 10% from baseline is generally considered significant and abnormal, signaling potential deficit or injury [3, 6]. Upon notification of these changes, indirect or unrelated causes, representing false-positive interpretation,

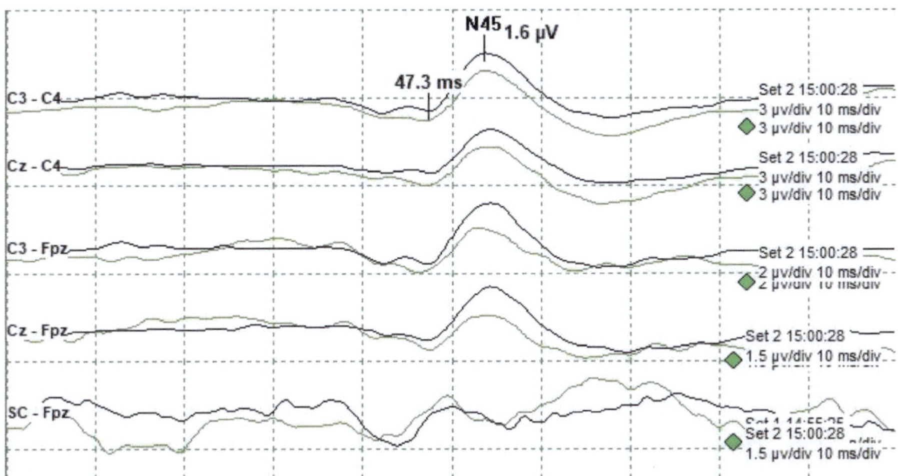


**Fig. 8.1** Baseline intraoperative somatosensory evoked potentials from left posterior tibial nerve stimulation demonstrating obligate peaks

should be ruled out. Equipment-related technical issues, hypotension, hypothermia, and anesthetic concerns should be expeditiously addressed with the neuromonitoring and anesthesia teams. If changes in SSEP signal are associated with a surgical maneuver, the surgeon should consider correcting or reversing the maneuver, augmentation of blood pressure to improve spinal cord perfusion, and/or steroid administration and allow time for signals to improve.

## Limitations

While SSEP neuromonitoring can provide a significant diagnostic advantage in the assessment of spinal cord integrity, its role as a therapeutic tool is not supported—that is, SSEP has not been shown to improve neurological function or outcome, nor has it been shown to reduce the rate of neurological injury during spine surgery [8].

In addition, spinal cord ischemic changes affecting the anterior horn motor nuclei and anterior spinal artery territory may be missed by SSEP alone [9]. Thus, focal motor deficits without changes in sensory or proprioception could theoretically occur without significant or abnormal changes in SSEP signals. SSEP also does not effectively monitor injury to a specific nerve root, and for this reason, multimodal intraoperative neuromonitoring with EMG is frequently employed.

Another disadvantage inherent to SSEP is the delay in the presentation of adverse signal changes related to temporal summation and the calculation of averaged evoked responses. As such, it may take upwards of 5–10 minutes for spinal cord injury to manifest on SSEP monitoring alone [10].

**Special Considerations in Anterior and Lateral Transpsoas Approaches**

The majority of anterior and lateral transpsoas approaches to the lumbar spine typically occur below the level of the conus medullaris, and here the contents of the thecal sac do not contain spinal cord, but rather lumbosacral nerves. Despite this, SSEP may still remain a prudent modality for intraoperative neuromonitoring [15, 20], and it is the authors' practice to routinely monitor SSEP during anterior and lateral transpsoas spinal instrumentation cases.

During anterior lumbar interbody fusion (ALIF), SSEP can play a unique role in monitoring for nerve root ischemia and correlation with lower extremity ischemic changes related to retraction and compression of the common iliac artery or vein. This may be particularly true for the L4–L5 level, when substantial mobilization of the left common iliac artery and vein is required for access to the disc space. Brau et al. describe a significant correlation between left lower extremity pulse oximeter $SaO_2$ decrease and loss of SSEP signals in 13 patients after exposure for an L4–L5 ALIF. All 13 patients subsequently experienced a return to normal left lower extremity $SaO_2$ and complete recovery of SSEP signals after retractor removal [15]. Since independent lower extremity pulse oximetry may be less commonly performed, these findings suggest the role for SSEP as an indirect monitoring modality for lower extremity ischemic changes during ALIF.

## *Electromyography*

**Background and Physiology**

Electromyography (EMG) is a real-time intraoperative neuromonitoring modality to detect injury to select nerve roots or neural elements during spine surgery. In the lower extremity, paired needle recording electrodes are typically inserted into the vastus medialis, tibialis anterior, biceps femoris, and gastrocnemius muscles to monitor the integrity of the L2 through S1 nerve roots.

EMG monitoring may be performed via continuous (also described as spontaneous or free-run) EMG, which provides a continuous direct observation of electrical activity between nerve root and myotome, or triggered EMG testing.

Triggered EMG employs an intraoperative probe that delivers pulses of current to a structure or tissue of interest. This modality has been classically used as an indirect method of assessing lumbar pedicle screw accuracy whereby the screw is stimulated with increasing current [10, 11]. Recording needle electrodes in the associated myotome measure compound muscle action potentials (CMAP), and assessment of the lowest threshold at which a CMAP is generated can provide information related to the likelihood of a medial pedicle wall breach. Triggered EMG is also useful during tethered cord release procedures in order to identify and distinguish filum terminale from surrounding lumbosacral nerves. In addition, triggered EMG monitoring incorporated into dilator (Fig. 8.2) and retractor systems for lateral

**Fig. 8.2** Intraoperative triggered EMG. Once the initial dilator has advanced through the psoas during a lateral lumbar interbody fusion, the stimulator clip is attached. Current is transmitted and recording electrodes in lower extremity muscle groups measure threshold EMG recordings

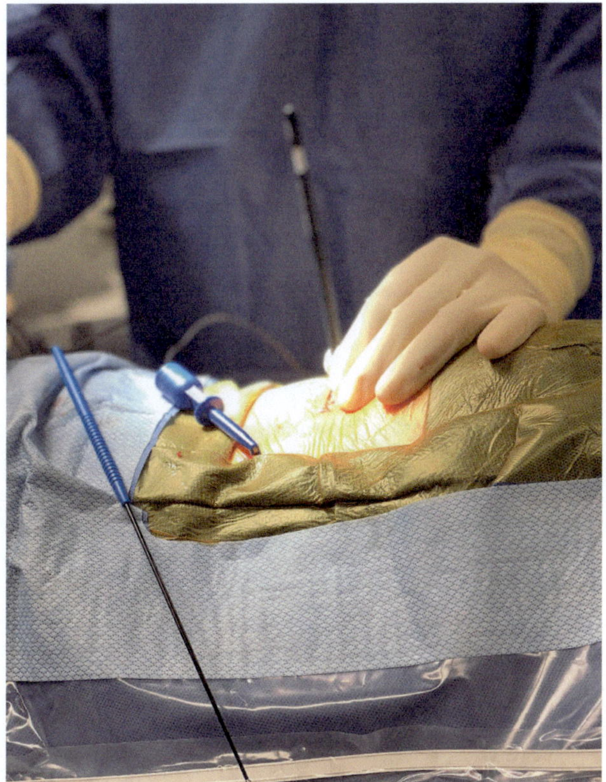

transpsoas approaches to the lumbar spine has vastly improved the safety of lateral access surgery [14, 16–19] and will be discussed separately below.

## Clinical Utility and Alarm Criteria

Today, both free-run and triggered EMG are regularly employed alongside SSEP and MEP in the multimodality neuromonitoring armamentarium to deliver high-sensitivity monitoring for nerve root injury and improve specificity for new postoperative neurological deficits. In addition to providing instantaneous feedback, free-run EMG affords precise correlation with specific nerve roots. In a retrospective review of patients undergoing multimodality neuromonitoring during intramedullary spinal cord tumor resection, Jin et al. found that the addition of free-run EMG led to earlier detection of abnormal signal alerts, preceding those from MEP in 72% [21]. Further Class II evidence for the diagnostic utility of free-run EMG is provided by Paradiso et al. in a prospective series of adults undergoing multimodality neuromonitoring during tethered cord release [22].

When excessive surgical manipulation occurs on or in close vicinity to a nerve root, there is deviation from the activity of the muscle at rest in the form of neurotonic discharges. Pulling, short-term compression, or mild stretch of a nerve root is associated with spike or burst EMG activity. More severe stretch or ongoing compression can cause train activity, which denotes sustained, repetitive EMG firing and indicates a greater likelihood of nerve root injury [10].

A triggered EMG stimulation threshold of less than 10 mA generally suggests a potential breach of the medial lumbar pedicle wall [23]. Variability in individual bone density and pedicle screw coating limit generalizability, but a threshold of greater than 15 mA is associated with a 98% likelihood of accurate or satisfactory screw positioning [6].

## Limitations

EMG intraoperative neuromonitoring is not without its own set of limitations. Free-run EMG on its own has a low specificity (23–65%) for postoperative nerve root injury [5, 24]. Another disadvantage of both free-run and triggered EMG is the relatively high rate of false-positive alerts [25, 26]. Signal artifact and interference from electrocautery or drilling can be mistaken for free-run EMG activity. Cold water irrigation may also falsely induce spontaneous EMG activity. In addition, EMG monitoring precludes the use of paralytics, and patients must have neuromuscular blockade fully reversed with four twitches on train-of-four testing for consistent monitoring.

In patients with a preoperative nerve root deficit, triggered EMG can yield a false-negative reading as impaired nerve conduction may result in higher stimulation thresholds required for myotome CMAP generation.

## Special Considerations in Anterior and Lateral Transpsoas Approaches

The authors routinely monitor free-run EMG for all anterior and lateral spine instrumentation cases. During ALIF, prolonged EMG activity after graft placement may signify new nerve root compression or disc space over-distraction with resultant nerve root stretch neuropraxia [27]. The same notion holds true for lateral lumbar interbody fusion (LLIF), and for these transpsoas approaches we also routinely monitor directional triggered EMG.

As the psoas muscle is traversed during a lateral approach to the lumbar spine, the lumbar plexus is uniquely at risk for injury. Safe passage of the dilator and retractor is paramount, and there should not be undue retraction of the lumbar plexus upon opening of the retractor blades. In addition to a comprehensive understanding of the lumbar plexus regional anatomy, the use of directional triggered EMG coupled with free-run EMG is essential for patient safety and has been shown to decrease the prevalence of lumbar plexus injury during lateral access surgery [14, 17–19].

Well-validated cadaveric studies have characterized the course of the lumbar plexus within the psoas muscle and identified safe zones from the L1–L2 to the

L4–L5 disc spaces [28–30]. Directional triggered EMG monitoring has been incorporated into modern dilator and retractor systems for minimally invasive lateral access. Unidirectional triggered EMG stimulation during dilator advancement provides instantaneous threshold readings in the vastus medialis, tibialis anterior, biceps femoris, and gastrocnemius muscles, from which the surgeon can indirectly assess the relative location and distance of the dilator to the intrapsoas plexus.

Typically, triggered EMG thresholds less than 5 mA suggest direct contact with a motor nerve bundle, and thresholds between 5 and 10 mA indicate unsafe close proximity between dilator and nerve with some intervening soft tissue (Fig. 8.3). Thresholds greater than 10 mA are generally safe, denoting adequate distance between dilator and nerve [19]. Ideally, high EMG thresholds are recorded anterior to the dilator with acceptably lower thresholds recorded posteriorly, representing the posterior position of the lumbar plexus to the dilator and subsequent retractor, which may be safely opened anteriorly (Fig. 8.4).

Sensory nerves of the lumbar plexus may not be detected by standard directional triggered EMG monitoring. Transient postoperative anterior thigh paresthesias and dysesthesias are a common finding associated with lateral access [31]. Despite the

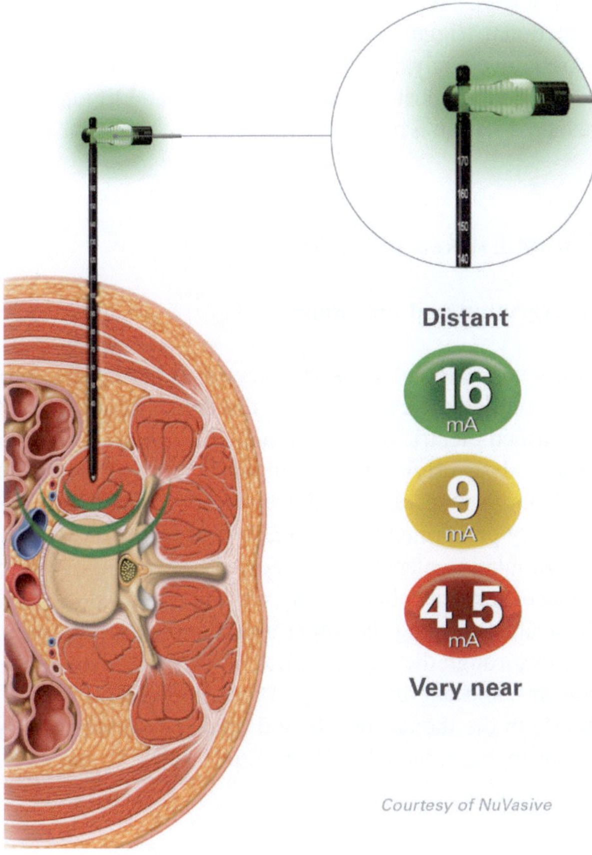


**Fig. 8.3** The NeuroVision system (NuVasive, Inc.) measures triggered EMG thresholds as the dilator traverses the psoas muscle. Color-coded readings denote safe or unsafe distance from the lumbar plexus. © NuVasive, Inc.

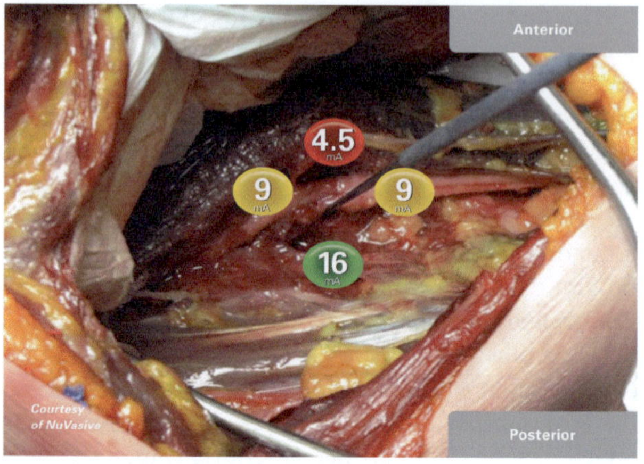

**Fig. 8.4** Cadaveric dissection study denoting unsafe EMG thresholds anteriorly as the dilator's anterior face comes into contact with the lumbar plexus. In this configuration, higher thresholds would be measured posterior to the dilator. © NuVasive, Inc.

use of free-running and directional triggered EMG, thigh weakness, pain, and dysesthesias were reported in 30% of patients undergoing lateral transpsoas interbody fusion for adult spinal deformity; these symptoms were transient in all but one patient [32]. The overall safety and complication profile of the lateral approach with directional triggered EMG neuromonitoring remains quite favorable. The largest prospective analysis of 600 patients yielded a 0.7% neurological complication rate, manifested by postoperative quadriceps and tibialis anterior weakness, all of which resolved within 3 months' time [16].

## *Motor Evoked Potentials*

### Background and Physiology

Transcranial motor evoked potential (MEP) intraoperative neuromonitoring provides immediate evaluation of the entire motor axis. Stimulation of MEP can be performed electrically or magnetically, and recording can be at the muscle, nerve, or directly overlying the spinal cord (D-wave monitoring for intramedullary spinal cord tumor resection). For degenerative spine pathology, electrical stimulation is typically performed transcranially and recorded at the myotome.

Stimulating electrodes are typically inserted in the scalp based upon the international electroencephalography system. A short pulse train current is initiated through the scalp overlying the upper and lower extremity motor homunculus. The current passes through the motor cortex, down the corticospinal tracts, into the alpha-motor neurons, and out the nerve root to the peripheral nerves. Recording electrodes commonly in the thenar muscle and tibialis anterior amplify and detect the subsequent electromyographic CMAP amplitude, latency, and waveform.

**Clinical Utility and Alarm Criteria**

Prior to implementation of MEP intraoperative neuromonitoring in the 1990s, the wake-up test was utilized to assess integrity of the corticospinal tract during spine surgery. Today, transcranial MEP monitoring has demonstrated sensitivity and specificity approaching 100% for the detection of postoperative motor deficits [9]. Level I evidence exists from recent guidelines to support MEP monitoring as a diagnostic adjunct for evaluation of spinal cord integrity [8]. When used together with SSEP and EMG multimodality neuromonitoring, MEP monitoring provides a powerful and reliable tool to enhance patient safety during spine surgery.

The complete loss of CMAP after transcranial stimulation heralds severe clinical significance and postoperative motor deficit, known as the all-or-nothing criterion. Additionally, an 80% decrease in signal amplitude at any recording site was also shown to be predictive of neurological deficit with greater than 90% sensitivity and specificity [33]. Further well-validated alarm criteria include an increase of more than 100 V in the maximum threshold stimulus required to generate a CMAP [34].

## *Limitations*

In patients with myelopathy or preexisting motor deficits, it may be difficult to establish baseline MEP signals. Another inherent disadvantage of MEP is the movement induced by the stimulation current. While tongue laceration from forced facial muscle contraction may be prevented by placement of a bite block, it remains a relatively common complication associated with MEP monitoring [35]. Since the data signal acquisition relies on electromyographic CMAP recording, MEP also precludes the use of neuromuscular blockade.

A significant limitation of MEP monitoring is the intermittent, noncontinuous nature of its assessment capabilities. Since MEPs are typically obtained at varying intervals intraoperatively, delayed recognition of neurological injury can result. In patients with cochlear implants or deep brain stimulators, MEP neuromonitoring is contraindicated; in patients with epilepsy, it is a relative contraindication due to the theoretical risk of seizure with transcranial electrical stimulation [36].

**Role in Anterior and Lateral Transpsoas Approaches**

MEP monitoring plays a limited role in anterior and lateral transpsoas approaches to the lumbar spine. The vast majority of ALIF and LLIF cases target lumbar levels below the termination of the conus medullaris. Since lumbosacral nerves and nerve roots are at risk, the neuromonitoring modality must be tailored to detect injury to these neural structures. MEP does not reliably detect nerve root lesions due to the significant overlap in myotome innervation [35]. The authors do not typically monitor MEP in routine one- to three-level spinal instrumentation cases involving anterior and/or lateral access.

Nevertheless, there is evidence of added benefit when transcranial MEP monitoring is utilized in addition to routine free-run and directional triggered EMG in lateral transpsoas approaches to the lumbar spine. In a prospective study, Berends et al. report a 50% decrease in MEP amplitude after breaking the table in seven (30%) cases. MEP changes were also noted during retractor positioning without correlating EMG changes. Although the clinical effect of the reported decrease in MEP amplitude was unclear, they recommend MEP and conclude that MEP monitoring during the lateral transpsoas approach can provide additional value by detecting unnoticed events on EMG [14].

In spinal deformity cases involving osteotomies and significant curvature correction during a combined anterior-posterior or lateral-posterior approach, consideration should be given for multimodal intraoperative neuromonitoring that includes MEP. These high-risk maneuvers are expected to induce global sagittal or coronal alteration of the thoracolumbar spinal column, and in doing so, the functional integrity of the spinal cord, particularly the corticospinal tracts, must be safeguarded with instantaneous feedback. Delayed alarm criteria on SSEP monitoring alone may not allow for timely correction or reversal of surgical manipulation [37]. Ischemia or infarction affecting only the anterior spinal artery territory may be missed by SSEP, with resultant devastating neurological outcomes. Since the spinal cord is exquisitely sensitive to ischemic changes, the advantage of MEP in its immediate detection of compromised signal quickly alerts the surgeon and anesthesia team to institute corrective measures.

## Cardiovascular Perfusion Monitoring

Placement of an arterial line for continuous monitoring of cardiovascular perfusion may be necessary for patients in whom intraoperative hemodynamic or neurological disturbances may occur. Patients with extensive cardiac or pulmonary comorbidities may also benefit from continuous intraoperative cardiovascular perfusion monitoring.

A common consideration for arterial line placement is when expected blood loss is predicted to be noteworthy, typically greater than 500 mL, with the aim to avoid a significant decrease in blood pressure from baseline. Strict blood pressure control together with corrective measures are essential in patients with preexisting neurological deficits or myelopathy, or when intraoperative injury occurs to the spinal cord or nerves.

The rationale for continuous cardiovascular perfusion monitoring during spine surgery can be adapted from guidelines related to treatment of acute spinal cord trauma. Current evidence recommends maintenance of mean arterial blood pressure at 85–90 mmHg after spinal cord injury to enhance cord perfusion [38–41]. Should surgical manipulation result in neuromonitoring changes with reasonable suspicion of neurological injury, an arterial line would provide the best second-to-second readout of blood pressure from which further decision-making can be made.

For routine anterior and lateral instrumentation cases for degenerative etiology, the authors do not typically place an arterial line. For complex cases involving extensive deformity correction, corpectomy, or tumor resection, an arterial line is placed after induction. Together with the anesthesia team, individualized recommendations are made based on the patient's cardiovascular risk factors and comorbidities, erring on the side of safety.

## Foley Catheterization

Urinary catheterization via insertion of a Foley catheter allows for accurate monitoring of fluid homeostasis during surgery. If the case length is estimated to be greater than 3 hours, it may be advantageous to place a Foley catheter to reduce the risk of bladder distension injury. In addition, for patients in whom immediate postoperative mobility is expected to be significantly impaired, Foley catheterization may reduce pain and discomfort associated with assisted mobilization.

Further consideration should be given to patients on whom greater than two levels of instrumentation are placed, those with a preexisting diagnosis of benign prostatic hypertrophy (BPH), and patients expected to receive a postoperative patient-controlled analgesia (PCA) pump. In a retrospective review, risk factors for postoperative urinary retention were elucidated in 397 elective spine surgery cases. These included a history of urinary retention, chronic constipation, BPH, postoperative PCA usage, and longer operative times [42]. A randomized study in Sweden did not find an increase in urinary tract infection or urinary complication rate in patients undergoing spinal fusion in whom an intraoperative Foley catheter was placed [43].

Published guidelines do not exist for the placement of a Foley catheter during lumbar spine surgery, and practice patterns may vary significantly amongst surgeons. The authors typically elect for placement of a Foley catheter after induction of anesthesia for all patients undergoing multilevel anterior and/or lateral spinal instrumentation. In single-level cases, individualized recommendations are made based on patient history and risk factors.

## Conclusion

The intraoperative care and safety of patients undergoing anterior and lateral spine surgery is enhanced by the decision to institute adjunctive measures including multimodality neuromonitoring, arterial line cardiovascular perfusion monitoring, and Foley catheterization. Preoperative preparation and interdisciplinary collaboration with the anesthesia and neuromonitoring teams is essential. A comprehensive understanding of the strengths and limitations of each specific modality is a valuable complement to each surgeon's technical skillset.

## References


1. Chang R, Reddy RP, Coutinho DV, et al. Diagnostic accuracy of SSEP changes during lumbar spine surgery for predicting postoperative neurological deficit. Spine (Phila Pa 1976). 2021;46(24):E1343–52. https://doi.org/10.1097/brs.0000000000004099.
2. Charalampidis A, Jiang F, Wilson JRF, Badhiwala JH, Brodke DS, Fehlings MG. The use of intraoperative neurophysiological monitoring in spine surgery. Global Spine J. 2020;10(1_Suppl):104S–14S. https://doi.org/10.1177/2192568219859314.
3. Padberg AM, Thuet ED. Intraoperative electrophysiologic monitoring: considerations for complex spinal surgery. Neurosurg Clin N Am. 2006;17(3):205–26. https://doi.org/10.1016/j.nec.2006.05.008.
4. Park J-H. Intraoperative neurophysiological monitoring in spinal surgery. World J Clin Cases. 2015;3(9):765. https://doi.org/10.12998/wjcc.v3.i9.765.
5. Quraishi NA, Lewis SJ, Kelleher MO, Sarjeant R, Rampersaud YR, Fehlings MG. Intraoperative multimodality monitoring in adult spinal deformity: analysis of a prospective series of one hundred two cases with independent evaluation. Spine (Phila Pa 1976). 2009;34(14):1504–12. https://doi.org/10.1097/BRS.0b013e3181a87b66.
6. Gonzalez AA, Jeyanandarajan D, Hansen C, Zada G, Hsieh PC. Intraoperative neurophysiological monitoring during spine surgery: a review. Neurosurg Focus. 2009;27(4):1–10. https://doi.org/10.3171/2009.8.FOCUS09150.
7. Griggs RC, Alcauskas M. Evidence-based guideline update: intraoperative spinal monitoring with somatosensory and transcranial electrical motor evoked potentials: report of the therapeutics and technology assessment subcommittee of the American Academy of Neurology and the American Clinical Neurophysiology Society. Neurology. 2012;79(3):292–4. https://doi.org/10.1212/WNL.0b013e3182637c24.
8. Hadley MN, Shank CD, Rozzelle CJ, Walters BC. In reply: guidelines for the use of electrophysiological monitoring for surgery of the human spinal column and spinal cord. Clin Neurosurg. 2018;83(2):E80–1. https://doi.org/10.1093/neuros/nyy207.
9. Hilibrand AS, Schwartz DM, Sethuraman V, Vaccaro AR, Albert TJ. Comparison of transcranial electric motor and somatosensory evoked potential monitoring during cervical spine surgery. J Bone Joint Surg Am. 2004;86(6):1248–53. https://doi.org/10.2106/00004623-200406000-00018.
10. Lall RR, Hauptman JS, Munoz C, et al. Intraoperative neurophysiological monitoring in spine surgery: indications, efficacy, and role of the preoperative checklist. Neurosurg Focus. 2012;33(5):1–10. https://doi.org/10.3171/2012.9.FOCUS12235.
11. Malhotra NR, Shaffrey CI. Intraoperative electrophysiological monitoring in spine surgery. Spine (Phila Pa 1976). 2010;35(25):2167–79. https://doi.org/10.1097/BRS.0b013e3181f6f0d0.
12. Melachuri SR, Stopera C, Melachuri MK, et al. The efficacy of somatosensory evoked potentials in evaluating new neurological deficits after spinal thoracic fusion and decompression. J Neurosurg Spine. 2020;33(1):35–40. https://doi.org/10.3171/2019.12.SPINE191157.
13. Nuwer MR, Dawson EG, Carlson LG, Kanim LEA, Sherman JE. Somatosensory evoked potential spinal cord monitoring reduces neurologic deficits after scoliosis surgery: results of a large multicenter survey. Electroencephalogr Clin Neurophysiol. 1995;96(1):6–11. https://doi.org/10.1016/0013-4694(94)00235-D.
14. Berends HI, Journée HL, Rácz I, van Loon J, Härtl R, Spruit M. Multimodality intraoperative neuromonitoring in extreme lateral interbody fusion. Transcranial electrical stimulation

as indispensable rearview. Eur Spine J. 2016;25(5):1581–6. https://doi.org/10.1007/s00586-015-4182-9.

15. Brau SA, Spoonamore MJ, Snyder L, et al. Nerve monitoring changes related to iliac artery compression during anterior lumbar spine surgery. Spine J. 2003;3(5):351–5. https://doi.org/10.1016/S1529-9430(03)00067-6.

16. Rodgers WB, Gerber EJ, Patterson J. Intraoperative and early postoperative complications in extreme lateral interbody fusion: an analysis of 600 cases. Spine (Phila Pa 1976). 2011;36(1):26–32. https://doi.org/10.1097/BRS.0b013e3181e1040a.

17. Tohmeh AG, Rodgers WB, Peterson MD. Dynamically evoked, discrete-threshold electromyography in the extreme lateral interbody fusion approach: clinical article. J Neurosurg Spine. 2011;14(1):31–7. https://doi.org/10.3171/2010.9.SPINE09871.

18. Uribe JS, Isaacs RE, Youssef JA, et al. Can triggered electromyography monitoring throughout retraction predict postoperative symptomatic neuropraxia after XLIF? Results from a prospective multicenter trial. Eur Spine J. 2015;24:378–85. https://doi.org/10.1007/s00586-015-3871-8.

19. Uribe JS, Vale FL, Dakwar E. Electromyographic monitoring and its anatomical implications in minimally invasive spine surgery. Spine (Phila Pa 1976). 2010;35(Suppl 26):368–74. https://doi.org/10.1097/BRS.0b013e3182027976.

20. Yaylali I, Ju H, Yoo J, Ching A, Hart R. Intraoperative neurophysiological monitoring in anterior lumbar interbody fusion surgery. J Clin Neurophysiol. 2014;31(4):352–5. https://doi.org/10.1097/WNP.0000000000000073.

21. Jin SH, Chung CK, Kim CH, Choi YD, Kwak G, Kim BE. Multimodal intraoperative monitoring during intramedullary spinal cord tumor surgery. Acta Neurochir. 2015;157(12):2149–55. https://doi.org/10.1007/s00701-015-2598-y.

22. Paradiso G, Lee GYF, Sarjeant R, Hoang L, Massicotte EM, Fehlings MG. Multimodality intraoperative neurophysiologic monitoring findings during surgery for adult tethered cord syndrome: analysis of a series of 44 patients with long-term follow-up. Spine (Phila Pa 1976). 2006;31(18):2095–102. https://doi.org/10.1097/01.brs.0000231687.02271.b6.

23. Clements DH, Morledge DE, Martin WH, Betz RR. Evoked and spontaneous electromyography to evaluate lumbosacral pedicle screw placement. Spine (Phila Pa 1976). 1996;21(5):600–4. https://doi.org/10.1097/00007632-199603010-00013.

24. Gunnarsson T, Krassioukov AV, Sarjeant R, Fehlings MG. Real-time continuous intraoperative electromyographic and somatosensory evoked potential recordings in spinal surgery: correlation of clinical and electrophysiologic findings in a prospective, consecutive series of 213 cases. Spine (Phila Pa 1976). 2004;29(6):677–84. https://doi.org/10.1097/01.BRS.0000115144.30607.E9.

25. Bose B, Sestokas AK, Schwartz DM. Neurophysiological detection of iatrogenic C-5 nerve deficit during anterior cervical spinal surgery. J Neurosurg Spine. 2007;6(5):381–5. https://doi.org/10.3171/spi.2007.6.5.381.

26. Jimenez JC, Sani S, Braverman B, Deutsch H, Ratliff JK. Palsies of the fifth cervical nerve root after cervical decompression: prevention using continuous intraoperative electromyography monitoring. J Neurosurg Spine. 2005;3(2):92–7. https://doi.org/10.3171/spi.2005.3.2.0092.

27. Dowlati E, Alexander H, Voyadzis JM. Vulnerability of the L5 nerve root during anterior lumbar interbody fusion at L5–S1: case series and review of the literature. Neurosurg Focus. 2020;49(3):1–9. https://doi.org/10.3171/2020.6.FOCUS20315.

28. Dakwar E, Vale FL, Uribe JS. Trajectory of the main sensory and motor branches of the lumbar plexus outside the psoas muscle related to the lateral retroperitoneal transpsoas approach. J Neurosurg Spine. 2011;14(2):290–5. https://doi.org/10.3171/2010.10.SPINE10395.

29. Uribe JS. Neural anatomy, neuromonitoring and related complications in extreme lateral interbody fusion: video lecture. Eur Spine J. 2015;24(S3):445–6. https://doi.org/10.1007/s00586-015-3950-x.

30. Uribe JS, Arredondo N, Dakwar E, Vale FL. Defining the safe working zones using the minimally invasive lateral retroperitoneal transpsoas approach: an anatomical study. J Neurosurg Spine. 2010;13(2):260–6. https://doi.org/10.3171/2010.3.SPINE09766.
31. Tormenti MJ, Maserati MB, Bonfield CM, Okonkwo DO, Kanter AS. Complications and radiographic correction in adult scoliosis following combined transpsoas extreme lateral interbody fusion and posterior pedicle screw instrumentation. Neurosurg Focus. 2010;28(3):1–7. https://doi.org/10.3171/2010.1.FOCUS09263.
32. Wang MY, Mummaneni PV. Minimally invasive surgery for thoracolumbar spinal deformity: initial clinical experience with clinical and radiographic outcomes. Neurosurg Focus. 2010;28(3):1–8. https://doi.org/10.3171/2010.1.FOCUS09286.
33. Langeloo DD, Lelivelt A, Journée HL, Slappendel R, De Kleuver M. Transcranial electrical motor-evoked potential monitoring during surgery for spinal deformity: a study of 145 patients. Spine (Phila Pa 1976). 2003;28(10):1043–50. https://doi.org/10.1097/00007632-200305150-00017.
34. Calancie B, Harris W, Broton JG, Alexeeva N, Green BA. "Threshold-level" multipulse transcranial electrical stimulation of motor cortex for intraoperative monitoring of spinal motor tracts: description of method and comparison to somatosensory evoked potential monitoring. J Neurosurg. 1998;88(3):457–70. https://doi.org/10.3171/jns.1998.88.3.0457.
35. Deletis V, Sala F. Intraoperative neurophysiological monitoring of the spinal cord during spinal cord and spine surgery: a review focus on the corticospinal tracts. Clin Neurophysiol. 2008;119(2):248–64. https://doi.org/10.1016/j.clinph.2007.09.135.
36. MacDonald DB. Intraoperative motor evoked potential monitoring: overview and update. J Clin Monit Comput. 2006;20(5):347–77. https://doi.org/10.1007/s10877-006-9033-0.
37. MacDonald DB, Janusz M. An approach to intraoperative neurophysiologic monitoring of thoracoabdominal aneurysm surgery. J Clin Neurophysiol. 2002;19(1):43–54. https://doi.org/10.1097/00004691-200201000-00006.
38. Kong CY, Hosseini AM, Belanger LM, et al. A prospective evaluation of hemodynamic management in acute spinal cord injury patients. Spinal Cord. 2013;51(6):466–71. https://doi.org/10.1038/sc.2013.32.
39. Walters BC, Hadley MN, Hurlbert RJ, et al. Guidelines for the management of acute cervical spine and spinal cord injuries: 2013 update. Neurosurgery. 2013;60(Suppl 1):82–91. https://doi.org/10.1227/01.neu.0000430319.32247.7f.
40. Ploumis A, Yadlapalli N, Fehlings MG, Kwon BK, Vaccaro AR. A systematic review of the evidence supporting a role for vasopressor support in acute SCI. Spinal Cord. 2010;48(5):356–62. https://doi.org/10.1038/sc.2009.150.
41. Hawryluk G, Whetstone W, Saigal R, et al. Mean arterial blood pressure correlates with neurological recovery after human spinal cord injury: analysis of high frequency physiologic data. J Neurotrauma. 2015;32(24):1958–67. https://doi.org/10.1089/neu.2014.3778.
42. Altschul D, Kobets AJ, Nakhla J, et al. Postoperative urinary retention in patients undergoing elective spinal surgery. J Neurosurg Spine. 2017;26(2):229–34. https://doi.org/10.3171/2016.8.SPINE151371.
43. Normelli H, Aaro S, Hedlund R, Svensson O, Strömberg L. Urethral catheterization in spinal surgery: a randomized prospective study. Eur Spine J. 1993;2(3):132–5. https://doi.org/10.1007/BF00301409.

# Chapter 9
# Incision Choice for Anterior Lumbar Access Surgery

Parth K. Patel and Jeffrey B. Weinreb

## Introduction

The anterior approach to the lumbar spine has been described for centuries, though the first recording of an anterior approach to be successfully carried out was in the early twentieth century [1, 2]. Done by Walter Müller in 1906, this technique would be utilized by other surgeons such as Norman Capaner and Hiromu Ito, serving its purpose of exposing aspects of the spine inaccessible by the conventional posterior approach [3–5]. However, incisions made on the anterior and lateral aspect of the abdomen for purposes accessing abdominal and retroperitoneal structures have also been described in the vascular, gynecologic/obstetric, urologic and, general surgery literature for indications including cesarean section, prostatectomies, appendectomies, inguinal hernia repairs, and sigmoid resection [6–11]. After the decision to approach the anterior or lateral lumbar spine is made, the exposure and/or spine surgeons must determine which specific incision will help them achieve the goals in the safest, most efficient, and, when possible, minimally invasive or cosmetic manner possible. The purpose of this chapter is to review the important considerations when deciding on an incision, including preoperative planning, local anatomy, various existing options, and potential complications.

P. K. Patel
The George Washington University School of Medicine, Washington, DC, USA

J. B. Weinreb (✉)
Department of Orthopaedic Surgery, The George Washington University, Washington, DC, USA

Department of Orthopaedic Surgery, The University of Maryland, Baltimore, MD, USA

© The Author(s), under exclusive license to Springer Nature Switzerland AG 2023
J. R. O'Brien et al. (eds.), *Lumbar Spine Access Surgery*, https://doi.org/10.1007/978-3-031-48034-8_9

# Preoperative Planning

The anterior approach requires several considerations preoperatively, collectively influencing the incision type utilized. As an overview, incisions are generally transverse, paramedian vertical, or midline vertical. An incision should be made in the direction of lines of skin cleavage (Langer's lines) when possible to result in minimal scar formation [12]. Sharp angles or portions of the incision that result in skin devitalization must be avoided. Once an incision is made, the approach to access the spine can be transperitoneal or retroperitoneal, depending on the specific planes entered. The structures deep to the incision change depending on the level of the approach: above the arcuate line the layers are skin, subcutaneous fat, anterior rectus sheath (which is comprised of the aponeuroses of the external and internal oblique muscles), rectus muscle, posterior rectus sheath (which is comprised of the aponeuroses of the internal oblique and transversus abdominis muscles), transversalis fascia, and the peritoneum, and below the arcuate line the posterior rectus sheath is absent and the rectus muscle overlies the peritoneum. The retroperitoneal approach has become the dominant technique due to lower postoperative complications including retrograde ejaculation and ileus [13]. Variation in retroperitoneal anatomy results in a risk differential depending on which critical structures are involved in surgical exposure of the spine. The more robust arterial structures, including the descending aorta and common iliac vessels are located on the patient's left, while the more delicate venous structures, including the inferior vena cava and common iliac veins, are located on the right. For this reason, the majority of modern surgeons approach via the left side. Historically, the right-sided retroperitoneal approach was more common, as many surgeons preferred to leave the left side untouched in case a revision or adjacent segment surgery was required [14]. Additionally, the level at which the aorta bifurcates must be taken into consideration. Aortic bifurcation typically occurs at L4, but it may divide into the common iliac arteries anywhere from L3 to L5 [15]. Furthermore, it is critical to evaluate every patient's abdominal surgical history and carefully examine preoperative imaging. A prior retroperitoneal or abdominal procedure might make a contralateral incision and approach more attractive, and excessive scarring seen on magnetic resonance imaging may change the surgical plan entirely. Generally, if there is a fat layer seen between the disc space or vertebral body and the large anterior vessels, they can be mobilized.

A surgeon must also consider patient positioning when choosing the incision. The anterior approach is performed with the patient supine with the possibility of induced hyperlordosis via a lumbar or sacral bolster or angulation of the operating table [1, 16–18]. Trendelenburg positioning may be employed to translate the peritoneal structures cranially and for better operative visualization and to better access the L4–L5 and L5–S1 levels as they tend to be the most lordotic [19]. While the anterior approach allows for optimal access to the lumbar spine, the thoracolumbar region between T12 and L2 can be accessed via an anterior or lateral retroperitoneal approach with the patient placed in a lateral decubitus position. Once a patient is positioned on the operating room table, fluoroscopy can be utilized to localize the incision. A blunt metal instrument, such as bariatric sponge forceps, can be pushed into the abdominal skin directed at the target disc space or spaces prior to sterile preparation and utilized to mark the optimal incision level under fluoroscopy. It is important to recognize that the incision must be centered where the trajectory of the disk level meets the skin rather than over the disc space itself [19].

Available retraction may also influence which incision is selected. A table-mounted retractor system allows for more rigid retraction than handheld retractors. A paramedian retroperitoneal approach requires retraction against the entire rectus musculature as opposed to a midline vertical retroperitoneal approach, which requires retraction against only half of the rectus musculature but might be associated with higher incisional hernia rates [20]. Lighted retractors may also be utilized to allow for improved visualization.

## Paramedian Incision

The paramedian incision is commonly used for a retroperitoneal lumbar approach. A longitudinal incision is made over either the lateral border or directly over the rectus abdominis with the latter reducing the risk of dead space creation above the fascia [1]. The incision can also be made in the midline [21]. The incision is typically performed on the left as to better mobilize and protect the more fragile venous vasculature. A right-sided incision is generally less common and considered in revision settings or to preserve left-sided access to adjacent levels for revisions [14]. As previously discussed, fluoroscopy can be utilized to localize the incision, which generally can be extensile and allow exposure of L2–S1. Once the anterior rectus sheath has been dissected, the rectus abdominis can either be retracted towards or away from midline, with the latter theoretically preserving the innervation to the muscle [22]. To access the retroperitoneum, the peritoneum is mobilized lateral to medial off the overlying posterior rectus sheath which is then divided cranially-caudally [22]. In the case where the patient has had prior abdominal surgery or is larger, a midline dissection may be indicated [1].

## Anterolateral

The anterolateral incision is similar to the paramedian approach and is also well described [22]. In this approach, the incision is also generally made on the left side for similar reasons to the paramedian approach but the incision begins more cranially and laterally. The incision may begin at the distal tip of the 11th or 12th rib and curves medially to the lateral rectus sheath and distally to the symphysis pubis when L5–S1 exposure is required [22]. The distal 2 cm of the rib may be osteotomized to provide access to retroperitoneal fat. The peritoneal layer is cleared from the undersurface of the transversalis abdominis and the external oblique muscle is split in line with the incision and followed by division of the internal oblique and transversalis muscles with electrocautery [22].

## Transverse Incision

The low transverse incision, also known as a Pfannenstiel incision, was initially described by German gynecologist Hermann Johannes Pfannenstiel in 1900 (Fig. 9.1) [23, 24]. In his original description, Pfannenstiel's stated goals were to improve access in gynecologic and obstetric procedures, improve cosmetic results, and reduce the risk of incisional hernias by relying on the robust anterior fascial sheath below the arcuate line [24]. For the spine, this incision is used in the approach to the lower lumbar to S1 region [25, 26]. The patient is placed in the supine position and the incision is made horizontally with a slight curvature between the umbilicus and pubic symphysis. Once subcutaneous flaps are made, the linea alba is divided with electrocautery. The left-sided rectus is elevated and retracted, and the retroperitoneum can be entered laterally [26].

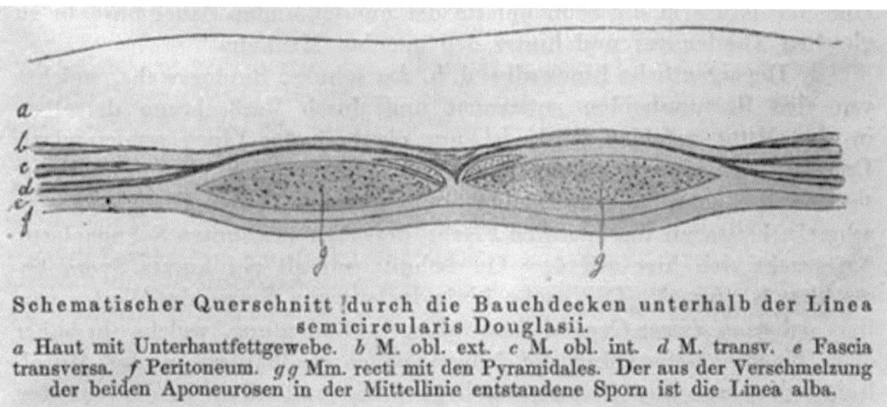



**Fig. 9.1** Figure from Pfannenstiel's original article demonstrating the lower abdominal wall anatomy. (**a**) Skin and fat, (**b**) oblique external abdominal muscle, (**c**) oblique internal abdominal muscle, (**d**) transverse abdominal muscle, (**e**) transversalis fascia, (**f**) peritoneal layer, (**g**) rectus, and pyramidalis muscles [24]

## Periumbilical Incision

The periumbilical incision was described in 2018 by Bassani et al. [27]. A 270° nearly circular cut is made with a diameter of 6 inches, the opening facing cranially, and is concentric with the patient's naval. After encountering subcutaneous fat, the dissection is carried radially at a 45° angle, creating a mound of subcutaneous fat around the umbilicus until the anterior rectus sheath is visualized. The resulting deep incision is therefore much larger than the skin incision [27]. From here, the procedure is continued similarly to the paramedian approach. The anterior rectus sheath is incised at its medial attachment to the linea alba, the left rectus is retracted laterally, the posterior sheath is entered at the lateral aspect of the arcuate line, and retroperitoneal dissection is continued. The periumbilical incision provides enough operative space to perform not just a single-level fusion but has also proven compatible with multilevel procedures from L3–S1 and has been reproduced by other authors [28].

## Lateral Incision

The lateral retroperitoneal approach to the lumbar spine was described by Pimenta in 2001 and popularized by Ogzur et al. in 2006 [29, 30]. It can generally be used to access the lower thoracic to L4–L5 levels. The original descriptions called for placing the patient in the right lateral decubitus position (left side up) and localizing the target level on fluoroscopy. A perfect lateral should be confirmed with cross-table anterior-posterior imaging with the spinous process perfectly centered between the pedicles and excellent view of the end plates. Through table positioning or bolster placement, the spine is flexed to open the space between the bottom of the rib cage and the iliac crest. Using crossed k-wires on a lateral view, the midpoint of the disc space is marked. A 2-cm-long second mark is made posterior to the planned initial mark between the erector spinae and abdominal oblique muscles [30]. This second incision is used to accommodate the surgeon's index finger to enter the retroperitoneal space and guide the direct lateral dilators into the primary lateral working portal. As the technique has been developed, most surgeons elect to utilize only a single lateral incision, as a finger can be utilized to sweep the peritoneum through this incision, and specialized localization tools are widespread. Additionally, a direct lateral approach with the patient in the prone position has become more widely utilized [31].

## Complications

Incisional complications include wound dehiscence, infection, hernia/bulging, and pain, which are all discussed in more detail in Chap. 22. Overall, the occurrence of these complications is well documented, but few studies compare complications with regards to specific incisional choice. The Pfannenstiel incision has been shown to have a very low rate of incisional hernia between 0% and 2% [6, 7, 24, 32]. However, there is a fairly high rate of postoperative nerve pain, which may represent entrapment of the iliohypogastric or ilioinguinal nerves [33]. Loos et al. conducted a study of 690 postoperative obstetric/gynecologic patients [34]. One-third of these patients had chronic pain at their incision site, and 17 of these were determined to have nerve entrapment. Eight patients underwent a 1% lidocaine injection, and two had long-term pain relief. In their study of 300 patients, Jagannathan et al. compared 180 patients who underwent a paramedian approach and 120 who underwent an anterolateral approach [22]. Abdominal bulging was the most common postoperative complaint with rates of 1.1% in the paramedian approach and 18% in the anterolateral group ($p = 0.04$). Abdominal bulging was associated with three or more surgical levels as well as significantly lower wound appearance and satisfaction scores and there were no statistical differences in reoperation rates [22]. Incisional hernia after a lateral approach is rare and limited to case studies in the literature [35–37]. A longitudinal incision has been theorized to have higher rates of rectus denervation and atonia [38].

## Conclusion

The decision of which incision to use when approaching the anterior or lateral lumbar spine can have important implications for surgical planning and execution. A variety of factors must be considered including surgeon experience, surgical goals, number of levels targeted, prior surgeries, patient anatomy, and potential complications. Ultimately, there are many described surgical incisions with specific risks, benefits, and postoperative considerations that may be utilized. Modern practitioners should be aware of the different options to best suit each individual surgical case to facilitate optimal patient outcomes.

## References


1. Huddleston PM, Zietlow S, Eck JC. Lumbar spine. In: Morrey BF, Morrey MC, editors. Master techniques in orthopaedic surgery: relevant surgical exposures. Philadelphia: Wolters Kluwer Health; 2018. p. 315–38.
2. Matur AV, Mejia-Munne JC, Plummer ZJ, et al. The history of anterior and lateral approaches to the lumbar spine. World Neurosurg. 2020;144:213–21.

3. Muller W. Transperitoneale freilegung der wirbelsaule bei tuberkuloser spondylitis. Dtsch Z Chir. 1906;85:128–35.
4. Ito H, Tsuchiya J, Asami G. A new radical operation for Pott's disease: report of ten cases. JBJS. 1934;16:499.
5. Capener N. Spondylolisthesis. Br J Surg. 1932;19(75):374–86.
6. Luijendijk RW, Jeekel J, Storm RK, et al. The low transverse Pfannenstiel incision and the prevalence of incisional hernia and nerve entrapment. Ann Surg. 1997;225:365.
7. Griffiths DA. A reappraisal of the Pfannenstiel incision. Br J Urol. 1976;48:469–74.
8. El-Boghdadly S, Abel K. Pfannenstiel incision for appendicectomy in females. Br J Clin Pract. 1984;38:17–9.
9. Saetta J, Abel K. The use of the Pfannenstiel incision in the female with presumed appendicitis. Br J Clin Pract. 1990;44:145–7.
10. Abarbanel J, Kimche D. Combined retropubic prostatectomy and preperitoneal inguinal herniorrhaphy. J Urol. 1988;140:1442–4.
11. Freundt I, Toolenaar T, Huikeshoven F, et al. A modified technique to create a neovagina with an isolated segment of sigmoid colon. Surg Gynecol Obstet. 1992;174:11–6.
12. Gardner JH, Holyoke EA, Giovacchini R. Cleavage lines of the visceral and parietal peritoneum. Anat Rec. 1957;127:247–55.
13. Bateman DK, Millhouse PW, Shahi N, et al. Anterior lumbar spine surgery: a systematic review and meta-analysis of associated complications. Spine J. 2015;15:1118–32.
14. Gumbs AA, Shah RV, Yue JJ, et al. The open anterior paramedian retroperitoneal approach for spine procedures. Arch Surg. 2005;140:339–43.
15. Deswal A, Tamang BK, Bala A. Study of aortic-common iliac bifurcation and its clinical significance. J Clin Diagn Res. 2014;8:AC06–8.
16. Bauer R, Kerschbaumer F, Poisel S. Spine, anterior approaches. In: Kerschbaumer F, Weise K, Wirth CJ, Vaccaro AR, editors. Operative approaches in orthopedic surgery and traumatology. New York: Thieme; 2015.
17. Majid K, Bains R-R. Thoracic and lumbar spine approaches. In: Chapman MW, James MA, editors. Chapman's comprehensive orthopaedic surgery. New Delhi: Jaypee Brothers Medial Publishers; 2019. p. 4134–44.
18. Steinmetz MP, Benzel EC. Benzel's spine surgery. 4th ed. Philadelphia: Elsevier; 2017.
19. Saadt E, Heller JG, Rhee JM. Anterior lumbar interbody fusion. In: Rhee JM, editor. Emory university spine illustrated tips and tricks in spine surgery. Philadelphia: Wolters Kluwer Health; 2020. p. 263–74.
20. Manunga J, Alcala C, Smith J, et al. Technical approach, outcomes, and exposure-related complications in patients undergoing anterior lumbar interbody fusion. J Vasc Surg. 2021;73:992–8.
21. Mobbs RJ, Phan K, Daly D, et al. Approach-related complications of anterior lumbar interbody fusion: results of a combined spine and vascular surgical team. Global Spine J. 2016;6:147–54.
22. Jagannathan J, Chankaew E, Urban P, et al. Cosmetic and functional outcomes following paramedian and anterolateral retroperitoneal access in anterior lumbar spine surgery. J Neurosurg Spine. 2008;9:454–65.
23. Kisielinski K, Conze J, Murken A, et al. The Pfannenstiel or so called "bikini cut": still effective more than 100 years after first description. Hernia. 2004;8:177–81.
24. Pfannenstiel HJ. Ober die Vorteile des suprasymphysaren Fascienquerschnitts fur die gynakologische Koliotomien zugleich ein Beitrag zu der Indikationsstellung der Operationswege. Samml Klin Vortr Gynakolog. 1900;97:1735–56.
25. Kernodle AB, Abularrage CJ. Spinal operative exposure. In: Rutherford's vascular surgery and endovascular therapy. Philadelphia: Elsevier; 2023. p. 762–70.
26. Mobbs RJ, Lennox A, Ho Y-T, et al. L5/S1 anterior lumbar interbody fusion technique. J Spine Surg. 2017;3:429–32.
27. Bassani R, Querenghi AM, Cecchinato R, et al. A new "keyhole" approach for multilevel anterior lumbar interbody fusion: the perinavel approach—technical note and literature review. Eur Spine J. 2018;27:1956–63.

28. Abdoli S, Sui J, Ziegler K, et al. The periumbilical incision for anterior lumbar interbody fusions. J Vasc Surg Cases Innov Tech. 2020;6:384–7.
29. Pimenta L. Lateral endoscopic transpsoas retroperitoneal approach for lumbar spine surgery. Minas Gerais: Belo Horizonte; 2001.
30. Ozgur BM, Aryan HE, Pimenta L, et al. Extreme Lateral interbody Fusion (XLIF): a novel surgical technique for anterior lumbar interbody fusion. Spine J. 2006;6:435–43.
31. Pimenta L, Taylor WR, Stone LE, et al. Prone transpsoas technique for simultaneous single-position access to the anterior and posterior lumbar spine. Oper Neurosurg (Hagerstown). 2020;20:E5–12.
32. Biswas KK. Why not Pfannenstiel's incision? Obstet Gynecol. 1973;41:303–7.
33. Sippo WC, Burghardt A, Gomez AC. Nerve entrapment after Pfannenstiel incision. Am J Obstet Gynecol. 1987;157:420–1.
34. Loos MJ, Scheltinga MR, Mulders LG, et al. The Pfannenstiel incision as a source of chronic pain. Obstet Gynecol. 2008;111:839–46.
35. Wakabayashi M, Miyazaki Y, Aoki K, et al. Incisional hernia after extreme lateral interbody fusion on the lumbar spine: a case report. Int J Surg Case Rep. 2021;78:130–2.
36. Galan TV, Mohan V, Klineberg EO, et al. Case report: incisional hernia as a complication of extreme lateral interbody fusion. Spine J. 2012;12:e1–6.
37. Gundanna M, Shah K. Delayed incisional hernia following minimally invasive trans-psoas lumbar spine surgery: report of a rare complication and management. Int J Spine Surg. 2018;12:126–30.
38. Kim Y-H, Ha K-Y, Rhyu K-W, et al. Lumbar interbody fusion: techniques, pearls and pitfalls. Asian Spine J. 2020;14:730.

# Chapter 10
# ALIF Retractor Options for Anterior Lumbar Access Surgery

Timothy R. Rasmusson

## Retractor Options: Fixed vs. Handheld

### Introduction

As improving technology and minimally invasive techniques have become more commonplace in most surgical specialties, similar advances are also being seen anterior lumbar spine surgery. The decision of when to incorporate newer methods versus utilizing more traditional approaches is an important one, perhaps even more so when exposing the anterior lumbar spine. Mitigation of risks specific to the anterior approach is critical when planning and performing surgery. The selection of a retractor and exposure technique must be tailored not only to the patient, but often to the surgeon or implant. Exposure options range from the mini-open approach with fixed vascular retraction to the traditional approach with handheld vascular retraction. The former is more widely utilized, but the latter still has indications and remains the preferred technique for some surgeons.

There are several complications associated with the exposure portion of anterior spine surgery. Across most reviews, the incidence of the comparatively minor complications, such as retrograde ejaculation, deep venous thrombosis, ileus, etc., is consistently low [1, 2]. In contrast, the incidence of vascular injuries ranges from 2% to 24%, with one study documenting a 3% incidence of "life-threatening" injuries [3, 4]. While the retractor selection or presence of an access surgeon is rarely mentioned, this disparity would suggest that one or both could be a factor worth considering when planning a procedure. Is this a case where one can set up a mini-open approach with fixed retraction and move on to another case, or is this a

T. R. Rasmusson (✉)
Surgical Associates of Western New York, Kenmore, NY, USA

© The Author(s), under exclusive license to Springer Nature Switzerland AG 2023

J. R. O'Brien et al. (eds.), *Lumbar Spine Access Surgery*,
https://doi.org/10.1007/978-3-031-48034-8_10

situation which requires a traditional handheld retractor and the continued presence of an access surgeon?

## *Fixed Retraction*

In the early days of anterior spine exposure, creating a "wall of steel" with fixed vascular retraction was the goal, providing a layer of protection between the discectomy/implant placement and the iliac vessels. This has evolved into the increasingly popular minimally invasive or "mini-open" approach, offering smaller incisions and the relative sparing of the abdominal wall musculature. Several companies now offer specialty systems with blades specifically designed for vascular retraction (Fig. 10.1).

This method does have its limitations, as it provides only a comparatively small working channel which may become an issue when dealing with challenging anatomy or vascular injury. There is also some data to suggest that an increased risk of arterial injury may be associated with fixed vascular retraction in some patients [4, 5].

## *Intermittent Vascular Retraction*

The traditional intermittent vascular retraction technique and associated retractors can still play an important role in exposure of the anterior lumbar spine, particularly in challenging cases. Handheld vascular retraction can also be used in conjunction with a fixed ring/arm retractor for soft tissue, with the larger working footprint potentially providing some risk mitigation. Another advantage, although difficult to quantify from an objective standpoint, is the presence of the access surgeon for the

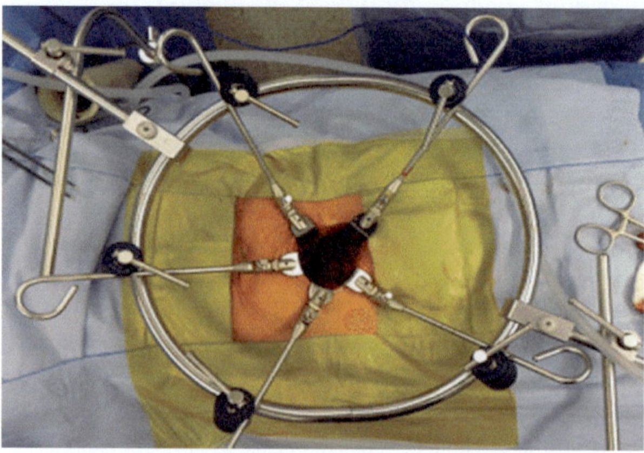

**Fig. 10.1** Fixed retraction system

**Fig. 10.2** Handheld retraction using Bookwalter retractor

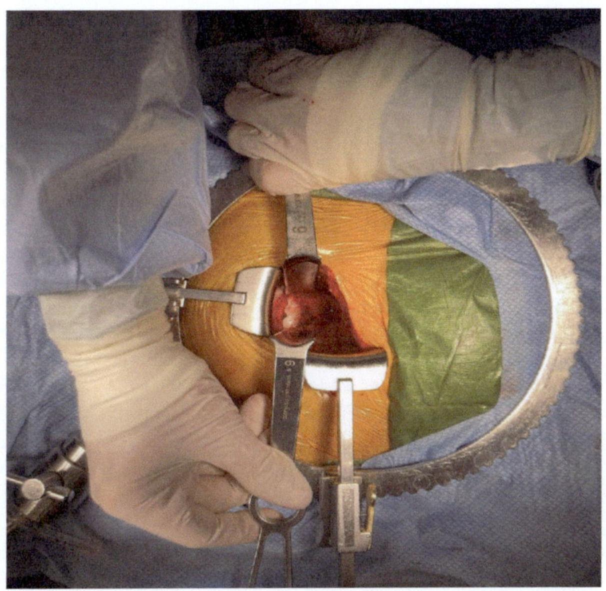

duration of the procedure. Two sets of eyes, as well as the ability to safely manipulate the retractors as needed, can be critical in difficult cases (Fig. 10.2).

## *Conclusion*

The learning curve for anterior spine exposure is steep, reflected in the wide range of vascular injuries described in numerous studies. As such, the mini-open technique with fixed vascular retraction should be left to those with experience, not only in the operating room, but in preoperative assessment and planning. A conventional open exposure should be considered if one is new to the anterior lumbar approach, with the utilization of handheld vascular retractors allowing the surgeon to gauge the compliance, or lack thereof, of the iliac vessels. The division of the ascending lumbar vein, or the dissection of the left iliac vein off of an osteophyte, both potentially memorable maneuvers, are also best attempted in an open approach setting until one has gained experience. While there are differences of opinion regarding the need for an access surgeon, when new to the procedure or working in a high-risk environment, the exposure afforded in an open approach with an access surgeon present to assist and monitor the procedure may be beneficial [6, 7].

# References


1. Ballard JL, Carlson G, Chen J, White J. Anterior thoracolumbar spine exposure: critical review and analysis. Ann Vasc Surg. 2014;28(2):465–9. https://doi.org/10.1016/j.avsg.2013.06.026.
2. Bateman DK, Millhouse PW, Shahi N, Kadam AB, Maltenfort MG, Koerner JD, Vaccaro AR. Anterior lumbar spine surgery: a systematic review and meta-analysis of associated complications. Spine J. 2015;15(5):1118–32. https://doi.org/10.1016/j.spinee.2015.02.040.
3. Chiriano J, Abou-Zamzam AM Jr, Urayeneza O, Zhang WW, Cheng W. The role of the vascular surgeon in anterior retroperitoneal spine exposure: preservation of open surgical training. J Vasc Surg. 2009;50(1):148–51. https://doi.org/10.1016/j.jvs.2009.01.007.
4. Brau SA, Delamarter RB, Schiffman ML, Williams LA, Watkins RG. Vascular injury during anterior lumbar surgery. Spine J. 2004;4(4):409–12. https://doi.org/10.1016/j.spinee.2003.12.003.
5. Kulkarni SS, Lowery GL, Ross RE, Ravi Sankar K, Lykomitros V. Arterial complications following anterior lumbar interbody fusion: report of eight cases. Eur Spine J. 2003;12(1):48–54. https://doi.org/10.1007/s00586-002-0460-4.
6. Mobbs RJ, Phan K, Daly D, Rao PJ, Lennox A. Approach-related complications of anterior lumbar interbody fusion: results of a combined spine and vascular surgical team. Global Spine J. 2016;6(2):147–54. https://doi.org/10.1055/s-0035-1557141.
7. Smith MW, Rahn KA, Shugart RM, Belschner CD, Stout KS, Cheng I. Comparison of perioperative parameters and complications observed in the anterior exposure of the lumbar spine by a spine surgeon with and without the assistance of an access surgeon. Spine J. 2011;11(5):389–94. https://doi.org/10.1016/j.spinee.2011.03.014.

# Part IV

# Operative Technique for Lumbar Spine Access Surgery

# Chapter 11
# Mini-Open Anterior Retroperitoneal Approach

Brian A. Kuhn, Joel Hlavaty, and Sashi Kilaru

## Introduction

Anterior lumbar interbody fusion (ALIF) was first described in 1932 by Capener and has been utilized for definitive treatment of spinal pathology [1]. The goal for the access surgeon is to provide adequate midline exposure to the lumbar spine so the spine surgeon can safely perform their intervention. The anterior retroperitoneal approach takes advantage of this space and can minimize potential complications seen with other approaches. This approach still requires manipulation of the peritoneal contents, ureter, and significant arterial and venous structures that could be injured. Increased understanding of spinal pathology and biomechanics, especially at the L5–S1 level, has made anterior spinal surgery appealing to many spine surgeons. The original exposure and morbidity of large incisions, significant blood loss, and operative time have also prevented some from adopting this approach. This chapter provides a detailed approach for a minimally invasive retroperitoneal exposure of the lumbar spine from L2 to S1.

## Positioning and Localization

The patient is placed in the supine position on the operating room table with the patient's arms out to the side. The table is typically a Jackson or other radiolucent table. A urinary catheter is inserted to avoid bladder distention which may obscure


B. A. Kuhn (✉) · J. Hlavaty
TriHealth/Good Samaritan Hospital, Cincinnati, OH, USA
e-mail: Brian_kuhn@trihealth.com

S. Kilaru
The Christ Hospital, Cincinnati, OH, USA



© The Author(s), under exclusive license to Springer Nature Switzerland AG 2023


J. R. O'Brien et al. (eds.), *Lumbar Spine Access Surgery*,
https://doi.org/10.1007/978-3-031-48034-8_11

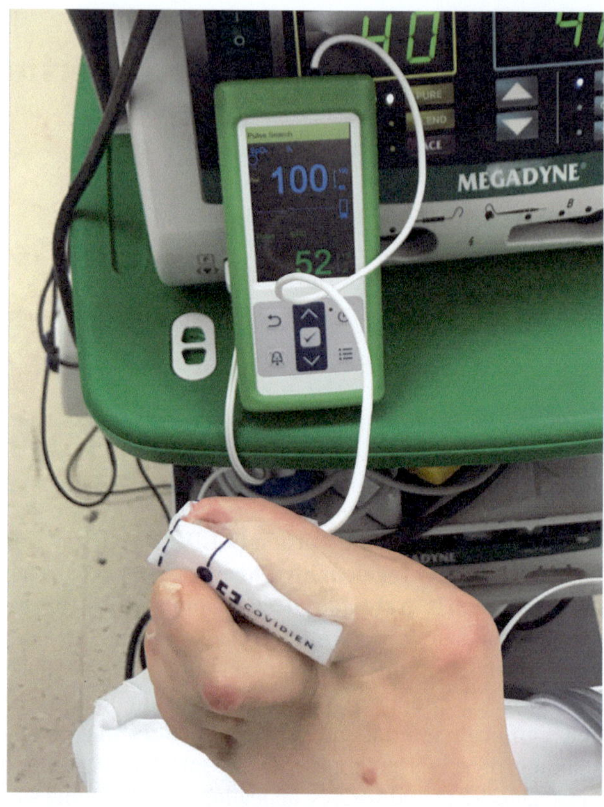

**Fig. 11.1** Pulse oximetry on left hallux

the operative field and predispose injury. The urinary catheter will also monitor urine output during the case and can be checked at the end of the case for blood which may indicate bladder or ureter injury. Pulse oximetry is then typically placed on the left hallux (Fig. 11.1) if a left retroperitoneal approach is going to be used and monitor located so it can be visualized throughout the case. If a right retroperitoneal approach is going to be used, this would be placed on the right hallux. The operative field is then shaved.

Fluoroscopy is then performed in the lateral position to mark the intended disk space for optimal exposure (Figs. 11.2 and 11.3). Once this has been determined, a skin marker is used for incision placement (Fig. 11.4). The amount of lordosis or kyphosis as well as depth of the spine is taken into consideration for incision placement. In general, the L5–S1 disk space has the most lordosis and the incision is caudal to the disk space. In contrast, the L2–L3 disk space has a more caudal angle

**Fig. 11.2** Fluoroscopy in lateral position to mark intended disk space

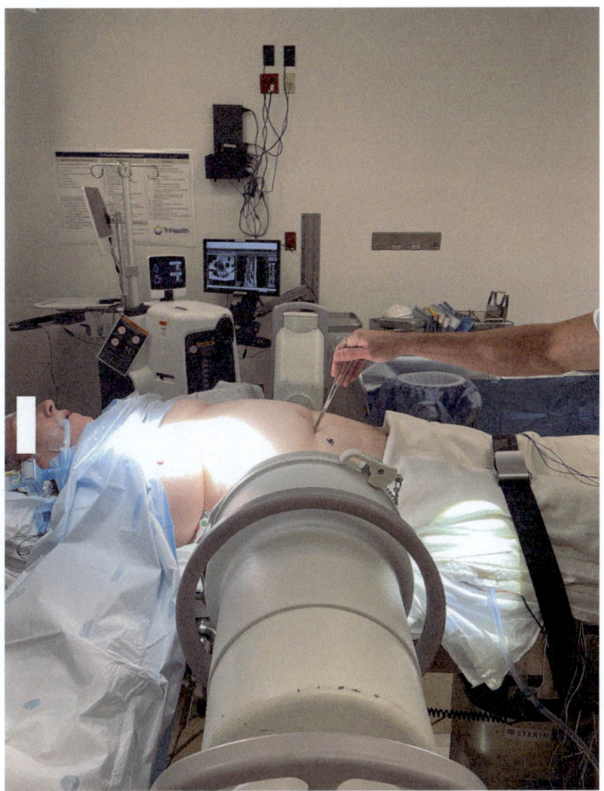

of entry into the disk space due to the natural lordotic curvature at this level and the incision is at or slightly cranial to this level for single-level exposure. If a multilevel exposure is being performed, the skin incision would split the difference between the multiple levels to allow for a minimally invasive incision.

The abdomen is then prepped and draped in a standard fashion. The patient is given full neuromuscular blockade by anesthesia during the exposure. The operative surgeon stands on the patient's right side and the assistant on the left. It is recommended that the operative exposing surgeon wears a headlight to allow for good illumination of the operative field. Surgical loupes, typically with 2.5× magnification, are also recommended to enhance visualization of the field. Multiple incision choices have been described and include transverse, longitudinal midline, paramedian, and oblique. In general, our preferred incision choice is mini-Pfannenstiel for the L5–S1 disk space and longitudinal for other single-level and multilevel exposures.

**Fig. 11.3** Lateral x-ray with operative level identified using radiopaque marker

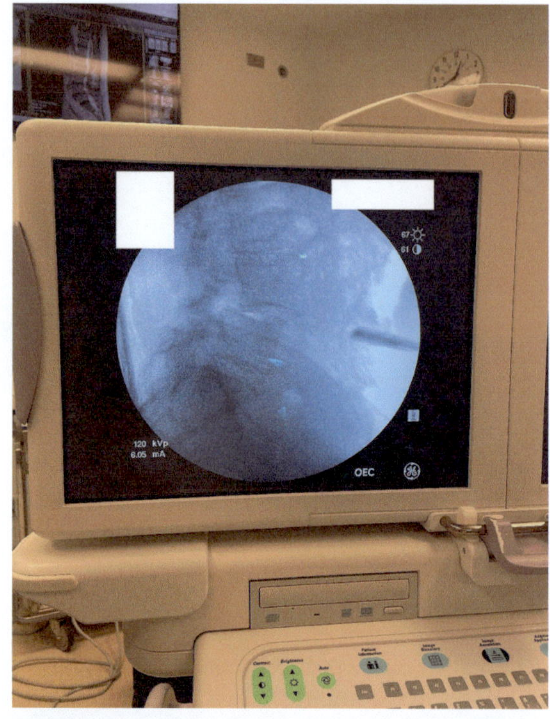

**Fig. 11.4** Skin marker used for incision placement

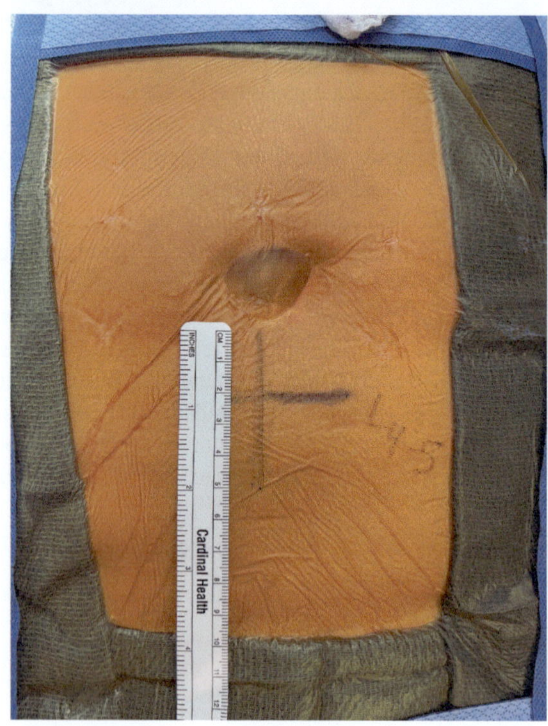

## Retroperitoneal Dissection and Vascular Mobilization

### *L5–S1*

A small transverse skin incision is made based on intraoperative localization. This is carried down through subcutaneous tissue and Scarpa's fascia to the anterior rectus sheath with electrocautery. The subcutaneous tissue is freed from the underlying anterior rectus sheath including the linea alba to allow for mobilization and longitudinal opening of the anterior rectus fascia left of the midline. Perforator vessels are cauterized and indicate that the dissection is off midline (Fig. 11.5). The anterior rectus sheath is then opened longitudinally 1 cm left of midline. It is then opened as far superiorly and inferiorly as possible by the operating surgeon while the assistant is retracting the skin with a handheld finger retractor as the surgeon works in each direction (Fig. 11.6). The medial aspect of the rectus muscle is then mobilized off midline the entire length of the fascial opening (Fig. 11.7). The assistant now uses a handheld Richardson retractor to elevate the left rectus muscle from the underlying

**Fig. 11.5** Anterior Rectus fascia identified left of midline

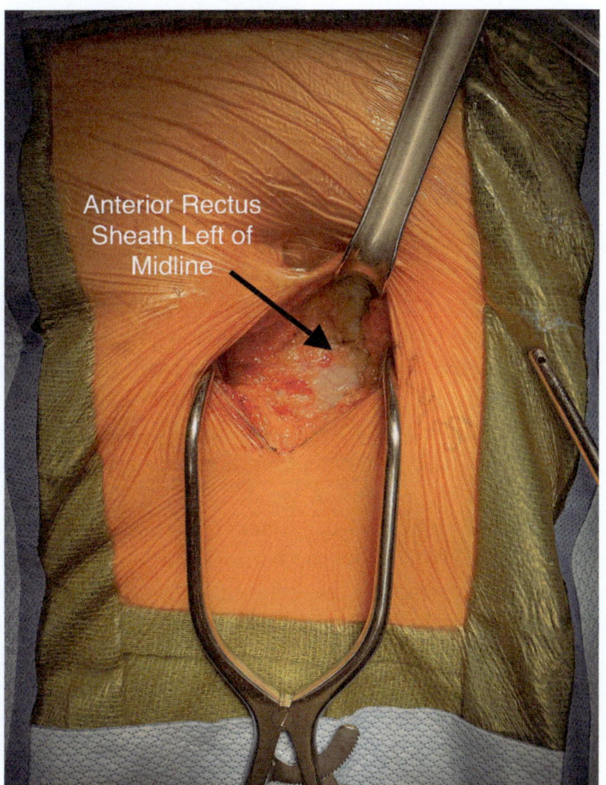

**Fig. 11.6** Anterior Rectus fascia opened off midline

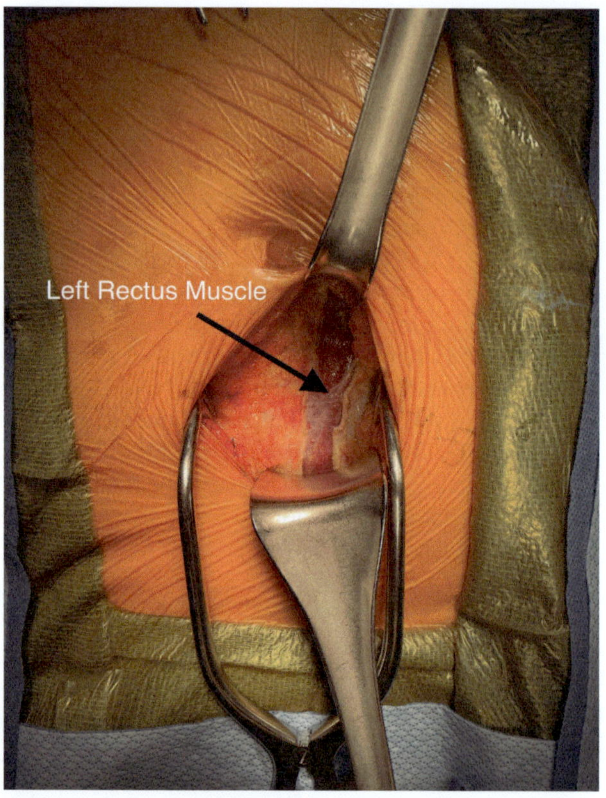


transversalis fascia and peritoneum (Fig. 11.8). At this level there is no posterior rectus sheath since the dissection is below the arcuate line. Blunt dissection is now performed posterior to the rectus muscle extending laterally. The inferior epigastric vessels are retracted anteriorly and any small branches can be cauterized (Fig. 11.9). The transversalis fascia is entered bluntly using either finger or Kittner dissection into the retroperitoneal space in the left lower quadrant making sure to keep the peritoneum intact. If a defect in the peritoneum is encountered, it is repaired with a running absorbable suture, typically a 2-0 Vicryl. During this maneuver the spermatic cord in men and the round ligament in women can be seen and should be swept inferiorly to allow the peritoneal contents to be mobilized medially. Caution should be used during this mobilization to avoid any unnecessary tension on the cord that could lead to postoperative testicular pain. It is usually not necessary, but the round ligament in women can be ligated and divided.

Once in the retroperitoneal space, the peritoneum is mobilized to the right (Fig. 11.10). The psoas muscle with the overlying genitofemoral nerve can be visualized. The left ureter should be mobilized to the right with the peritoneal contents (Fig.

**Fig. 11.7** Rectus muscle mobilized off midline

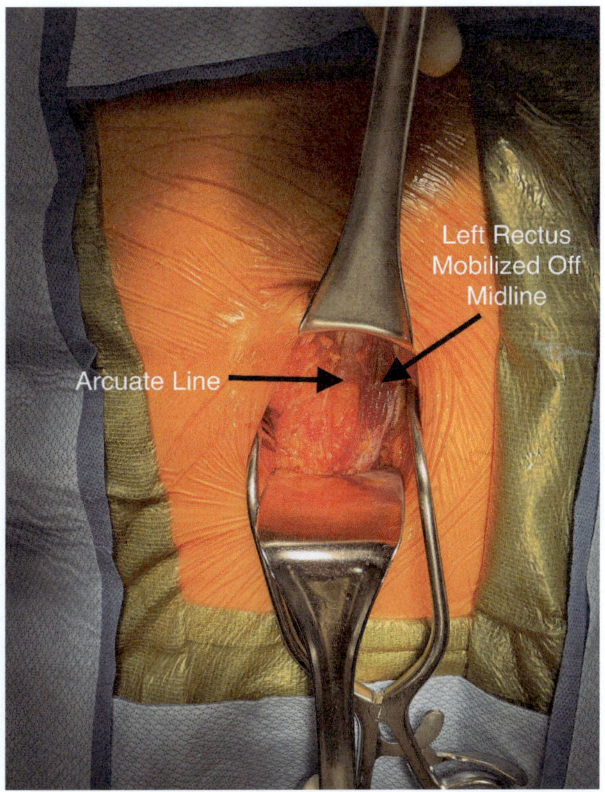


11.11). This mobilization is performed with a few fingers and in deeper patients is done with handheld Wiley retractors by the surgeon while the assistant holds the rectus muscle and subcutaneous tissue to the patient's left. As the surgeon moves the peritoneal contents and ureter to the right, the assistant relaxes tension on their retractor to allow for this to happen through the small incision. The left common iliac artery is then encountered, and dissection kept just anterior to this. At this point, the sacral promontory can be palpated, and the handheld Wiley can be used to sweep the presacral fat and superior hypogastric plexus to the right exposing the underlying middle sacral vessels. The L5–S1 disk space typically is located between both common iliac arteries and veins just posterior to the middle sacral vessels. A table-mounted retractor with radiolucent blades is then used to retract the iliac vessels away from the disk space. The first narrow blade is placed on the patient's left side to retract the left common iliac artery and vein. Next, the second narrow blade will be placed to the right which will retract the peritoneal contents, ureter, and right common iliac artery and vein to the right of the disk space. A third narrow blade

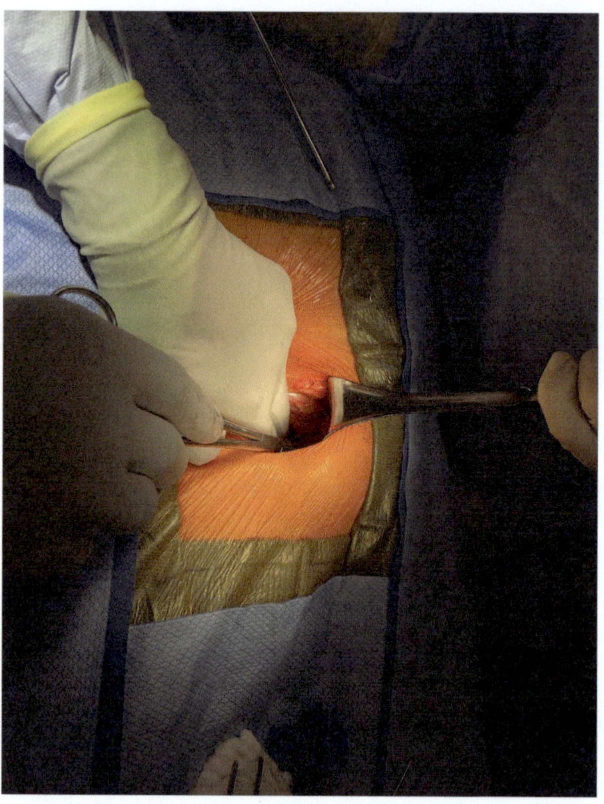

**Fig. 11.8** Elevation of left rectus muscle to start the retroperitoneal dissection

retractor is placed superiorly to help identify the underlying proximal left common iliac vein. Small clips are then used proximally and distally on the middle sacral artery, and it is divided with scissors. The middle sacral veins are cauterized with bipolar cautery to avoid any injury to the hypogastric plexus and divided. A Kittner is then used to sweep away the remaining soft tissue exposing the anterior longitudinal ligament and the entire anterior surface of the L5–S1 disk space. The proximal left common iliac vein commonly must be bluntly moved with a Kittner cranially and to the left to fully expose the underlying disk. Retractor blades are then placed to keep both common iliac veins lateral to the disk space and a superior blade is readjusted deeper to protect and retract the iliac venous bifurcation and inferior vena cava (IVC) (Fig. 11.12). A pin is then placed in the midline of the disk space and fluoroscopy is used to confirm the correct level and midline location (Fig. 11.13). Occasionally, a fourth narrow retractor blade is needed inferiorly to keep any creeping peritoneal contents out of the operative field.

**Fig. 11.9** Identification of inferior epigastric vessels

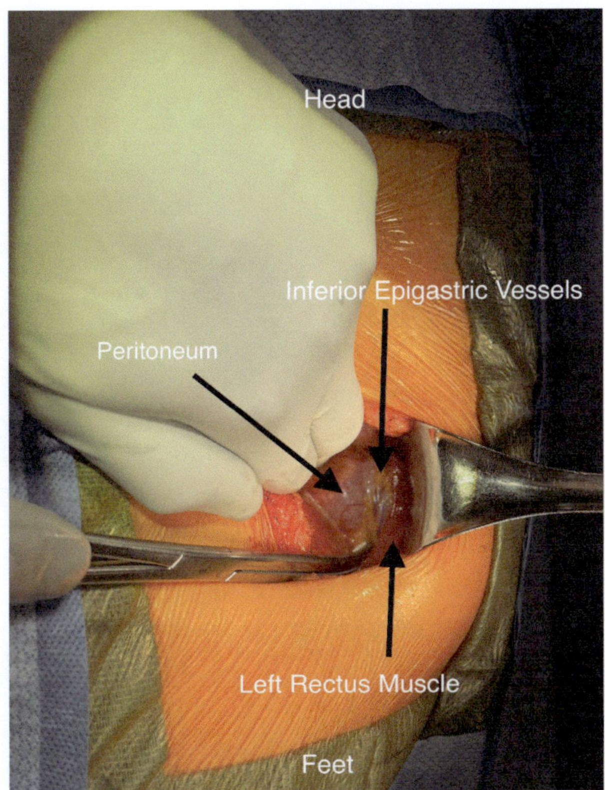


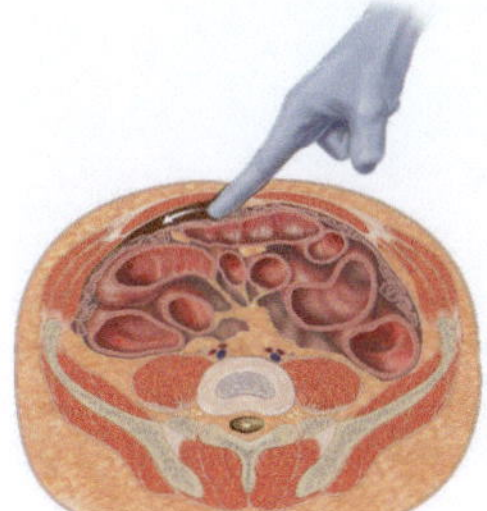
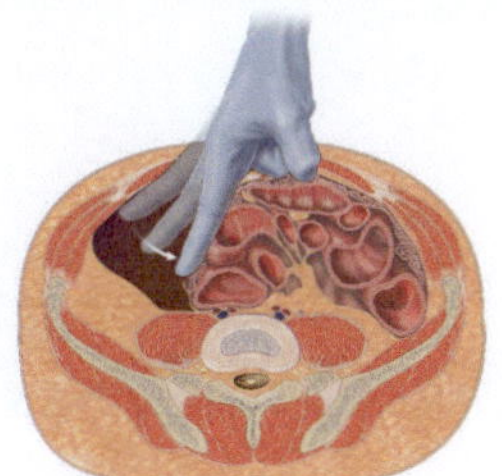
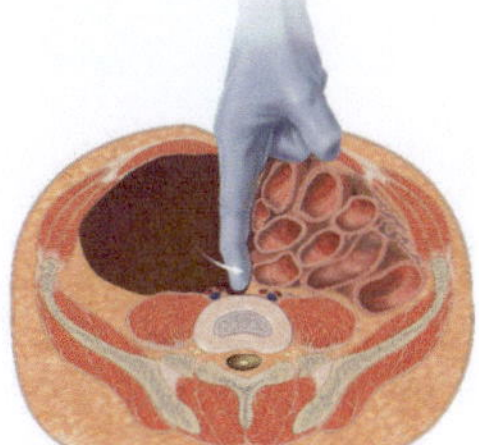

**Fig. 11.10** Blunt dissection of left retroperitoneum

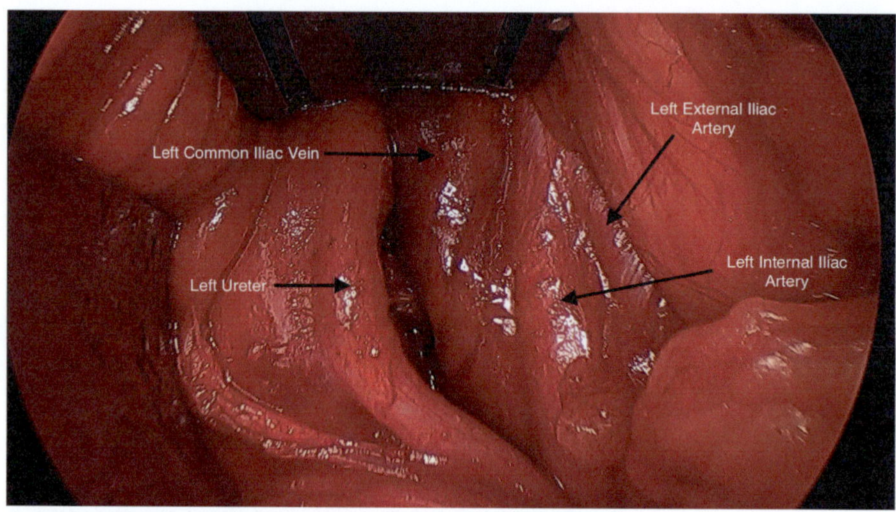


**Fig. 11.11** Left ureter and viscera mobilized to the right

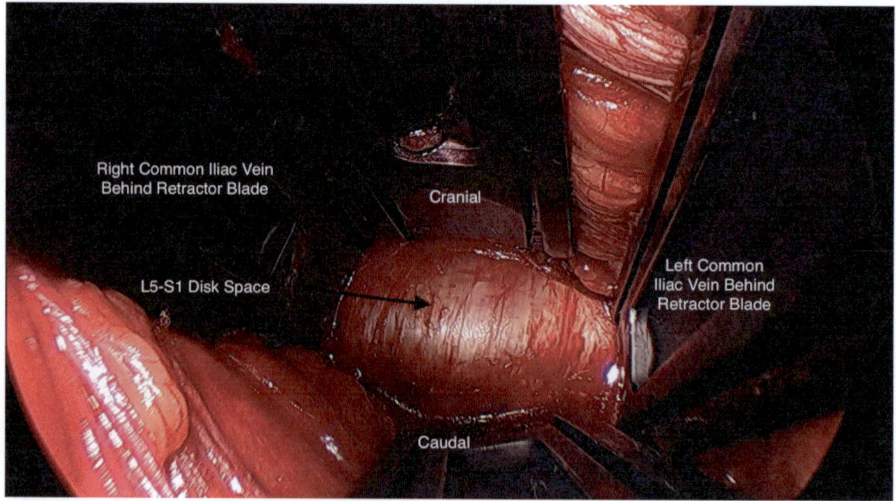


**Fig. 11.12** L5-S1 disk space exposed

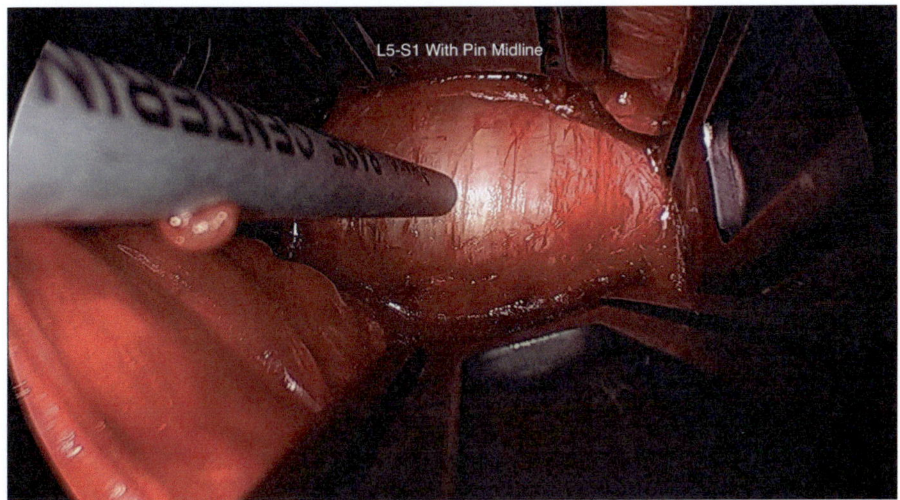


**Fig. 11.13**  L5-S1 with pin midline

## *L4–L5*

A small incision is made based on intraoperative localization and initial dissection is performed as detailed above. If the L4–L5 level is caudal to the arcuate line, the retroperitoneum can be entered as described above for L5–S1. Alternatively, if the L4–L5 disk space is superior to the arcuate line, the posterior rectus sheath is carefully and sharply incised about 4–5 mm with a scalpel or Metzenbaum scissors near the lateral edge of the rectus muscle. This can be done with the assistant retracting the rectus muscle laterally. The underlying peritoneum will now be visualized. Each side of the posterior rectus sheath can be grasped and the underlying peritoneum can be gently swept off the posterior sheath with blunt finger dissection or a Kittner. This lateral opening is important to help keep the peritoneum intact as it becomes thinner and more tenuous the closer one gets to the midline. Once the peritoneum is dissected free, the posterior sheath is opened with scissors as far superiorly and inferiorly as possible. This is usually done in a progressive manner alternating between dissecting the peritoneum and opening the posterior sheath. The retroperitoneum is entered as described above.

The lateral edges of the left common and external iliac arteries are exposed and released with bipolar cautery as far superiorly and inferiorly as possible. This allows the artery to be rolled to the right exposing the underlying left common iliac vein. The lymphatics present in this area can be clipped and transected for visualization. The lateral edge of the left common iliac vein should now be identified. A combination of bipolar cautery, sharp dissection with scissors, and blunt mobilization with a Kittner help identify the iliolumbar vein (Fig. 11.14). The iliolumbar vein typically crosses the lateral body of L5 and dives into the left paraspinous area. Multiple variations exist in the anatomy of the left common iliac vein and iliolumbar vein (Fig. 11.15). Great care is taken when performing this portion of the dissection to

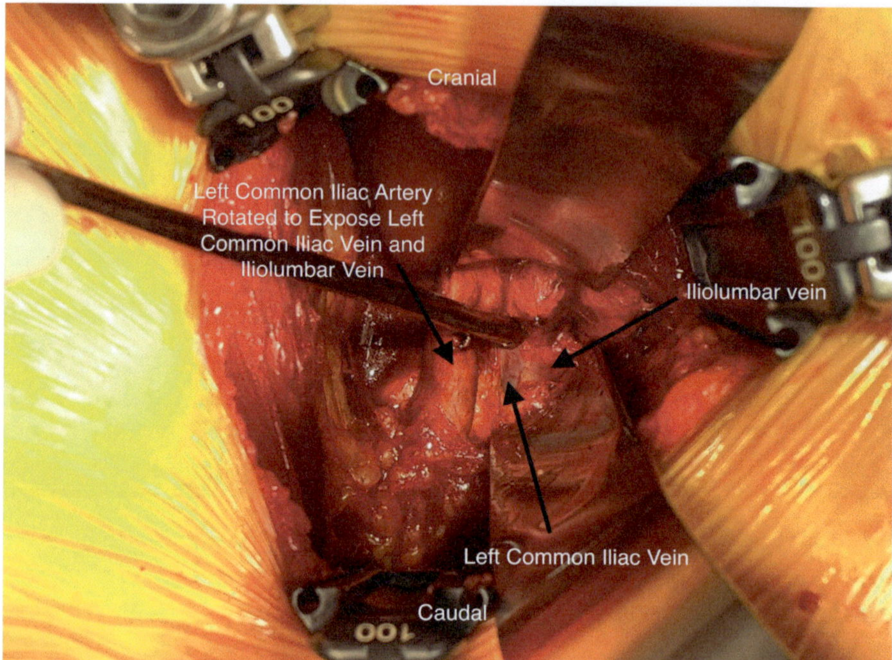



**Fig. 11.14** Iliolumbar vein identification during exposure of L4-L5

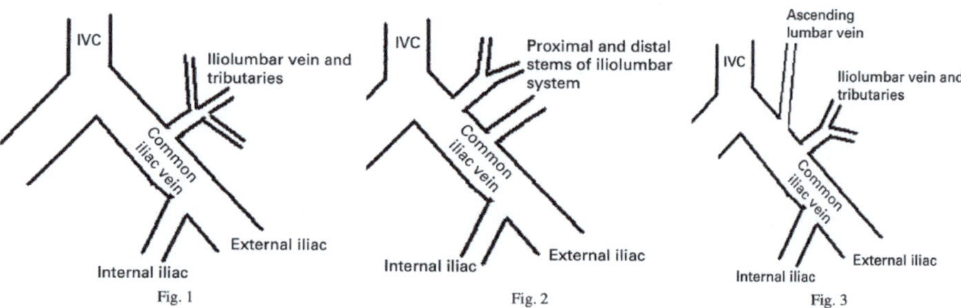



**Fig. 11.15** Iliolumbar vein anatomical variations

avoid any accidental injury. Some previous descriptions of this dissection considered it mandatory to ligate and divide the iliolumbar vein [2]. We have found it mandatory to look for this vein and identify it, but due to the multiple anatomic variations in the venous system and spine anatomy, we do not always ligate and divide it. If there is any question about tension on this vein during the dissection, it is ligated with a 2-0 silk suture and then clipped proximally and distally and then transected. The clips just beyond the tie help prevent the silk suture from inadvertently becoming loose or falling off during further mobilization of the vein. Occasionally, the iliolumbar vein can be short and wide based. In these cases, after the vein is divided, the base of the vein on the lateral edge of the left common iliac vein is oversewn with a running 4-0 Prolene suture on an RB-1 needle to prevent the silk suture and clips falling off during further mobilization. Tension on the left common iliac vein needs to be fully considered during the mobilization as well as the increased tension that will be placed on the vein once the lumbar height has been restored with instrumentation, which can lead to tears and avulsions and subsequent hemorrhage. The left common iliac vein can now be separated away from the spine using gentle dissection with a Kittner. In most patients the vein will peel away from the anterior surface of the spine. In some patients, however, there is inflammatory tissue in this plane making dissection difficult. This is particularly true when osteophytes are present. As the vein is mobilized to the right, lumbar veins and arteries might be encountered, especially superiorly, that can be clipped and transected for full exposure to the right side of the spine. During this dissection of the vein, the sympathetic trunk will be identified and preserved running on the lateral edge of the lumbar spine. This occasionally needs to be bluntly mobilized to the left for full disk exposure but should not be injured to avoid sympathetic dysfunction and warm leg phenomenon.

The left retractor blade is now placed at the level of the disk space deeper to help retract the sympathetic chain laterally. The right retractor blade is often replaced with a longer narrow blade and used to retract the left common iliac artery and vein to the right of the spine. The tip of the blade should fall over the right side of the disk to allow for full exposure. If there is any tension suspected on the vein at this time, further dissection and mobilization is mandatory. The superior blade is then placed so the tip is on the L4 vertebral body just cranial to the disk space. There should be no gaps at the blade tips which could lead to inadvertent tissue or vein creep. A pin is then placed in the midline of the disk space and fluoroscopy is used to confirm the correct level and midline location (Figs. 11.16, 11.17 and 11.18).

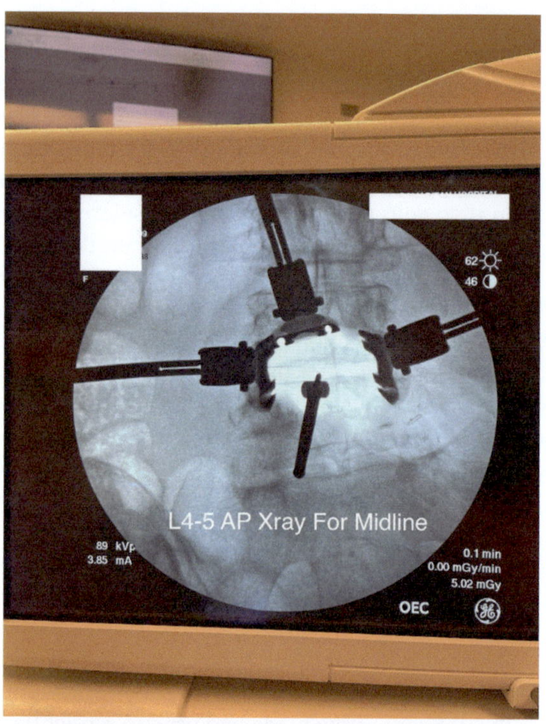


**Fig. 11.16** AP x-ray at L4-L5 to confirm midline

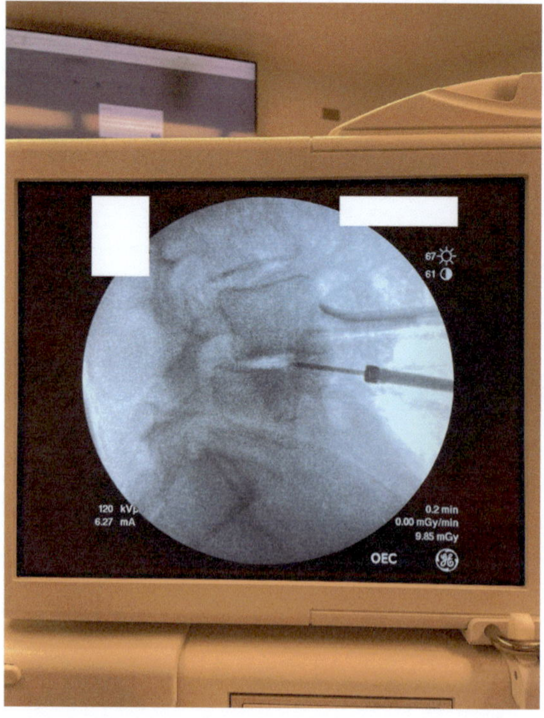

**Fig. 11.17** Lateral x-ray at L4-L5 to confirm the correct disk space

**Fig. 11.18** Lateral x-ray at L4-L5 with implant and height restoration

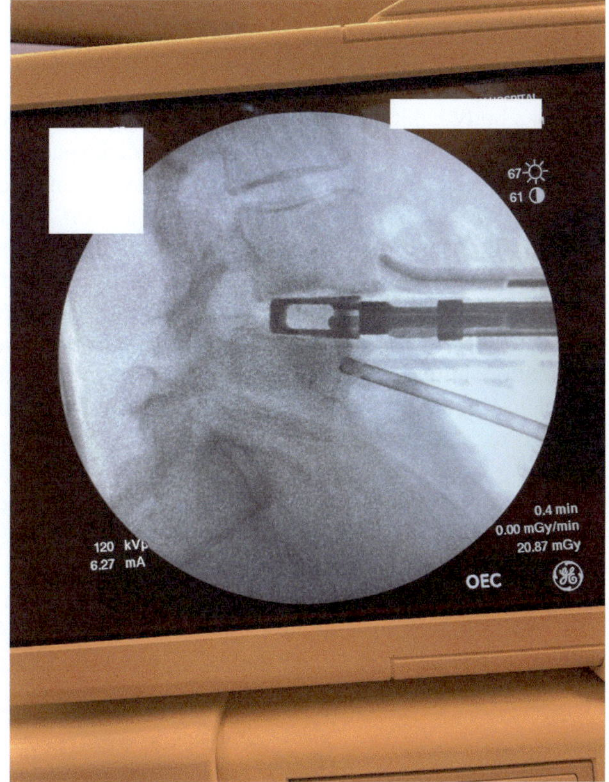

# *L3–L4*

A small incision is made based on intraoperative localization and dissection is conducted as detailed above. During mobilization of the aorta at this level, there typically will be segmental crossing lumbar arteries and veins. These can be clipped and divided to allow for mobilization of the aorta to the right. Once the tension has been released from the artery, it can be rotated to the right. The sympathetic chain should be identified and preserved. The narrow blade on the right side can now be replaced with a longer blade to retract the aorta to the right lateral edge of the L3–L4 disk space. The superior blade tip can also now be placed deeper with the tip directly on the L3 vertebral body since the aorta has been rotated to the right. Any remaining soft tissue over the L3–L4 disk space can now be swept free and the sympathetic chain can also be bluntly mobilized to the left if necessary. The narrow blade on the patient's left can be repositioned with the tip on the left lateral edge of the disk space to protect the sympathetic chain. A pin is then placed in the midline of the disk space and fluoroscopy is used to confirm the correct level and midline location. Exposure at this level is more straightforward due to less venous mobilization compared to L4–L5.

## *L2–L3*

The L2–L3 level warrants a few general considerations prior to exposure. The patient's body habitus and abdominal anatomy should be closely examined prior to an anterior approach. Typically, the L2–L3 disk space has a more caudal angle than any of the other lumbar disk spaces that have been discussed. An approach at this level may not be feasible in patients with a short abdominal segment, obesity, or kyphotic deformity. Additionally, the peritoneum is less robust compared to the lower lumbar levels and can be more prone to tearing during mobilization. During the retroperitoneal dissection, the left ureter can also be placed under significant tension when mobilizing it to the right and should be closely monitored to avoid any unintentional injuries. Preoperative imaging should be closely evaluated for vascular anomalies including the left renal artery (normally located at L1–L2), large accessory left renal arteries, duplicated IVC, or any low-lying left renal veins that could be retro- or circumaortic (Fig. 11.19). Preoperative recognition of these anatomic variants is helpful during mobilization and can change the surgical approach entirely.

The incision is placed directly over the L2–L3 disk space and the retroperitoneum is entered and mobilized as discussed for the L3–L4 level. During the approach, the surgical working angle should be kept in mind with adequate exposure and mobilization cranially for full visualization. A pin is then placed in the midline of the disk space and fluoroscopy is used to confirm the correct level and midline location.

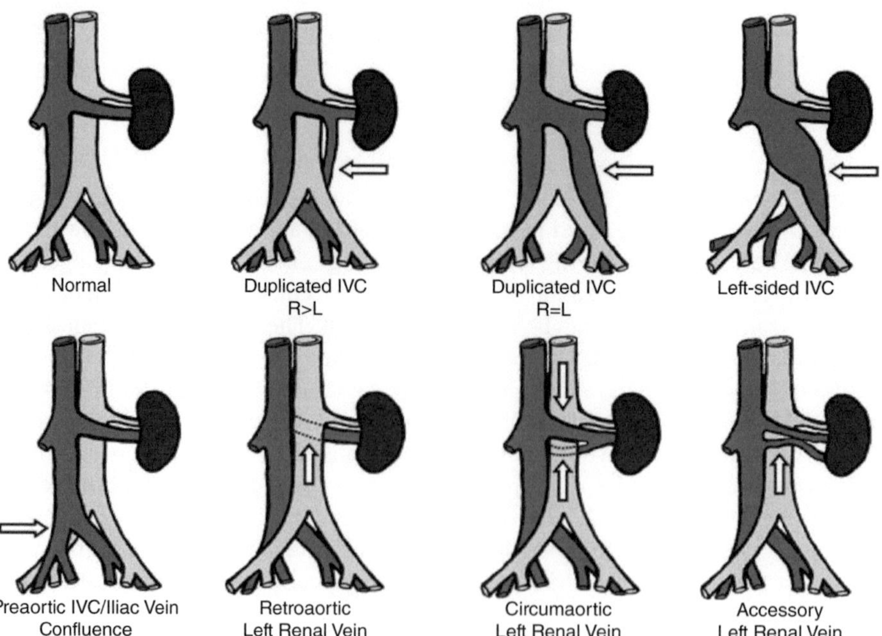


**Fig. 11.19** Venous anomalies encountered in the retroperitoneum

## Intraoperative Monitoring and Injury Avoidance

During surgery, various forms of monitoring can be utilized. Neuromonitoring with somatosensory evoked potentials (SSEPs) and motor evoked potentials (MEPs) are left to the discretion of the spine surgeon. We recommend neuromuscular blockade during exposure which does not allow for any MEP monitoring, but SSEPs can still be monitored. Pulse oximetry can also be monitored on the left hallux during exposure and retraction for any signs of decreased perfusion and ischemia. Oxygen saturation below 90% can be a sign of temporary ischemia. It has been demonstrated that close to 60% of patients can have both temporary changes in SSEP and desaturation of pulse oximetry with exposure of L4–L5 and retraction of the left iliac vessels. Despite these temporary changes with retraction, permanent changes and ischemia are uncommon [3]. It is important to perform a vascular exam before and after the procedure on both lower extremities with the exam documented in the patient's chart. Bilateral pedal pulses are documented prior to incision and after anterior abdominal closure. If the pedal pulses are not palpable, a Doppler exam and ankle brachial index are then performed before and after surgery. The exams and documentation can help with any postoperative changes and identify an acutely ischemic limb.

Intraoperative vascular and visceral injury can occur during the spine surgeon's intervention following exposure. Manipulation within the surgical field may lead to previously protected vascular and visceral structure to become threatened. Intermittent operative field checks by the access surgeon during the spine surgeon's intervention could potentially avoid unintentional visceral, ureteral, or vascular injury. The dynamics of the spine and height restoration are important for the vascular structures being retracted, especially at the L4–L5 level (Fig. 11.17). In severely degenerative cases and when significant height restoration is being performed, the retracted left common iliac vein can be injured by the retractor blade due to the increased stretch and tension from height restoration. This might not be recognized until the retractor blade is released and significant bleeding is encountered. Finally, the implants can entrap surrounding tissue that might creep into the operative field during implantation. Trial implants are often designed with smoother surfaces for easier introduction and explanting, and spine and access surgeons should be aware that the final implant may be more likely to entrap surrounding tissue by virtue of its design.

## *Post Implant Operative Field Evaluation*

After the spine intervention has been performed, it is important to evaluate the operative field to confirm hemostasis and rule out any visceral or ureteral injury (Figs. 11.20 and 11.21). Lymphatic leaks should be identified and clipped or suture ligated to prevent postoperative lymph leak or lymphocele. If there is any concern for ongoing fluid or lymphatic leakage, a flat Jackson-Pratt drain can be left in the

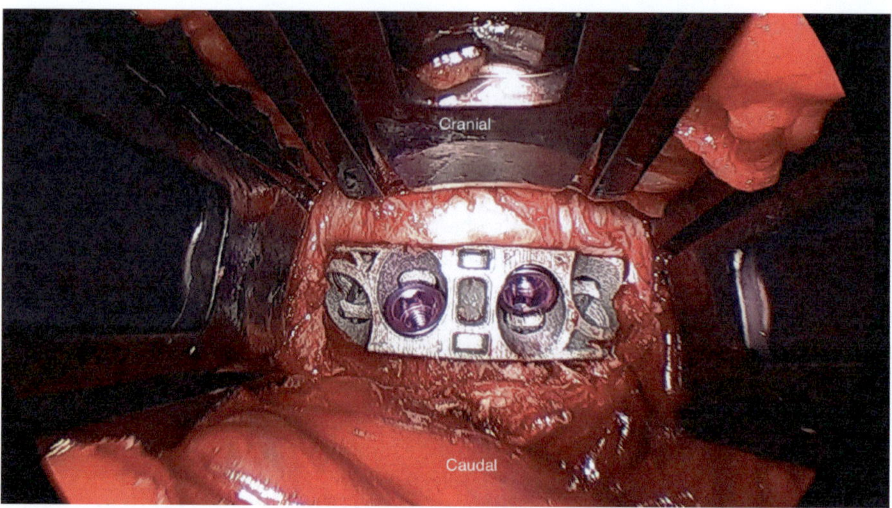


**Fig. 11.20** L5-S1 operative field post implant

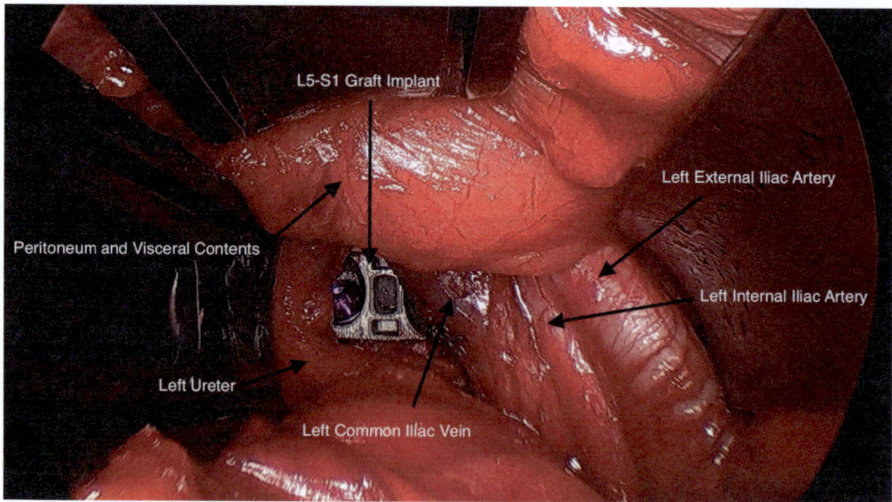


**Fig. 11.21** L5–S1 operative field examination after releasing the retractor blades

retroperitoneum. The retractor blades are released in the opposite order they were placed. In general, the superior retractor blade is gently released to identify any bleeding or injury. The same is then performed for the right and left retractor blades. Each level should be examined carefully prior to closure. If a visceral or ureteral injury is identified, it should be addressed immediately. The vascular structures that were retracted should be examined for bleeding and thrombosis. Any peritoneal defect identified during this time should be repaired with a running 2-0 Vicryl if possible. If the peritoneal defect is too large or there are many small "Swiss cheese"-type defects that cannot be repaired, one large peritoneal defect should be made to prevent any source for bowel to herniate or obstruct. The anterior rectus fascia is then closed with PDS or Prolene. The subcutaneous tissue is closed with a 2-0 or 3-0 Vicryl to close dead space and the skin closed with a subcuticular suture such as 4-0 Monocryl and a dry sterile occlusive dressing applied. Finally, a final lower extremity vascular exam is performed and documented.

## Conclusion

Mini-open anterior retroperitoneal lumbar spine exposure can be performed safely using sound surgical principles and attention to detail in the pre-, intra-, and postoperative phases. Complications may be avoided by utilizing the above surgical approach and technique. The anterior corridor for lumbar spine surgery has numerous advantages for multiple pathologies and should be available when needed for these patients.

## References


1. Capener N. Spondylolisthesis. Br J Surg. 1932;19:374–86.
2. Brau SA. Mini-open approach to the spine for anterior lumbar interbody fusion: description of the procedure, results and complications. Spine J. 2002;2:216–23.
3. Brau SA, Spoonamore MJ, Snyder L, Gilbert C, Rhonda G, Williams LA, Watkins RG. Nerve monitoring changes related to iliac artery compression during anterior lumbar spine surgery. Spine J. 2003;3:351–5.

# Chapter 12
# Anterior Transperitoneal Approach to the Lumbar Spine

Doru I. E. Georgescu and Benjamin C. Dorenkamp

## Introduction

While current surgical techniques and literature support and recommend a retroperitoneal approach to the lumbar spine, this is not always possible. It is important to have multiple techniques that allow a surgeon to successfully expose the lumbar spine in the setting of previous abdominal surgery.

## History

The transperitoneal approach was the first published approach allowing anterior access to the lumbar vertebra for treatment of spinal pathology. The first reports of a transperitoneal approach are credited to Müller in 1906 who utilized it to treat Pott's disease [1]. However, the approach fell out of favor due to complications. The approach was again described by Capener in 1932 and later successfully adopted and published by Burns in 1933 and subsequently Mercer in 1936 where the transperitoneal approach added new techniques for spinal surgeons in the treatment of spondylolisthesis [1–5]. It was not until 1948 when this new technique was applied to degenerative conditions by Lane and Moore. In addition to being the first to treat degenerative lumbar pathology, Lane and Moore also pushed the limits and reported the ability to reach L3–L5 with this technique [5, 6].

D. I. E. Georgescu (✉)
Center of Surgical Specialists, PC, Thornton, CO, USA
e-mail: drg@cssdenver.com

B. C. Dorenkamp
Michigan Orthopedic Center, Clinical Faculty Michigan State University,
East Lansing, MI, USA

© The Author(s), under exclusive license to Springer Nature Switzerland AG 2023
J. R. O'Brien et al. (eds.), *Lumbar Spine Access Surgery*,
https://doi.org/10.1007/978-3-031-48034-8_12

Meanwhile, in 1944, Iwahara was working on perfecting the extraperitoneal approach to the lumbar spine, later publishing a series of 58 patients in 1963 [7]. In the late 1960s, more surgeons were utilizing the anterior approach, but the technique had transitioned to primarily using an extraperitoneal approach. The transperitoneal approach at this point was only being used for patients with previous abdominal surgery where an extraperitoneal approach was not feasible [5, 8].

## Advantages

Though the transperitoneal approach to the lumbar spine has largely been replaced with the retroperitoneal approach, there are advantages in utilizing a transperitoneal exposure. This exposure involves a familiar surgical field for both general surgeons and vascular surgeons and tends to be easily adapted into an access surgeon's skillset for exposure of the lumbar spine. This approach is particularly advantageous for patients with known or potential scar tissue, adhesions, or fascial mesh in the retroperitoneal plane. Not surprisingly, Scaduto et al. had no vascular injuries while using the transperitoneal approach in 10 of their 88 patients, all of whom had previous abdominal surgeries and a high possibility of adhesions [9]. Previous literature, in conjunction with the authors' personal experiences, supports the idea that the transperitoneal approach minimizes scar tissue dissection and provides a safe corridor to access the lumbar spine in select patients.

A midline approach and dissection carried directly posteriorly to the spine offers several advantages. As the ureters run in the abdominal segment of the retroperitoneal space, they course lateral and anterior to the transverse processes of the lumbar spine. As they cross into the pelvic section, they remain retroperitoneal. However, they cross anterior and medial to the vascular anatomy at approximately the bifurcation of the common iliac artery and run medial to the vascular structures as they continue to course distally [10]. By utilizing the transperitoneal approach, the ureters remain lateral to the surgical field, thus decreasing risk for injury. This is especially advantageous when there is scar tissue in the retroperitoneal space. Also, the arcuate line does not need to be crossed in this approach and decreases need for dissection above this area. The inferior epigastric vessels are also protected during this approach as they stay lateral to the exposure and do not have to be identified and protected.

Anecdotally, we have encountered less retroperitoneal fluid collections following the transperitoneal approach. We theorize this is due to entry into the retroperitoneal space through the posterior peritoneum creating an avenue for drainage. However, we do not routinely image patients in the immediate postoperative period which limits our evaluation. Additionally, this approach allows for exposure of the lumbar spine in cases where a colostomy would prevent a retroperitoneal approach (Table 12.1).

**Table 12.1** Advantages

| | |
|---|---|
| 1. | Easy to learn with familiar surgical field for vascular and general surgeons |
| 2. | No need to mobilize the ureters |
| 3. | Lower risk for retroperitoneal collections |
| 4. | No need to develop a plane above the arcuate line |
| 5. | No concern of injury to inferior epigastric vessels |

## Disadvantages

While debated in the literature, the risk of retrograde ejaculation is thought to be increased in patients undergoing a transperitoneal approach to the lumbar spine. Specifically, there seems to be an increased risk in patients undergoing an approach to L5–S1; however, it has also been reported during exposure of the L4–L5 disc space [11]. In 1984, Flynn and Price performed a worldwide survey of 20 surgeons and did not find any difference between the transperitoneal or retroperitoneal approach regarding retrograde ejaculation [12]. In 1995, Tiusanen et al. reported on 40 male patients who underwent anterior lumbar surgery with either a retroperitoneal or transperitoneal approach. Retrograde ejaculation only occurred with a transperitoneal approach which led them to recommend against this approach in male patients [13].

More recently, Sasso et al. utilized prospective data from a U.S. Food and Drug Administration investigational device exemption study to analyze retrograde ejaculation after anterior lumbar interbody fusion (ALIF) transperitoneal versus retroperitoneal approaches [11, 14]. The authors identified a tenfold increase in retrograde ejaculation with a transperitoneal approach. Birch and Shaw responded to the Sasso et al. publication challenging their findings, citing their personal case series of 46 men of whom 17 underwent a retroperitoneal approach and 29 who underwent a transperitoneal approach by a single surgeon. They reported no patients who experienced any form of ejaculatory disturbance [15]. Men should be counseled on the risk of retrograde ejaculation and its consequences in male sexual function and fertility.

An increased risk of prolonged ileus has been reported with a transperitoneal approach due to bowel manipulation. This has been confirmed in both the spine and vascular surgery literature with some articles reporting a fivefold increased risk of prolonged ileus with a transperitoneal approach [9, 16]. In addition, the incidence of prolonged ileus and small bowel obstruction can lead to increased hospital stay and cost [16]. There is also inherent increased risk of bowel injury due to direct exposure [17].

Access above L4 can be difficult when utilizing the transperitoneal approach [18]. If exposure above L4 is attempted, special attention should be given to the takeoff of the inferior mesenteric artery (IMA) as this can limit the left to right dissection. Injury to the IMA can lead to left colon ischemia. Furthermore, L3–L4 exposure can necessitate exposing the intervertebral disc space between the vena cava and aorta. Placing retractors between these two vascular structures carries increased risk for vascular injury, especially during spine instrumentation. When exposing L4–L5 via this approach, the surgeon must be aware of the increased risk of ureteral injuries, particularly when it is necessary to mobilize the distal aspect of the common and external iliac arteries using blunt dissection. If the ureter is in the way during this maneuver, an alternative would be to dissect between the left iliac artery and vein, being aware that this is more difficult and carries increased risk. In the authors' experience, obese patients tend to be more difficult to expose via a transperitoneal approach. The increased mesenteric and retroperitoneal adipose tissue can make identification of posterior structures more difficult. Manipulation of the bowel can be difficult because of the increased weight and stiffness of short mesenteries. Additionally, vascular injuries can be difficult to control and repair while bowel and mesentery are exposed. This technique also requires additional time to pack the bowel and repair the posterior peritoneum (Table 12.2).

## Indications

While a retroperitoneal approach remains the workhorse of the anterior exposure, it is important to understand the indications for a transperitoneal approach. The approach is best suited for exposure of L4–L5 and L5–S1. It is important to note that while exposure at higher levels has been described, it can be more difficult and has an increased risk of vascular injury. In cases where there has been a prior retroperitoneal approach to the lumbar spine, the transperitoneal approach can offer a safer exposure. This approach is also useful when there has been prior abdominal surgery with placement of mesh in the preperitoneal space or along the anterolateral wall of the abdomen. Also, prior urologic surgery or radiation can obscure the retroperitoneal plane with scar tissue making the transperitoneal approach a good alternative (Table 12.3).

**Table 12.2** Disadvantages

| | |
|---|---|
| 1. | Retrograde ejaculation |
| 2. | Prolonged ileus |
| 3. | Small bowel obstruction |
| 4. | Increased risk of bowel injury |
| 5. | Difficult exposure above L4 |
| 6. | Manipulation of the bowel may cause mesenteric ischemia secondary to injury to the IMA |
| 7. | Difficult vascular repair |

**Table 12.3**  Indications

| | |
|---|---|
| 1. | Prior retroperitoneal exposure |
| 2. | Scar tissue in the preperitoneal space |
| 3. | Scar tissue in the retroperitoneal space |
| 4. | Large mesh in the preperitoneal space |

**Table 12.4**  Contraindications (relative)

| | |
|---|---|
| 1. | Approach above L4 |
| 2. | History of pelvic peritonitis |
| 3. | Prior abdominal surgeries describing severe adhesions |
| 4. | Previous open aortoiliac bypass or aortoiliac stents |
| 5. | Large aortic or iliac aneurysms |
| 6. | History of urinary bladder or ureteral surgeries |
| 7. | A very low confluence of the iliac vein that covers L5/S1 |

## Contraindications

While there are no absolute contraindications for a transperitoneal approach to the lumbar spine, there are relative contraindications that are similar to those for a retroperitoneal approach. In addition, there are relative contraindications that are specific to a transperitoneal approach. The main relative contraindications that are similar to a retroperitoneal approach include obesity (body mass index >40), severe atherosclerosis, aneurysms/open aneurysm repair preventing vascular mobilization, aberrant vascular anatomy (such as a low bifurcating aorta or vena cava for L5–S1 approach), and untreated paraspinal infections (in the setting of elective spine surgery) [17]. A history of ureteral or urinary bladder surgery should also be considered.

For a transperitoneal approach, access to L1–L2 and L2–L3 can be difficult and should be considered a relative contraindication, as the renal vessels at this level would typically prevent exposure. Any previous abdominal surgery or infection that has caused adhesions should be attempted with great caution and only if retroperitoneal access is not possible (Table 12.4).

                                      

## Preoperative Planning

The spine and access surgeons should coordinate preoperative planning prior to the procedure. This should include a thorough history and physical exam of the abdomen and a detailed surgical history including any previous small bowel obstructions, relevant surgeries, radiation, or history of pelvic or abdominal inflammatory disorders. In patients with prior surgeries, effort should be made to obtain a detailed operative report of prior procedures, being careful to look for evidence of abdominal adhesions and abdominal mesh placement.

Preoperative computed tomography angiography (CTA) is beneficial for defining patient-specific vascular anatomy. A study by Datta et al. showed that routine CTA changed surgical decision-making in 21% of patients [19]. This challenged previous teaching that conventional magnetic resonance imaging is sufficient in the majority of patients and that angiography should only be used in uncertain cases [20]. Gstottner et al. published a retrospective study of 28 patients and reported CTA did not change the preoperative plan. They concluded the risk of high-dose radiation and future cancer risk outweighs routine use of this imaging study [21]. Literature regarding CTA necessity for a transperitoneal approach is lacking. Given that a transperitoneal approach is typically only used in complicated revision settings, it is the authors' practice to obtain routine preoperative CTA. Although a CTA does not mandate changing the operative plan or approach, it does offer significant benefits in improving the safety of the procedure by detailing the relationships between the vascular structures and the spine. It is also beneficial for the spine surgeon for preoperative templating and identifying possible vascular dissection limitations.

While bowel preparation has traditionally been performed for anterior lumbar surgeries, it is not clear if it improves outcomes. Mayer advocated that patients should undergo routine mechanical bowel preparation (MBP) and take strong laxatives starting 24 h prior to ALIF surgery [20]. Since that time there have been numerous publications in the general, colorectal, urologic, and gynecologic fields that have failed to demonstrate any benefit of routine MBP [22–24]. Jeon et al. published a retrospective case-control study looking at MBP in 48 patients undergoing ALIF. They demonstrated that the MBP group had more discomfort and decreased blood pressure compared to the control group. They also noted there was no difference in difficulty of the procedure or time to return of bowel function following surgery. It was their conclusion that MBP can be omitted in ALIF procedures [25]. Acknowledging the recent literature and its limitations, it continues to be the authors' practice to have the patient on a clear liquid diet for 24 h prior to surgery. The patient is also given one dose of 300 mg magnesium citrate the day prior to surgery as well as polyethylene glycol and psyllium.

## Operative Technique

Patients are positioned supine on a radiolucent flat table. Arms are positioned out to the sides at 90° and well padded. A foley catheter is placed in all cases for bladder decompression. We then place a pillow under the knees to slightly flex the hips which allows relaxation of the psoas and makes deep retraction easier. Brackets are then placed on the radiolucent bedframe at the patient's mid left thigh and right axilla. Then, utilizing lateral fluoroscopy, the intervertebral disc space is marked on the skin for each operative level. The patient's abdomen is then shaved from the pubis to the xyphoid process and prepped in a standard sterile fashion. In revision cases we also prep the patient's groin into the field to allow access to the femoral artery and vein in the event of a vascular injury.

The incision is based on levels exposed. For surgeries involving L4–L5 and above, or multiple levels (L4–S1), a longitudinal midline incision is utilized. When only L5–S1 exposure is needed, a more cosmetic Pfannenstiel (transverse) incision is utilized. Dissection is then carried down through the superficial layers to the linea alba with electrocautery (the authors prefer this to be at 60/60 for cut and coagulation). When a longitudinal midline approach is utilized, a vertical incision is made through the linea alba once it is encountered. In cases where a transverse incision is used, the fascia is incised in a transverse direction and elevated, allowing it to be separated from the rectus muscle. In some cases, it is necessary to take down the linea alba. The peritoneal sac is then approached between the rectus muscles.

Once at the peritoneal sac, electrocautery is decreased by half (It is the authors' preference to decrease to 30/30 at this point), and this is maintained during vascular dissection. DeBakey forceps are used to lift the peritoneum anteriorly, away from the underlying bowel, to prevent injury. At this point, the peritoneum is sharply incised, and the bowel is exposed. The patient is then placed in a slight Trendelenburg position to aid in packing the bowel. The cecum is then bluntly retracted with a lap sponge to the patient's right, sigmoid to the left, and small bowel superiorly with Wylie and Sweetheart retractors held by the surgical assistant [26]. The sacral promontory is palpable as a reference prior to peritoneal incision. To avoid injury to the ureters, the posterior peritoneum is identified and sharply incised or opened with low-voltage electrocautery in the midline between the iliac arteries (Fig. 12.1). Also, in a thinner patient, it is possible to visualize the ureters through the transparency of the posterior peritoneum. This becomes critical when attempting to expand the dissection distally as the ureters may cross the iliac vessels at the distal aspect of the exposure, increasing risk of injury (Fig. 12.2).

When exposing L5–S1, the typical course of the hypogastric plexus is classically to the left of midline between the iliac vessels overlying the surface of the sacral promontory [27, 28]. To avoid injury to this structure, the dissection should be carried down through the peritoneum on the right side of the bifurcation. The presacral tissue is carefully bluntly dissected to avoid injury to the superior hypogastric plexus. After the tissues are swept from the front of the disc space, the middle sacral artery and presacral vein are visualized and, depending on the size, are ligated or

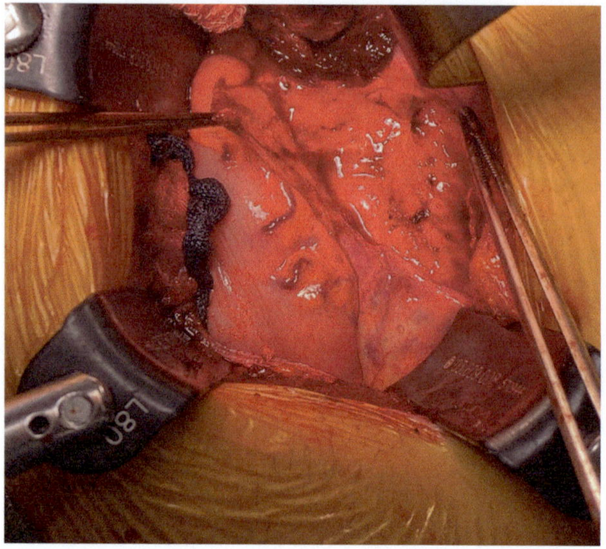

**Fig. 12.1** Intraoperative photograph from the head of the patient. To the left, the sigmoid colon is exposed, and a long incision of the posterior parietal peritoneum is demonstrated exposing the great vessels

clipped and divided using bipolar electrocautery. The tissue is then elevated from the sacral cortex as a block, avoiding any dissection through the plexus. It is important to limit cautery and transverse cutting at this stage [15, 29].

After exposure of the vertebral disc, an 18-gauge spinal needle is placed into the disc space and the surgical level is confirmed via lateral fluoroscopy. Once the surgical level is confirmed, a self-retaining retractor is attached to the bedframe and positioned in the abdomen with laparotomy sponges protecting the exposed bowel between the retractor blades, and the discectomy and interbody fixation can be performed.

When exposure of L4–L5 is required, bowel packing is carried out in a similar manner. However, vascular dissection is done by dissecting the lateral wall off the left common iliac or terminal end of the aorta. In very rare cases in which the vessels bifurcate above the L4–L5 disc space, this level can be approached between the iliac vessels. If the iliac vessels must be mobilized from left to right instead of going between the bifurcation, the surgeon accesses the spine on the left side of the aorta and iliac vessels. In doing this, care is taken to identify the iliolumbar vein that can tether the left common iliac vein. If an iliolumbar vein is found within 1–2 cm of the disc space of L4–L5, it should be carefully dissected and divided with ligatures and clips, allowing mobilization of the iliac vein.

The lumbar sympathetic chain is located anterior to the medial boarder of the psoas muscle and lateral to the vertebral body and is typically contained in dense tissue. This should be swept lateral when exposing L4–L5 and above. Injury to the sympathetic structures can result in abnormal vascular function and unopposed vasodilation, resulting in a warmer extremity and a comparatively cooler unaffected lower extremity [27, 30].

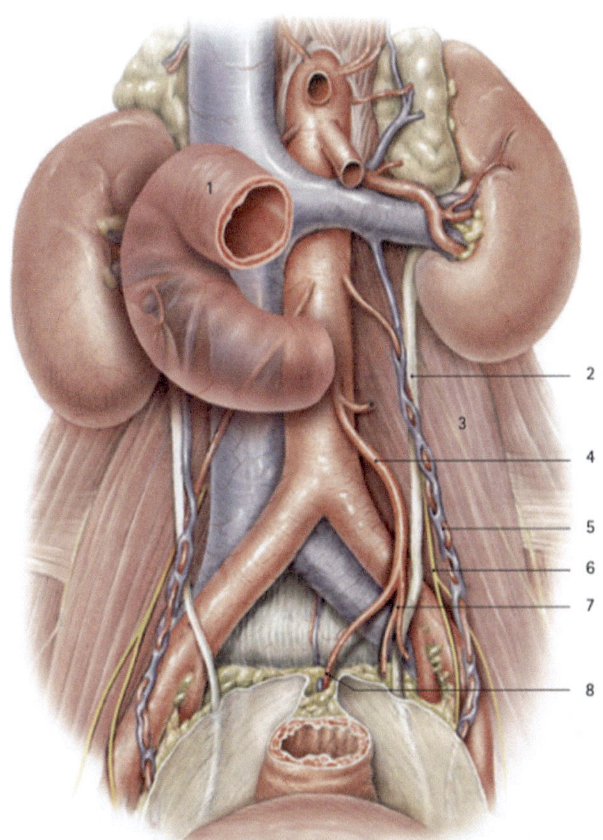

**Fig. 12.2** Demonstrates the relationship of the ureter (2) to the left common iliac vessels. This illustrates the risk of ureter injury with distal dissection at L5–S1 as the ureter courses from lateral to medial at this level anterior to the iliac vessels. The inferior mesenteric artery (4) is also noted here and must be considered with an approach to L3–L4 to avoid inadvertent injury and resultant colonic ischemia. Labeled structures: duodenum (1), ureter (2), psoas (3), inferior mesenteric artery (4), testicular/ovarian artery and vein (5), genitofemoral nerve, femoral and genital branches (6), sigmoid arteries (7), and superior rectal artery (8). Permissions for reproduction and use of the image obtained on 10/6/2021 from John Wiley & Sons—Books [10]

When exposing L3–L4, it is important to be aware of the takeoff of the IMA which could limit mobilization of the vessels from left to right. Injury to the IMA could lead to colonic ischemia. Transperitoneal exposure of the L3–L4 disc space may require dissection between the aorta and inferior vena cava (Figs. 12.2 and 12.3).

After instrumentation, a synthetic soft tissue patch or a biologic placental implant is placed and secured over the top of the exposed level. These are placed between the iliac vessels and the vertebral body and implant to protect the vessels from possible hardware erosion and lower the risk of scar tissue in the event of revision surgery. Retractors are carefully released one at a time while evaluating the vascular structures for any signs of bleeding. The vessels are then allowed to fall back over the top of the surgical level. The posterior peritoneum is identified and repaired with a 2-0 Vicryl stitch and the bowel is allowed to drape over the closed posterior peritoneum (Fig. 12.4).

The anterior wall of the abdomen is closed based on the type of incision utilized. For a transverse (Pfannenstiel) incision, it is necessary to first close the anterior peritoneum with 2-0 Vicryl followed by reapproximation of the rectus muscle with

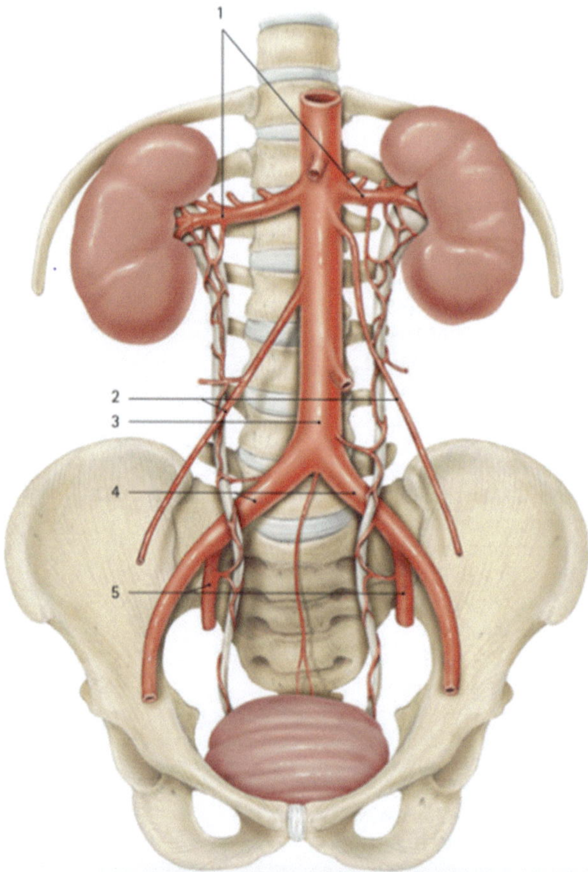


**Fig. 12.3** Illustrates the relationship of the vascular anatomy and ureter to the lumbar spine. The renal arteries are illustrated demonstrating their relationship to the upper lumbar spine and the difficulty as described with mobilizing the aorta left or right when exposing L1–L3 (1). Ovarian/testicular arteries (2). Aorta (3). Common iliac arteries (4). Internal Iliac arteries (5). Inferior mesenteric artery noted to be approximately at L3–L4 disc space (6). Permissions for reproduction and use of the image obtained on 10/6/2021 from John Wiley & Sons—Books [10]

0 Vicryl. This is particularly important in obese patients in order to avoid rectus diastasis with bulging of the peritoneal sac between the muscle fibers. After this, the anterior fascia is reapproximated with looped polydioxanone (PDS) suture.

For a longitudinal (midline) incision, the fascia and linea alba are reapproximated with a looped 0 PDS suture, being careful to not inadvertently injure the underlying bowel. For both incisions, the subcutaneous tissues and skin are then closed per surgeon preference, usually with a subcuticular stich for shorter incision.

## Postoperative Care

Postoperative care for a patient undergoing a transperitoneal approach to the lumbar spine does not differ significantly when compared to a retroperitoneal approach. Mobilization and spinal precautions are not changed by the approach and should be directed at the discretion of the spinal surgeon. Overall, we advocate for early

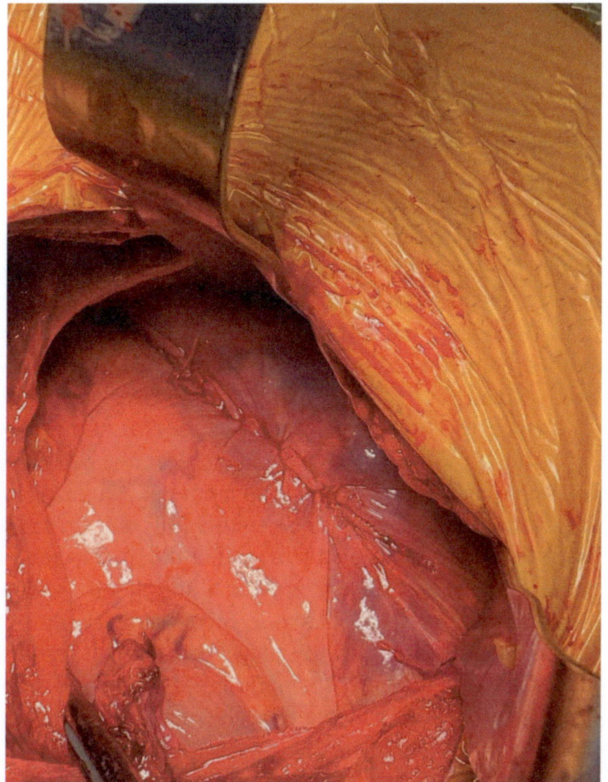

**Fig. 12.4** Intraoperative photograph demonstrating closure of the posterior parietal peritoneum with a running 2-0 Vicryl stitch. During this step, care is taken to avoid injury to the underlying ureter during suture passes

mobilization and a multimodal pain control regimen. Typically, unless there are special circumstances, postoperative bracing is not indicated.

Risk factors for venous thromboembolism (VTE) after thoracolumbar surgery were evaluated in a retrospective review of 43,777 patients which did not show any statistical difference in VTE rates between anterior and posterior thoracolumbar surgery [31]. However, when additional literature is analyzed there seems to be an increase in VTE events in patients undergoing anterior spinal surgery [32, 33]. Vint et al. in the International Journal of Spine Surgery in 2021 looked at their VTE prophylaxis protocol for patients undergoing ALIF. In their analysis, they found that the antithrombotic regimen was safe and effective [34]. However, these articles contradict NASS guidelines published in 2009 which cite only inconclusive evidence for chemical prophylaxis. According to NASS guidelines, chemoprophylaxis may be considered for long anterior-posterior spinal fusions or in patients with risk factors but otherwise does not recommend anticoagulation [35]. Although there are arguments for both prophylaxis and no prophylaxis in the current literature the authors reserve prophylaxis for only those with increased risk factors for VTE.

One of the main downfalls with the transperitoneal approach is the increased risk of postoperative ileus, which must be discussed with patients prior to surgery. Postoperative ileus can be extremely uncomfortable to the patient and can increase overall costs by extending the patient's hospital stay or increasing readmission rates [36].

In patients struggling with postoperative ileus, careful examination of electrolytes should be done and corrected as needed. Postoperative analgesia should be evaluated, and non-opioid therapies should be maximized. Acetaminophen is a safe and effective first-line treatment and should be used for baseline pain management. Nonsteroidal anti-inflammatories (NSAIDs) are also effective in postoperative pain management. In one trial, celecoxib (selective COX-2 inhibitor), but not diclofenac, reduced the risk of prolonged postoperative ileus, but did not accelerate early recovery of bowel function [37]. Opioid avoidance and the use of newer agents such as tramadol, which has fewer gastrointestinal (GI) symptoms, may also be beneficial. With smaller incisions, either local or regional anesthetics can be beneficial and help with minimizing opioid medication consumption.

Nasogastric (NG) tube insertion is almost never necessary, especially when exposure of only one level is required. Routine use of NG tubes has been associated with significantly higher risk of pneumonia, atelectasis, fever, and prolonged return of GI function and should be avoided [38–40]. Prokinetic agents, such as metoclopramide, have been shown to decrease the time to return of bowel function. It is the authors' preference to start a clear liquid diet the day of surgery and then advance the diet on postoperative day one, followed by oral magnesium hydroxide and intravenous metoclopramide until bowel function returns. However, there is some debate in the literature about metoclopramides' effect on return of bowel function [40–42]. It has also been shown that gum chewing can improve GI function but it is unclear what the optimal regimen is [43]. Early resumption of diet significantly decreases the duration of ileus, which helps prevent electrolyte imbalances, fluid imbalances, and infectious complications [43]. Every effort should be made to resume an oral diet after the transperitoneal approach to the spine.

## Conclusion

In appropriately selected patients, the transperitoneal approach to the lumbar spine can be safe and effective. Although the retroperitoneal approach has become the predominant choice for anterior access to the lumbar spine, patient factors, such as patient anatomy, vascular anatomy, or previous surgery, may necessitate a transperitoneal approach. This approach warrants its own considerations for intraoperative and postoperative care, but it may be a valuable tool for treating patients who require an anterior approach to the lumbar spine.

# References


1. Matur AV, Mejia-Munne JC, Plummer ZJ, Cheng JS, Prestigiacomo CJ. The history of anterior and lateral approaches to the lumbar spine. World Neurosurg. 2020;144:213–21.
2. Capener N. Spondylolisthesis. Br J Surg. 2005;19(75):374–86.
3. Burns BH. An operation for spondylolisthesis. Lancet. 1933;221(5728):1233.
4. Mercer W. Spondylolisthesis: with a description of a new method of operative treatment and notes of ten cases. Edinb Med J. 1936;43(9):545–72.
5. Bassani R, Gregori F, Peretti G. Evolution of the anterior approach in lumbar spine fusion. World Neurosurg. 2019;131:391–8.
6. Lane JD, Moore ES. Transperitoneal approach to the intervertebral disc in the lumbar area. Ann Surg. 1948;127(3):537–51.
7. Iwahara T, Ikeda K, Hirabayashi K. Results of anterior spine fusion by extraperitoneal approach for spondylolysis and spondylolisthesis. Nihon Seikeigeka Gakkai Zasshi. 1963;36:1049–67.
8. Hodgson AR, Wong SK. A description of a technic and evaluation of results in anterior spinal fusion for deranged intervertebral disk and spondylolisthesis. Clin Orthop Relat Res. 1968;56:133–62.
9. Scaduto AA, Gamradt SC, Yu WD, Huang J, Delamarter RB, Wang JC. Perioperative complications of threaded cylindrical lumbar interbody fusion devices: anterior versus posterior approach. J Spinal Disord Tech. 2003;16(6):502–7.
10. Fröber R. Surgical anatomy of the ureter. BJU Int. 2007;100(4):949–65.
11. Sasso RC, Kenneth Burkus J, LeHuec J-C. Retrograde ejaculation after anterior lumbar interbody fusion: transperitoneal versus retroperitoneal exposure. Spine (Phila Pa 1976). 2003;28(10):1023–6.
12. Flynn JC, Price CT. Sexual complications of anterior fusion of the lumbar spine. Spine (Phila Pa 1976). 1984;9(5):489–92.
13. Tiusanen H, Seitsalo S, Osterman K, Soini J. Retrograde ejaculation after anterior interbody lumbar fusion. Eur Spine J. 1995;4(6):339–42.
14. Kim Y-H, Ha K-Y, Rhyu K-W, Park H-Y, Cho C-H, Kim H-C, et al. Lumbar interbody fusion: techniques, pearls and pitfalls. Asian Spine J. 2020;14(5):730–41.
15. Birch N, Shaw M. Retrograde ejaculation after anterior lumbar interbody fusion. Spine (Phila Pa 1976). 2004;29(1):106–7.
16. Sicard GA, Reilly JM, Rubin BG, Thompson RW, Allen BT, Flye MW, et al. Transabdominal versus retroperitoneal incision for abdominal aortic surgery: report of a prospective randomized trial. J Vasc Surg. 1995;21(2):174–81; discussion 181–183.
17. Wiesel SW, editor. Operative techniques in orthopaedic surgery. 2nd ed. Philadelphia: Wolters Kluwer; 2016.
18. Meng B, Bunch J, Burton D, Wang J. Lumbar interbody fusion: recent advances in surgical techniques and bone healing strategies. Eur Spine J. 2021;30(1):22–33.
19. Datta JC, Janssen ME, Beckham R, Ponce C. The use of computed tomography angiography to define the prevertebral vascular anatomy prior to anterior lumbar procedures. Spine. 2007;32(1):113–9.
20. Mayer HM. The ALIF concept. Eur Spine J. 2000;9(Suppl 1):S35–43.
21. Gstöttner M, Glodny B, Petersen J, Thaler M, Bach CM. CT angiography for anterior lumbar spine access: high radiation exposure and low clinical relevance. Clin Orthop Relat Res. 2011;469(3):819–24.
22. Güenaga KF, Matos D, Wille-Jørgensen P. Mechanical bowel preparation for elective colorectal surgery. Cochrane Database Syst Rev. 2011;2011(9):CD001544.
23. Deng S, Dong Q, Wang J, Zhang P. The role of mechanical bowel preparation before ileal urinary diversion: a systematic review and meta-analysis. Urol Int. 2014;92(3):339–48.
24. Cao F, Li J, Li F. Mechanical bowel preparation for elective colorectal surgery: updated systematic review and meta-analysis. Int J Color Dis. 2012;27(6):803–10.

25. Jeon C-H, Lee H-D, Chung N-S. Does mechanical bowel preparation ameliorate surgical performance in anterior lumbar interbody fusion? Global Spine J. 2019;9(7):692–6.
26. Laratta JL, Davis EG, Glassman SD, Dimar JR. The transperitoneal approach for anterior lumbar interbody fusion at L5-S1: a technical note. J Spine Surg. 2018;4(2):459–60.
27. Kim DH. Surgical anatomy & techniques to the spine. 2nd ed. Elsevier Saunders: Philadelphia; 2013.
28. Johnson RM, McGuire EJ. Urogenital complications of anterior approaches to the lumbar spine. Clin Orthop Relat Res. 1981;154:114–8.
29. Frymoyer JW, editor. The adult spine: principles and practice. Philadelphia: Lippincott-Raven; 1997.
30. Mahatthanatrakul A, Itthipanichpong T, Ratanakornphan C, Numkarunarunrote N, Singhatanadgige W, Yingsakmongkol W, et al. Relation of lumbar sympathetic chain to the open corridor of retroperitoneal oblique approach to lumbar spine: an MRI study. Eur Spine J. 2019;28(4):829–34.
31. Sebastian AS, Currier BL, Kakar S, Nguyen EC, Wagie AE, Habermann ES, et al. Risk factors for venous thromboembolism following thoracolumbar surgery: analysis of 43,777 patients from the American College of Surgeons National Surgical Quality Improvement Program 2005 to 2012. Global Spine J. 2016;6(8):738–43.
32. Qureshi R, Puvanesarajah V, Jain A, Shimer AL, Shen FH, Hassanzadeh H. A comparison of anterior and posterior lumbar interbody fusions: complications, readmissions, discharge dispositions, and costs. Spine. 2017;42(24):1865–70.
33. Pateder DB, Gonzales RA, Kebaish KM, Antezana DF, Cohen DB, Chang J-Y, et al. Pulmonary embolism after adult spinal deformity surgery. Spine. 2008;33(3):301–5.
34. Vint H, Mawdsley MJ, Coe C, Jensen CD, Kasis AG. The incidence of venous thromboembolism in patients undergoing anterior lumbar interbody fusion: a proposed thromboprophylactic regime. Int J Spine Surg. 2021;15(2):348–52.
35. Bono CM, Watters WC, Heggeness MH, Resnick DK, Shaffer WO, Baisden J, et al. An evidence-based clinical guideline for the use of antithrombotic therapies in spine surgery. Spine J. 2009;9(12):1046–51.
36. Vather R, Bissett I. Management of prolonged post-operative ileus: evidence-based recommendations. ANZ J Surg. 2013;83(5):319–24.
37. Wattchow DA, De Fontgalland D, Bampton PA, Leach PL, Mclaughlin K, Costa M. Clinical trial: the impact of cyclooxygenase inhibitors on gastrointestinal recovery after major surgery - a randomized double blind controlled trial of celecoxib or diclofenac vs. placebo. Aliment Pharmacol Ther. 2009;30(10):987–98.
38. Cheatham ML, Chapman WC, Key SP, Sawyers JL. A meta-analysis of selective versus routine nasogastric decompression after elective laparotomy. Ann Surg. 1995;221(5):469–78.
39. Nelson R, Edwards S, Tse B. Prophylactic nasogastric decompression after abdominal surgery. Cochrane Database Syst Rev. 2007;2007(3):CD004929.
40. Seta ML, Kale-Pradhan PB. Efficacy of metoclopramide in postoperative ileus after exploratory laparotomy. Pharmacotherapy. 2001;21(10):1181–6.
41. Chan D-C, Liu Y-C, Chen C-J, Yu J-C, Chu H-C, Chen F-C, et al. Preventing prolonged postoperative ileus in gastric cancer patients undergoing gastrectomy and intra-peritoneal chemotherapy. World J Gastroenterol. 2005;11(31):4776–81.
42. Venara A, Neunlist M, Slim K, Barbieux J, Colas PA, Hamy A, et al. Postoperative ileus: pathophysiology, incidence, and prevention. J Visc Surg. 2016;153(6):439–46.
43. Boelens PG, Heesakkers FFBM, Luyer MDP, van Barneveld KWY, de Hingh IHJT, Nieuwenhuijzen GAP, et al. Reduction of postoperative ileus by early enteral nutrition in patients undergoing major rectal surgery: prospective, randomized, controlled trial. Ann Surg. 2014;259(4):649–55.

# Chapter 13
# Biomechanics of Anterior, Oblique, and Lateral Approaches to the Lumbosacral Spine

G. Bryan Cornwall (D), William R. Walsh (D), Ralph Mobbs (D), Claire van Ekdom, and Joseph O'Brien (D)

## Introduction

The anterior column of the lumbosacral spine provides the majority of load transfer and stability during normal activities. When spinal pathologies advance to a clinically relevant degree and surgery is required, anterior, lateral, and oblique approaches to the anterior lumbar spine provide powerful techniques for both addressing the pathology and providing stabilization (Fig. 13.1). Numerous clinical indications, including deformity, degenerative disc disease with instability, and spondylolisthesis, involve replacing the disc with a bone graft or an implant. The aim of this surgery is to restore the stability and alignment of the spine while reducing pain and neurological symptoms. The biomechanics of ALIF are complex, involving the interplay of multiple structures, including the intervertebral disc, the vertebral bodies, and the implant. Classic textbooks [2, 3] and a new textbook [4] are dedicated to the biomechanics of the spine. Interested readers are encouraged to delve into these resources. The purpose of this chapter is to provide an overview of the biomechanical concepts pertinent to the anterior, oblique, and lateral approaches to spine surgery and structural reconstruction. The goals of stabilizing the anterior column

G. B. Cornwall (✉)
University of San Diego, San Diego, CA, USA

W. R. Walsh
UNSW Sydney, Sydney, NSW, Australia
e-mail: w.walsh@unsw.edu.au

R. Mobbs
NeuroSpineClinic, Sydney, NSW, Australia

C. van Ekdom · J. O'Brien
OrthoBethesda, Bethesda, MD, USA

© The Author(s), under exclusive license to Springer Nature Switzerland AG 2023

J. R. O'Brien et al. (eds.), *Lumbar Spine Access Surgery*,
https://doi.org/10.1007/978-3-031-48034-8_13

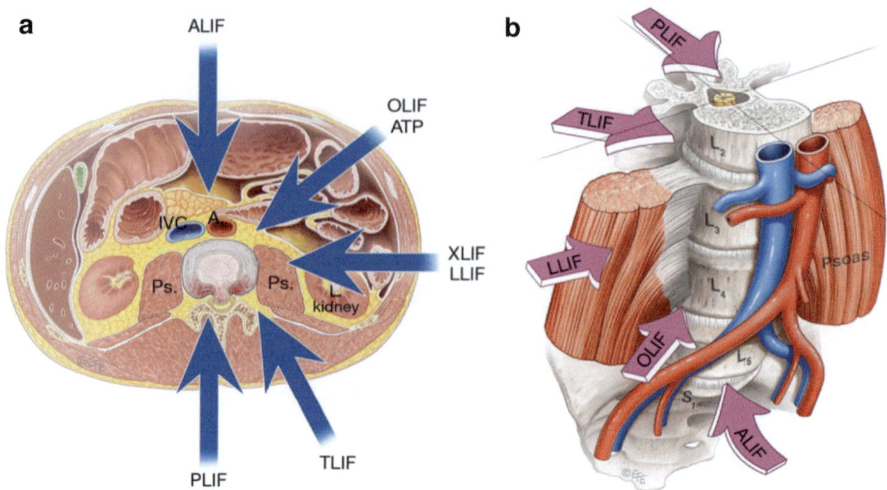


**Fig. 13.1** (**a**) Axial view of the lumbar spine indicating various approaches. (**b**) Three-dimensional isometric view of the lumbosacral spine indicating various approaches [1]

could be through fusion or with motion preservation. There are different biomechanical considerations for each construct philosophy (fusion or motion).

The degree of stability required after surgery depends upon numerous patient- and approach-related factors such as weight, alignment, previous surgeries, degree of instability, comorbidities, and iatrogenic tissue removal to address the pathology [1, 5, 6]. Stability can be provided through the anterior column with many options of fixation devices for fusion and total disc replacement devices for preserving motion. This chapter will provide a comprehensive summary of the biomechanics of ALIF, including the anatomy and function of the lumbar spine, the biomechanical changes that occur following ALIF, and the alignment considerations associated with these procedures.

## The Anatomy and Function of the Lumbosacral Spine

The lumbar spine is comprised of five vertebrae (L1–L5) that are separated by intervertebral discs. The intervertebral discs are composed of a gel-like nucleus pulposus surrounded by a more fibrous and robust annulus fibrosus. The vertebral bodies are connected by ligaments and muscles that provide both mobility and stability to the lumbosacral spine. The lumbar spine supports the load of the body and distributes those forces through the pelvis to the legs. There are six degrees of motion that can occur in the lumbar spine including bending (flexion and extension), twisting or side bending (lateral bending), and rotation (axial rotation) along with displacements along the three principal planes: sagittal, coronal, and axial.

The lumbar spine provides approximately 55° of flexion and 15° of extension motion in healthy individuals, though these approximate values change with gender, race, and age [7]. The anterior column supports the majority of the load transferred through the spine [8]. In biomechanics research, a functional spinal unit is defined as a cranial vertebral body, disc (including both the annulus and nucleus), and a caudal vertebral body as shown in Fig. 13.2.

The relative strength of the lumbar ligaments which contribute to the flexibility and the stability of the lumbosacral spine was summarized by White and Panjabi (Table 13.1) [3]. A more recent study sequentially removing stabilizing structures confirmed these findings with additional observations about relative contribution [6]. The order of sequential removal of lumbar spine stabilizing structures is illustrated in Fig. 13.3. The anterior longitudinal ligament (ALL) contributes the most stability to the functional spinal unit in extension and lateral bending. The posterior longitudinal ligament (PLL) and ligamentum flavum (LF) contribute to stability in flexion. The intertransverse, supraspinous, and interspinous ligaments contribute relatively little to the stability of the spine.

The amount of load transmitted through the anterior column was measured *in vivo* through changes in intradiscal pressure in various positions from lying down to sitting, standing, and lifting weights. Original studies performed by Nachemson in Sweden in the 1960s and 1970s were repeated by Wilke *et al.* in Germany in the late 1990s [8–12]. The results were similar between the studies; Fig. 13.4 summarizes the relative increase in intradiscal pressure (implying increased loads) on the disc with different postures and exercises.

## Lumbar Surgery Biomechanics

Numerous custom machines and robotic devices have been designed for spinal biomechanical testing [8, 13–15]. The most common way to perform range of motion testing is with the application of a pure moment at the top of the functional spinal

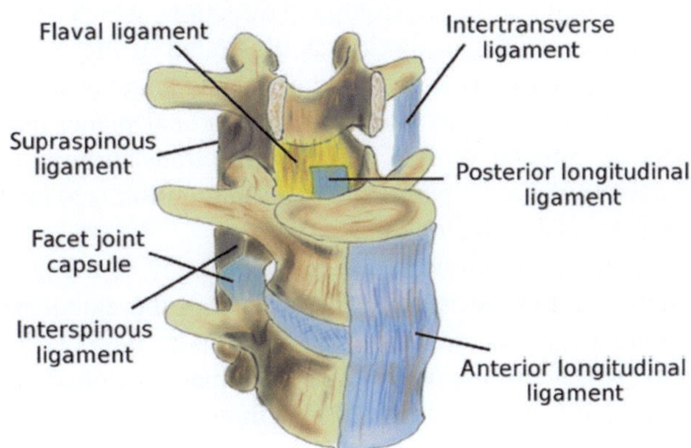


**Fig. 13.2** Lumbar ligaments from an oblique perspective of a functional spinal unit [8]

**Table 13.1** The relative strength of the lumbar ligaments which contribute to the flexibility and the stability of the lumbosacral spine

| Ligament | Load (N) | | Deformation (mm) | | Stress (MPa) | | Strain (%) | |
|---|---|---|---|---|---|---|---|---|
| | Average | Range | Average | Range | Average | Range | Average | Range |
| ALL | 450 | 390–510 | 15.2 | 7–20 | 11.6 | 2.4–21 | 36.5 | 16–57 |
| PLL | 324 | 264–384 | 5.1 | 4.2–7.0 | 11.5 | 2.9–20 | 26.0 | 8–44 |
| LF | 285 | 230–340 | 12.7 | 12.0–14.5 | 8.7 | 2.4–15 | 26.0 | 10–46 |
| CL | 222 | 160–284 | 11.3 | 9.8–12.8 | 7.6 | 7.6 | 12.0 | 12.0 |
| ISL | 125 | 120–130 | 13.0 | 7.4–17.8 | 3.2 | 1.8–4.6 | 13.0 | 13.0 |
| SSL | 150 | 100–200 | 25.9 | 22.1–28.1 | 5.4 | 2.0–8.7 | 32.5 | 26–39 |

*ALL* anterior longitudinal ligament, *PLL* posterior longitudinal ligament, *LF* ligamentum flavum, *CL* capsular ligament, *ISL* interspinous ligament, *SSL* supraspinous ligament

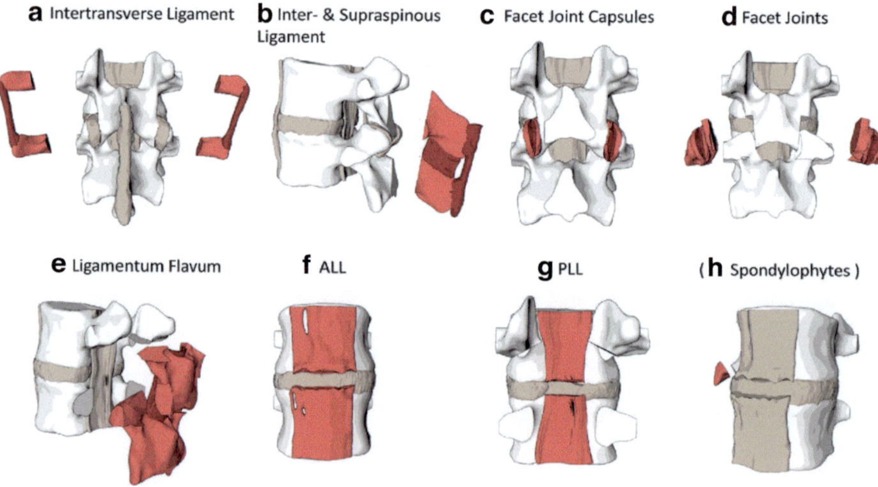


**Fig. 13.3** Transection of stabilizing elements in eight sequential steps [5]

unit or multi-segment spine specimen as shown in Fig. 13.5a. Pure moments are applied in the three physiological directions which can result in six degrees of freedom, or six types of motion as illustrated in Fig. 13.5b. In the sagittal plane, the resulting motion is flexion and extension angular motion, or anterior and posterior translation along the x-axis. In the coronal plane, the resulting motion is lateral bending angular motion and possible translation to the right and left along the y-axis. In the axial plane, the resulting motion is axial rotation or possible cranial/caudal translation along the z-axis.

As the pure moments are applied in any of the physiologic planes, a resulting nonlinear, hysteresis curve demonstrates the extent of motion in each direction. Figure 13.6 illustrates the example of pure moment testing of a functional spinal unit [18]. The amount of torque or moment is plotted on the x-axis and the resulting motion in angles is measured by a three-dimensional marker system and plotted on

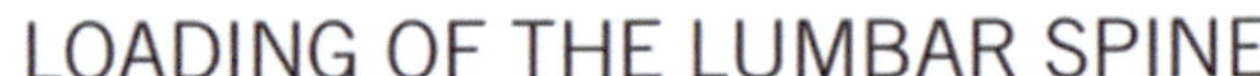

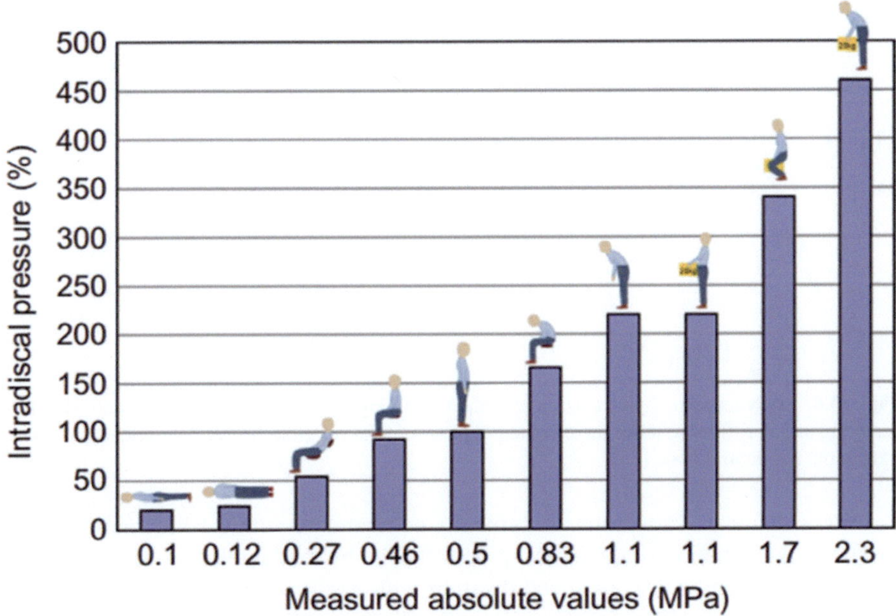


**Fig. 13.4** Intradiscal pressure was measured *in vivo* in the L4–L5 lumbar disc for different postures and activities with a special pressure transducer [8]

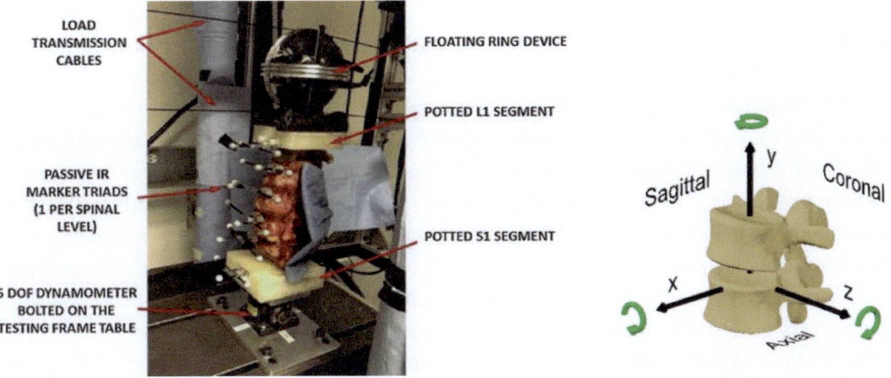


**Fig. 13.5** (**a**) Example of a custom design and built spine biomechanic testing applying pure moments and measuring the response of the vertebral bodies with passive IR markers [16]. (**b**) Functional spinal unit illustrating the six degrees of motion of the lumbar spine. *DOF* degrees of freedom [17]

the y-axis (Fig. 13.6a). The extent of motion in the physiologic planes is illustrated in Fig. 13.6b. The neutral zone (NZ) is the region of the curve where the spine has the least stiffness.

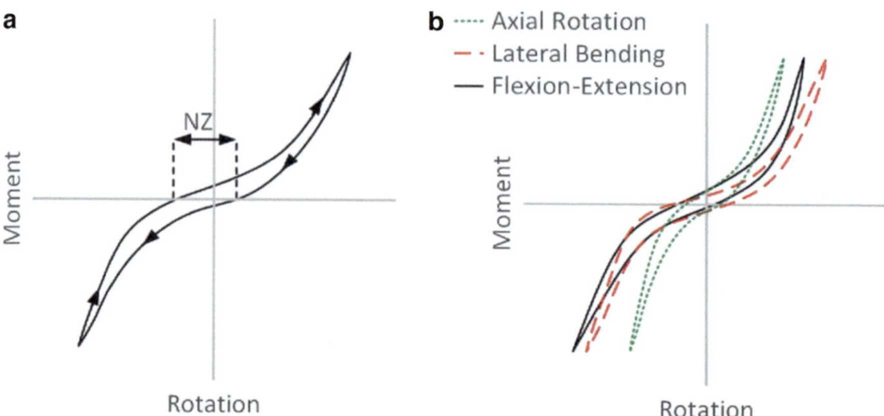

Fig. 13.6 (a) Nonlinear, hysteresis curve when applying pure moments to the spine. (b) The resulting angular motion in the three principal planes: axial rotation, lateral bending, and flexion/extension. *NZ* neutral zone [18]

Biomechanical evaluations are typically comparative with the kinematic (angular motion) evaluation of the intact spine followed by methodologies for measuring destabilization and subsequent stabilization with various surgical options [19–22]. Typically, human cadaver functional spinal units are preferred although there can be variability in the bone quality and soft tissue stability depending upon the age, gender, and degree of disc degeneration or other pathologies. Animal models and simulated spine analogues can also be used which theoretically provide more consistent tissue properties between specimens [22, 23]. Animal models may require different implant designs and synthetic models are relatively new with more studies characterizing their properties.

A biomechanical evaluation of different ALIF fixation options examined standalone ALIF, ALIF with three or four integrated screws, ALIF with an anterior plate, ALIF with bilateral pedicle screws, and finally ALIF with three integrated screws and a posteriorly placed spinous process plate; the results are summarized in Fig. 13.7 [24]. The results of each subsequent fixation option were compared with the range of motion of the intact spine described as 100%. The stand-alone ALIF cage provided some degree of stabilization in flexion/extension and lateral bending, but it was less stable than the intact spine in axial rotation. The most stable constructs were ALIF with bilateral pedicle screws and ALIF with three integrated screws supplemented with a posterior spinous process plate. The team from the Surgical Orthopaedic Research Lab from the University of New South Wales performed a similar study comparing lateral lumbar interbody fusion (LLIF) options with the final construct removing the ALL and fixating with an anterior plate in synthetic (analogue) spines; they found similar results and relative stabilization [22].

In LLIF, various authors have evaluated different fixation schemes compared with the intact spine. Cappuccino *et al.* compared numerous fixation options to the intact spine including stand-alone lateral implants, lateral implants with lateral

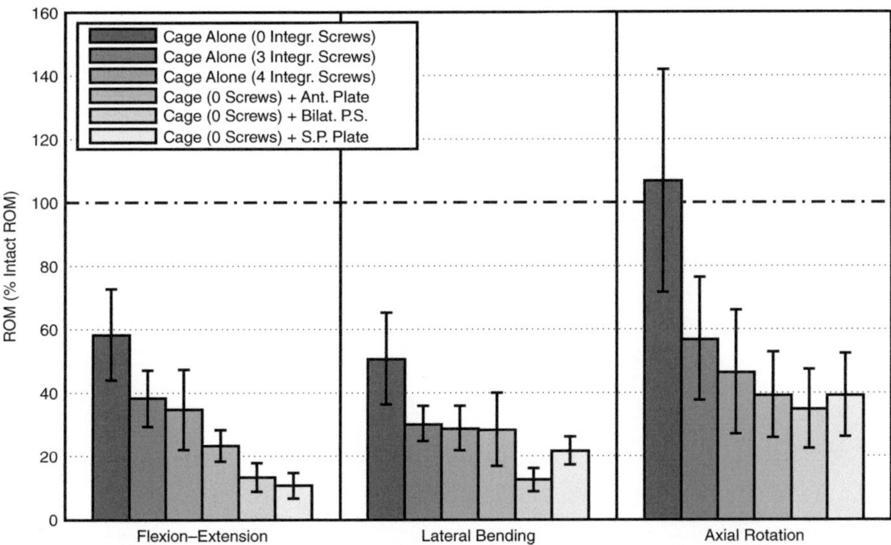


**Fig. 13.7** Comparison of range of motion (ROM) of various fixation schemes relative to the intact spine at 100% ROM [24]

plates, lateral implants with unilateral pedicle screws, and lateral implants with bilateral pedicle screws in the three planes of motion [25]. A summary of the results and comparison with other fixation options (ALIF and TLIF) is shown in Fig. 13.8.

Subsidence is affected by the quality of bone, the quality of the endplate, the location of the implant with weaker support in the center, and stronger bone with increased subsidence resistance at the periphery [26]. Figure 13.9 illustrates the variation of indentation load in a map of locations around the endplate. Biomechanics evaluations of subsidence can be performed with cadavers although the variability of bone quality can influence results. The relative location of bone within the endplate is also a significant influence on the subsidence resistance with the weakest bone towards the center of the vertebral body [27]. The lateral periphery of the vertebral body is most resistant to compression, thus giving laterally placed interbody cages that span the ring apophysis an advantage in resisting compression [26, 28].

Subsidence is also influenced by cage design, especially the surface area contacting bone, the material of the interbody implant, and the structural design of the implant [29]. Figure 13.10 demonstrates four different ALIF interbody implant designs. It is important for the surgeon to note that subsidence can affect both interbody cages and total disc replacement implants. Biomechanical comparisons of subsidence of different implant designs and materials can also be performed in simulated bone foam [29, 30]. This is the recommendation of standardized testing based upon the reproducibility of the material and the possibility of simulating bone of different densities [27–38].

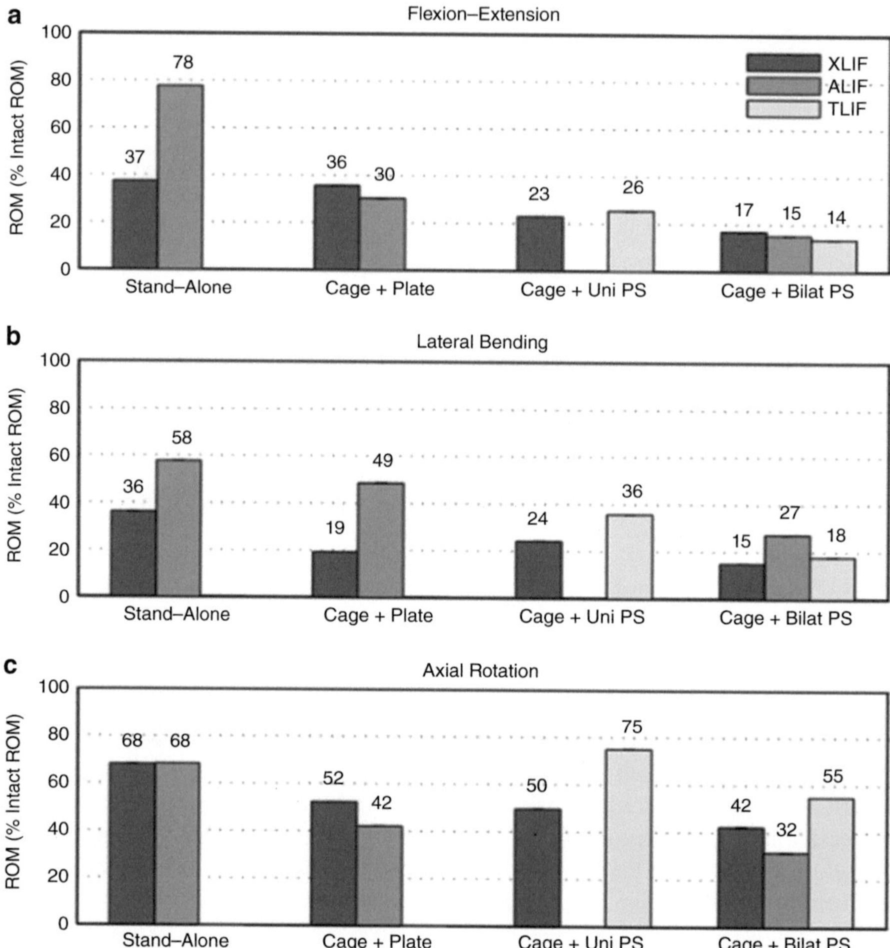


**Fig. 13.8** Comparison of biomechanical stability in LLIF, ALIF, and TLIF: (**a**) flexion-extension, (**b**) lateral bending, and (**c**) axial rotation [25]

The goal of lumbar total disc replacement is the restoration of stability while maintaining the biomechanics and kinematics of the lumbar spine [39–42]. It has been hypothesized that restoring this motion at the operative level would reduce the compensatory loads at adjacent levels.

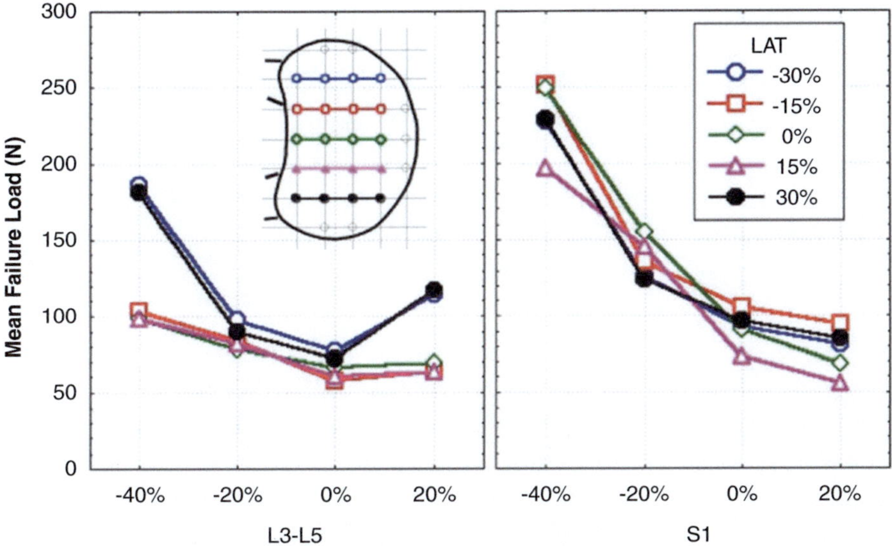



**Fig. 13.9** Indentation testing map illustrating location and relative mean failure load at different endplate locations [26]

## Lumbosacral Alignment Considerations

The final biomechanical principle to discuss in this chapter is a brief overview of lumbosacral alignment in adults. Some surgeons have postulated the importance of considering alignment in every surgery including single-level degenerative cases. Spinal alignment changes as we age [43–45]. Further, the relationship between the global spinal alignment and the pelvis has important implications for gait and other compensatory mechanisms, including knee bending to maintain the "cone of economy"—a geometric estimation of the range of global alignment within which an adult uses energy efficiently. Outside this cone, subjects become increasingly debilitated [46–48].

Anterior column realignment (ACR) has been proposed as a minimally invasive approach to modifying sagittal alignment [47, 49–51]. This is accomplished with a lateral approach, carefully resecting the ALL, and inserting a hyperlordotic lateral interbody cage. One of the surgical implications of sagittal alignment is that the location of introducing lordosis into the lumbar spine is important given most of the lumbar lordosis is between L4 and S1 (approximately 40°), while approximately 12° of lordosis occurs between L1 and L4. Furthermore, better sagittal alignment has been linked to favorable patient-reported outcomes compared with larger values describing poor global sagittal alignment [43–45, 48, 52–56].

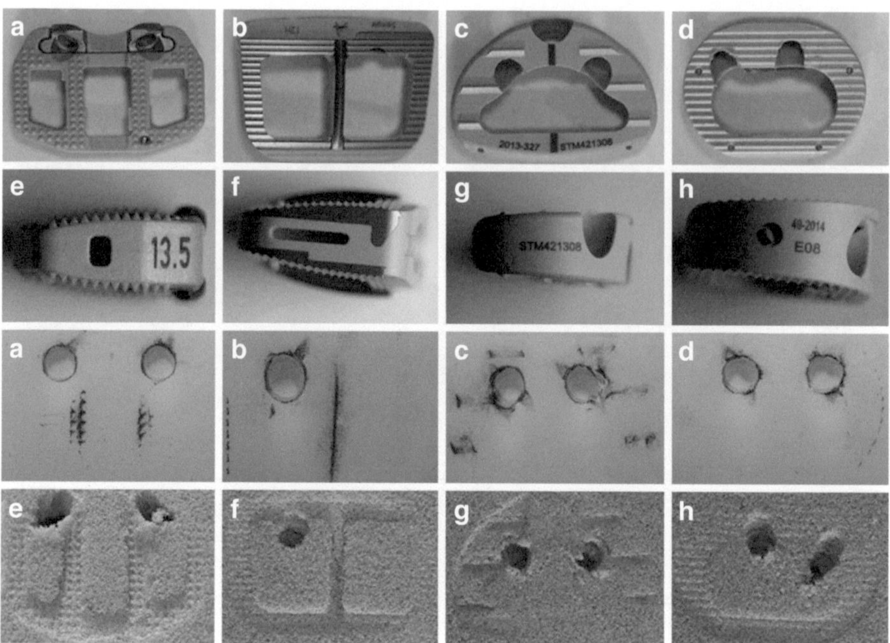

**Fig. 13.10** Four different ALIF interbody implant designs (Figs: **a-d** represent axial views & Figs: **e-h** represent sagittal views of the four designs) and the pressure film footprint after inserting screws (Figs: **a-d** third row) and the relative subsidence after compression (Figs. **e-h** fourth row) and post-rotational testing [29]

## Conclusion

Anterior approaches to the lumbar spine including ALIF, OLIF, and LLIF are clinically important spinal procedures with good outcomes and relatively few complications. In addition to a thorough understanding of the lumbar anatomy, it is important for the surgeon to understand the relative stability provided by various fixation options. The surgeon decides how much stability the patient may need depending upon the alignment, degree of instability from pathology, or iatrogenic destabilization from approach-related decompression.

## References


1. Mobbs R, Phan K, Malham G, et al. Lumbar interbody fusion: techniques, indications and comparison of interbody fusion options including PLIF, TLIF, MI-TLIF, OLIF/ATP, LLIF and ALIF. J Spine Surg. 2015;1(1):2–18. https://doi.org/10.3978/j.issn.2414-469X.2015.10.05.
2. White A, Panjabi M, editors. Clinical biomechanics of the spine. Philadelphia: Lippincott; 1990.
3. Benzel C, editor. Biomechanics of spine stabilization. New York: Thieme; 2001.

4. Galbusera F, Wilke, H.-J. (Eds.). Biomechanics of the spine: basic concepts, spinal disorders, and treatments. London: Academic Press; 2018.
5. Widmer J, Cornaz F, Scheibler G, Spirig JM, Snedeker JG, Farshad M. Biomechanical contribution of spinal structures to stability of the lumbar spine—novel biomechanical insights. Spine J. 2020;20(10):1705–16. https://doi.org/10.1016/J.SPINEE.2020.05.541.
6. Teng I, Han J, Phan K, Mobbs R. A meta-analysis comparing ALIF, PLIF, TLIF and LLIF. J Clin Neurosci. 2017;44:11–7. https://doi.org/10.1016/j.jocn.2017.06.01.
7. Trudelle-Jackson E, Ann Fleisher L, Borman N, Morrow JR, Frierson GM. Lumbar spine flexion and extension extremes of motion in women of different age and racial groups. Spine (Phila Pa 1976). 2010;35(16):1539. https://doi.org/10.1097/BRS.0B013E3181B0C3D1.
8. Wilke H-J, Volkheimer D. Basic biomechanics of the lumbar spine. In: Galbusera F, Wilke H-J, editors. Biomechanics of the spine: basic concepts, spinal disorders, and treatments. London: Academic Press; 2018. p. 51–67.
9. Nachemson A. The effect of forward leaning on lumbar intradiscal pressure. Acta Orthop. 1965;35(1–4):314–28. https://doi.org/10.3109/17453676508989362.
10. Nachemson A, Morris J. Lumbar discometry. Lumbar intradiscal pressure measurements in vivo. Lancet. 1963;1(7291):1140–2. https://doi.org/10.1016/S0140-6736(63)91806-3.
11. Nachemson AL, Schultz AB, Berkson MH. Mechanical properties of human lumbar spine motion segments. Influence of age, sex, disc level, and degeneration. Spine. 1979;4(1):1–8. https://doi.org/10.1097/00007632-197901000-00001.
12. Wilke HJ, Neef P, Caimi M, Hoogland T, Claes LE. New in vivo measurements of pressures in the intervertebral disc in daily life. Spine. 1999;24(8):755–62. https://doi.org/10.1097/00007632-199904150-00005.
13. Noble LD, Colbrunn RW, Lee D-G, van den Bogert AJ, Davis BL. Design and validation of a general purpose robotic testing system for musculoskeletal applications. J Biomech Eng. 2010;132(2):025001. https://doi.org/10.1115/1.4000851.
14. Rohlmann A, Neller S, Claes L, Bergmann G, Wilke HJ. Influence of a follower load on intradiscal pressure and intersegmental rotation of the lumbar spine. Spine (Phila Pa 1976). 2001;26(24):E557–61. https://doi.org/10.1097/00007632-200112150-00014.
15. Volkheimer D, Malakoutian M, Oxland TR, Wilke H-J. Limitations of current in vitro test protocols for investigation of instrumented adjacent segment biomechanics: critical analysis of the literature. Eur Spine J. 2015;24(9):1882–92.
16. Orías A, He J, Wang M. Biomechanical testing of the intact and surgically treated spine. In: Zdero R, editor. Experimental methodist orthopedic biomechanics. London: Elsevier; 2017. p. 133–47.
17. McCombe P, Diwan A, Wilke H-J. Biomechanics of motion preservation technologies. In: Boden S, editor. Lumbar spine online textbook. Towson, MD: International Society for the Study of the Lumbar Spine. Data Trace Publishing; 2023.
18. Newell N, Little JP, Christou A, Adams MA, Adam CJ, Masouros SD. Biomechanics of the human intervertebral disc: a review of testing techniques and results. J Mech Behav Biomed Mater. 2017;69:420–34. https://doi.org/10.1016/J.JMBBM.2017.01.037.
19. Wilke H-J, Jungkunz B, Wenger K, Claes LE. Spinal segment range of motion as a function of in vitro test conditions: effects of exposure period, accumulated cycles, angular-deformation rate, and moisture condition. Anat Rec. 1998;251(1):15–9. https://doi.org/10.1002/(SICI)1097-0185(199805)251:1<15::AID-AR4>3.0.CO;2-D.
20. Galbusera F, Volkheimer D, Wilke H-J. In vitro testing of cadaveric specimens. In: Galbusera F, Wilke H-J, editors. Biomechanics of the spine: basic concepts, spinal disorders, and treatments. London: Academic Press; 2018. p. 203–21.
21. Lee BS, Walsh KM, Healy AT, Colbrunn R, Butler RS, Goodwin RC, Steinmetz MP, Mroz TE. Biomechanics of L5/S1 in long thoracolumbosacral constructs: a cadaveric study. Global Spine J. 2018;8(6):607–14. https://doi.org/10.1177/2192568218759037.
22. Wang T, Ball JR, Pelletier MH, Walsh WR. Biomechanical evaluation of a biomimetic spinal construct. J Exp Orthop. 2014;1(1):3. https://doi.org/10.1186/s40634-014-0003-.

23. Wilke H-J, Kettler A, Claes LE. Are sheep spines a valid biomechanical model for human spines? Spine (Phila Pa 1976). 1997;22(20):2365–74. https://doi.org/10.1097/00007632-199710150-00009.
24. Kornblum MB, Turner AWL, Cornwall GB, Zatushevsky MA, Phillips FM. Biomechanical evaluation of stand-alone lumbar polyether-ether-ketone interbody cage with integrated screws. Spine J. 2013;13(1):77–84. https://doi.org/10.1016/j.spinee.2012.11.013.
25. Cappuccino A, Cornwall GB, Turner AWL, Fogel GR, Duong HT, Kim KD, Brodke DS. Biomechanical analysis and review of lateral lumbar fusion constructs. Spine. 2010;35(Suppl):S361–7. https://doi.org/10.1097/BRS.0b013e318202308b.
26. Oxland TR. Fundamental biomechanics of the spine—what we have learned in the past 25 years and future directions. J Biomech. 2016;49(6):817–32. https://doi.org/10.1016/J.JBIOMECH.2015.10.035.
27. Jost B, Cripton PA, Lund T, Oxland TR, Lippuner K, Jaeger P, Nolte LP. Compressive strength of interbody cages in the lumbar spine: the effect of cage shape, posterior instrumentation and bone density. Eur Spine J. 1998;7(2):132–41. https://doi.org/10.1007/S005860050043.
28. Marchi L, Abdala N, Oliveira L, Amaral R, Coutinho E, Pimenta L. Radiographic and clinical evaluation of cage subsidence after stand-alone lateral interbody fusion. J Neurosurg Spine. 2013;19(1):110–8. https://doi.org/10.3171/2013.4.SPINE12319.
29. Assem Y, Pelletier MH, Mobbs RJ, Phan K, Walsh WR. Anterior lumbar interbody fusion integrated screw cages: intrinsic load generation, subsidence, and torsional stability. Orthop Surg. 2017;9(2):191–7. https://doi.org/10.1111/OS.12283.
30. Yee-Yanagishita C, Fogel G, Douglas B, Essayan G, Poojary B, Martin N, Williams GM, Peng Y, Jekir M. Biomechanical comparison of subsidence performance among three modern porous lateral cage designs. Clin Biomech (Bristol, Avon). 2022b;99:105764. https://doi.org/10.1016/j.clinbiomech.2022.10576.
31. Agarwal N, White MD, Zhang X, Alan N, Ozpinar A, Salvetti DJ, Tempel ZJ, Okonkwo DO, Kanter AS, Hamilton DK. Impact of endplate-implant area mismatch on rates and grades of subsidence following stand-alone lateral lumbar interbody fusion: an analysis of 623 levels. J Neurosurg Spine. 2020;6:1–5. https://doi.org/10.3171/2020.1.SPINE19776.
32. Campbell PG, Cavanaugh DA, Nunley P, Utter PA, Kerr E, Wadhwa R, Stone M. PEEK versus titanium cages in lateral lumbar interbody fusion: a comparative analysis of subsidence. Neurosurg Focus. 2020;49(3):1–9. https://doi.org/10.3171/2020.6.FOCUS20367.
33. Choi JY, Sung KH. Subsidence after anterior lumbar interbody fusion using paired stand-alone rectangular cages. Eur Spine J. 2006;15(1):16–22. https://doi.org/10.1007/S00586-004-0817-Y.
34. Godolias P, Tataryn ZL, Plümer J, Cibura C, Freyvert Y, Heep H, Dudda M, Schildhauer TA, Chapman JR, Oskouian RJ. Cage subsidence—a multifactorial matter! Orthopadie (Heidelb). 2023;52(8):662–9. https://doi.org/10.1007/S00132-023-04363-9.
35. Parisien A, Wai EK, Elsayed MSA, Frei H. Subsidence of spinal fusion cages: a systematic review. Int J Spine Surg. 2022;16(6):1103–18. https://doi.org/10.14444/8363.
36. Tempel ZJ, McDowell MM, Panczykowski DM, Gandhoke GS, Kojo Hamilton D, Okonkwo DO, Kanter AS. Graft subsidence as a predictor of revision surgery following stand-alone lateral lumbar interbody fusion. J Neurosurg Spine. 2018;28(1):50–6. https://doi.org/10.3171/2017.5.SPINE16427.
37. Theologis AA, Patel S, Burch S. Radiographic comparison of L5–S1 lateral anterior lumbar interbody fusion cage subsidence and displacement by fixation strategy: anterior plate versus integrated screws. J Neurosurg Spine. 2023;38(1):126–30. https://doi.org/10.3171/2022.7.SPINE22436.
38. Wu H, Shan Z, Zhao F, Cheung JPY. Poor bone quality, multilevel surgery, and narrow and tall cages are associated with intraoperative endplate injuries and late-onset cage subsidence in lateral lumbar interbody fusion: a systematic review. Clin Orthop Relat Res. 2022;480(1):163–88. https://doi.org/10.1097/CORR.0000000000001915.

39. Auerbach JD, Wills BPD, McIntosh TC, Balderston RA. Evaluation of spinal kinematics following lumbar total disc replacement and circumferential fusion using in vivo fluoroscopy. Spine. 2007;32(5):527–36. https://doi.org/10.1097/01.brs.0000256915.90236.17.
40. Bao QB, McCullen GM, Higham PA, Dumbleton JH, Yuan HA. The artificial disc: theory, design and materials. Biomaterials. 1996;17(12):1157–67. https://doi.org/10.1016/0142-9612(96)84936-2.
41. Frelinghuysen P, Huang RC, Girardi FP, Cammisa FP. Lumbar total disc replacement part I: rationale, biomechanics, and implant types. Orthop Clin North Am. 2005;36(3):293–9. https://doi.org/10.1016/j.ocl.2005.02.014.
42. Galbusera F, Bellini CM, Zweig T, Ferguson S, Raimondi MT, Lamartina C, Brayda-Bruno M, Fornari M. Design concepts in lumbar total disc arthroplasty. Eur Spine J. 2008;17(12):1635–50. https://doi.org/10.1007/S00586-008-0811-X/METRICS.
43. Mac-Thiong JM, Roussouly P, Berthonnaud É, Guigui P. Sagittal parameters of global spinal balance: normative values from a prospective cohort of seven hundred nine caucasian asymptomatic adults. Spine (Phila Pa 1976). 2010;35(22):E1193–8. https://doi.org/10.1097/BRS.0B013E3181E50808.
44. Sardar ZM, Cerpa M, Hassan F, Kelly M, Le Huec JC, Bourret S, Hasegawa K, Wong HK, Liu G, Dennis Hey HW, Riahi H, Lenke L. Age- and gender-based global sagittal spinal alignment in asymptomatic adult volunteers: results of the Multiethnic Alignment Normative Study (MEANS). Spine. 2022;47(19):1372–81. https://doi.org/10.1097/BRS.0000000000004413.
45. Yokoyama K, Kawanishi M, Yamada M, Tanaka H, Ito Y, Kawabata S, Kuroiwa T. Age-related variations in global spinal alignment and sagittal balance in asymptomatic. Neurol Res. 2017;39(5):414–8. https://doi.org/10.1080/01616412.2017.1296654.
46. Garbossa D, Pejrona M, Damilano M, Sansone V, Ducati A, Berjano P. Pelvic parameters and global spine balance for spine degenerative disease: the importance of containing for the well being of content. Eur Spine J. 2014;23(6):S616–27. https://doi.org/10.1007/S00586-014-3558-6/METRICS.
47. Klineberg E, Schwab F, Smith JS, Gupta MC, Lafage V, Bess S. Sagittal spinal pelvic alignment. Neurosurg Clin N Am. 2013;24(2):157–62. https://doi.org/10.1016/j.nec.2012.12.003.
48. Roussouly P, Nnadi C. Sagittal plane deformity: an overview of interpretation and management. Eur Spine J. 2010;19(11):1824–36. https://doi.org/10.1007/s00586-010-1476-9.
49. Hosseini P, Mundis GM, Eastlack RK, Bagheri R, Vargas E, Tran S, Akbarnia BA. Preliminary results of anterior lumbar interbody fusion, anterior column realignment for the treatment of sagittal malalignment. Neurosurg Focus. 2017;43(6):E6. https://doi.org/10.3171/2017.8.FOCUS17423.
50. Mundis GM, Turner JD, Kabirian N, Pawelek J, Eastlack RK, Uribe J, Klineberg E, Bess S, Ames C, Deviren V, Nguyen S, Lafage V, Akbarnia BA. Anterior column realignment has similar results to pedicle subtraction osteotomy in treating adults with sagittal plane deformity. World Neurosurg. 2017;105:249–56. https://doi.org/10.1016/J.WNEU.2017.05.122.
51. Pimenta L, Fortti F, Oliveira L, Marchi L, Jensen R, Coutinho E, Amaral R. Anterior column realignment following lateral interbody fusion for sagittal deformity correction. Eur J Orthop Surg Traumatol. 2015;25:29–33. https://doi.org/10.1007/s00590-015-1642-1.
52. Saigal R, Mundis GM, Eastlack R, Uribe JS, Phillips FM, Akbarnia BA. Anterior Column Realignment (ACR) in adult sagittal deformity correction: technique and review of the literature. Spine. 2016;41(Suppl 8):S66–73. https://doi.org/10.1097/BRS.0000000000001483.
53. Glassman SD, Bridwell K, Dimar JR, Horton W, Berven S, Schwab F. The impact of positive sagittal balance in adult spinal deformity. Spine. 2005;30(18):2024–9. https://doi.org/10.1097/01.BRS.0000179086.30449.96.
54. Durand WM, Lafage R, Hamilton DK, Passias PG, Kim HJ, Protopsaltis T, Lafage V, Smith JS, Shaffrey C, Gupta M, Kelly MP, Klineberg EO, Schwab F, Gum JL, Mundis G, Eastlack R, Kebaish K, Soroceanu A, Hostin RA, et al. Artificial intelligence clustering of adult spi-

nal deformity sagittal plane morphology predicts surgical characteristics, alignment, and outcomes. Eur Spine J. 2021;30(8):2157–66. https://doi.org/10.1007/s00586-021-06799-z.
55. Sheikh Alshabab B, Gupta MC, Lafage R, Bess S, Shaffrey C, Kim HJ, Ames CP, Burton DC, Smith JS, Eastlack RK, Klineberg EO, Mundis GM, Schwab FJ, Lafage V. Does achieving global spinal alignment lead to higher patient satisfaction and lower disability in adult spinal deformity? Spine. 2021;46(16):1105–10. https://doi.org/10.1097/BRS.0000000000004002.
56. Sugrue PA, McClendon J, Smith TR, Halpin RJ, Nasr FF, O'Shaughnessy BA, Koski TR. Redefining global spinal balance: normative values of cranial center of mass from a prospective cohort of asymptomatic individuals. Spine. 2013;38(6):484–9. https://doi.org/10.1097/BRS.0B013E318273A1C0.

# Chapter 14
# Direct Lateral Transpsoas Approach

**Ryan DenHaese**

## Introduction

Surgical safety and effectiveness are dependent on surgeon experience and comfort with anatomy, which develop over time. This is uniquely true with the direct lateral transpsoas approach to the lumbar spine. Lateral surgery at the time of this writing is two decades old [1, 2]. Biomechanical studies, technological advances, and collective surgical experience have led to a deeper understanding of this approach, and it continues to become more widespread [3–5].

As this technique becomes more streamlined, including improved preoperative planning, patient positioning, retractor selection, instrument specialization, radiology technician experience, and general workflow, the surgeon can decrease time spent within the psoas and thereby decrease nerve retraction time. Retractor time in early transpsoas approaches could take over an hour compared to under 15 min for modern approaches with the goal of minimizing postoperative complications.

## Indications

Indications for a lateral approach to the lumbar spine include spondylolisthesis, anterior longitudinal ligament release, pseudoarthrosis, hardware removal, deformity, corpectomy, tumor, trauma, infection, and adjacent segment failure.

Contraindications may include prior lateral surgery or anatomy that is not amenable to the approach due to either high iliac crests, low ribs, or lumbosacral plexus proximity.

R. DenHaese (✉)
Axis Neurosurgery and Spine, Buffalo, NY, USA

© The Author(s), under exclusive license to Springer Nature Switzerland AG 2023

J. R. O'Brien et al. (eds.), *Lumbar Spine Access Surgery*,
https://doi.org/10.1007/978-3-031-48034-8_14

## Advantages

The direct lateral approach allows for near complete disc access, facilitating efficient discectomy and cartilage removal, thereby promoting fusion. Access to both sides of the apophyseal ring allows correction of sagittal and coronal deformity, helps prevent subsidence, and allows indirect decompression of both the central canal and neural foramina. The psoas muscle is left intact, which belies the minimally invasive nature of the approach, and on postoperative magnetic resonance imaging (MRI), muscle atrophy is rarely seen. The optimal direct lateral disc access allows for large cage insertion and therefore larger graft windows, theoretically increasing fusion rates and reducing subsidence risk, all while preserving stabilizing structures of the spine and minimizing blood loss.

## Disadvantages

Disadvantages of this approach primarily relate to postoperative thigh pain, which has been reported at 14.3% to 20% [6, 7]. More serious complications, including motor and sensory disturbances (0.7–33.6% and 0–75%, respectively) as well as femoral nerve palsies, have also been reported [8]. As the lumbosacral plexus moves from dorsal to ventral more caudally, injury becomes more likely, especially below the L4 level [9].

## Anatomy

Understanding the surgical anatomy is paramount to successful completion of the direct lateral approach in a reproducible manner.

The window to the retroperitoneum can be identified caudal to the 12th rib. A line from the midpoint of the 12th rib to the iliac crest halfway to the anterior superior iliac spine on the lateral portion of the ilium demarcates the retroperitoneal space while the patient is in the lateral decubitus position. The retroperitoneal space is defined anteriorly by the parietal peritoneum and posteriorly by the transversalis fascia. The thoracic cavity is located above the 11th rib.

Muscle layers encountered from superficial to deep include the external obliques, internal obliques, the attachment of the latissimus dorsi, and finally the transversus abdominus before entering the retroperitoneum. The transversus abdominus fascia is a more robust fascial layer.

Superficial sensory nerves are avoided by understanding their location as they are often not visualized. The lateral femoral cutaneous nerve (LFCN) (L2, L3) is in the retroperitoneal fat and ascends over the iliac crest to the lateral thigh. The LFCN is avoided by limiting aggressive fat dissection upon entry into the retroperitoneum, especially at L4–L5, and avoiding direct dissection over the iliac crest. The ilioinguinal (L1) and iliohypogastric (L1) nerves course on the back wall of the retroperitoneal cavity and are almost never visualized. They are most prone to injury as they course through the oblique musculature and dissection through these muscles with monopolar cautery is avoided. The genitofemoral (GF) (L1–L2) nerve can be seen via the direct lateral approach at L2–L3 or L3–L4 within the substance of the psoas muscle prior to its final position anterior-superiorly on the surface of the psoas at L4–L5. Multiple passes through the psoas at L4–L5 are thus discouraged. If the GF nerve is encountered within the substance of the psoas, it must be protected.

The femoral nerve is comprised of the L2, L3, and L4 nerves. It provides innervation to the quadriceps and psoas muscles, as well as sensation to the anterior thigh. Beginning with L2, the femoral nerve is posterior to the L2–L3 disc space and rarely a surgical concern at this level. L3 joins with L2 and moves more ventral at L3–L4 and is usually well behind the midpoint of the L3–L4 disc space. After the femoral nerve gains final contribution from L4, it can cross at the midpoint of the L4–L5 disc space.

The vascular anatomy is variable, but the most common variant is the bifurcation of the vena cava and aorta at the L4 vertebral body, which gives rise to the iliac vessels. The iliac vessels become more lateral on the side of the spine, leaving from their anteriorly situated parent vessels. The degree of laterality varies and is directly related to the bifurcation level: the higher the bifurcation, the earlier the iliac vessels can become laterally situated. The direct lateral surgeon should be aware of the location of these vessels to avoid injury ipsilateral or contralateral to the approach. Segmental vessels are paired arteries and veins that course in the valley of the midpoint of the vertebral body. The artery of Adamkiewicz can be as caudal as the L2 vertebral body, and for corpectomy one should obtain diagnostic angiography. The iliolumbar vein is situated at the most posterior aspect of the disc space adjacent to the foramen and is vulnerable to injury with posterior retraction.

## Surgical Technique and Patient Positioning

The patient is positioned in a lateral decubitus position with an axillary roll and a roll under the iliac crest centered at the greater trochanter of the femur. A pillow is placed between the legs with the ipsilateral thigh flexed to take tension off the psoas. All boney prominences are padded. A three-inch silk tape is used to secure the patient over the chest, the iliac crest, from the iliac crest to the end of the bed on the left and right, and over the knees (Fig. 14.1).

Fluoroscopy is utilized to mark the boundaries of the target disc space, and an incision is made after sterile preparation. Dissection is carried down through the subcutaneous fat to the lateral margin of the obliques. The junction between the lumbar extensors (quadratus lumborum and longissimus) and the obliques is palpated and the posterior margin of the oblique muscle is either bluntly or sharply dissected to avoid transecting traversing the iliohypogastric and ilioinguinal nerves.

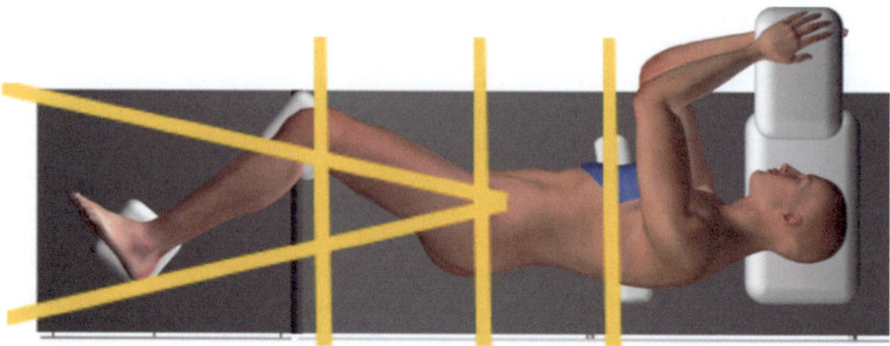

**Fig. 14.1** A lateral view demonstrating tape locations (yellow lines)

**Fig. 14.2** An axial view demonstrating sweeping the retroperitoneum off the psoas muscle

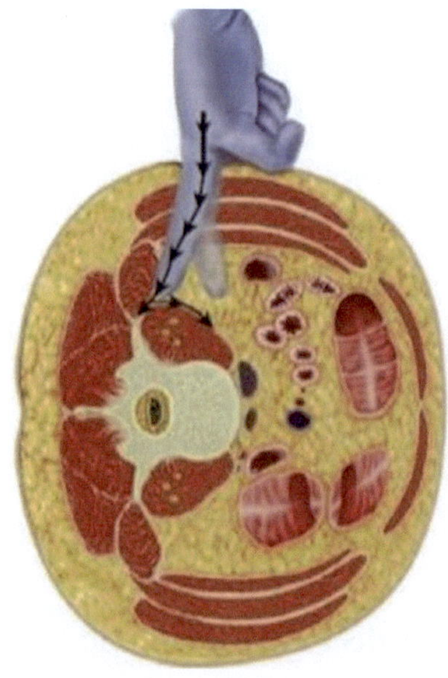

The approach is then continued through the layers of the oblique muscles to the transversalis fascia. The fascial layer is more robust and can be opened sharply or with digital dissection. The fascia is then parted in a cranial-caudal fashion, and digital dissection is carried down to the retroperitoneal space. The retroperitoneal fat can be felt anteriorly and has little resistance (Fig. 14.2).

At this point, the finger can be walked posteriorly to the transverse processes to ensure there is no interposed tissue. The psoas recess and iliac crest (L4–L5) or the 12th rib (L2–L3) may also be felt depending on the surgical level.

Once in the retroperitoneal space, a finger can be used to guide the initial dilator to the lateral margin of the psoas muscle. The dilator is then placed into the substance of the psoas muscle using neuromonitoring to avoid the lumbosacral plexus. Following instrumentation, the dilator should be removed slowly to visualize any bleeding vessels that may have been temporarily occluded by the retractors to prevent postoperative hematoma formation.


## Fluoroscopic Imaging

The lateral approach relies on excellent imaging for successful surgery and complication avoidance. The cross-table anterior-posterior (AP) X-ray requires considerable "wig-wag" to visualize parallel endplates, midline spinous processes, and equidistant pedicles. Table-mounted retractors may obscure imaging, so the attachment may be placed at the head of the bed adjacent to the arms or at the foot of the bed by the legs. Prior to sterile preparation, the surgeon must check adequate X-ray visualization of the operative level, which must be in the center of the fluoroscopic image to avoid parallax. The fluoroscope may be left in the 0° and 90° positions and the table can be rotated to obtain optimal imaging.


## Neuromonitoring

Neuromonitoring is the standard of care for a direct lateral approach. The use of somatosensory evoked potentials (SSEPs), motor evoked potentials, and triggered electromyography is routinely employed throughout direct lateral surgery. These modalities allow nerve avoidance and provide safe passage through the psoas. It is imperative that anesthesia provided is free of paralytics and hence a lack of neuromuscular blockade. Saphenous nerve SSEP can be used if available to monitor the femoral nerve, although this is not yet routine in direct lateral surgery.


## Pearls and Pitfalls

- Timing in the psoas affects outcomes and less than 15 min of retractor time in the psoas muscle is the goal.
- Understand the nuances of psoas anatomy on MRI as accurate prediction of femoral nerve location will mitigate prolonged compression.
- Flexing the hip will allow for less tension on the femoral nerve and psoas and prevent anterior translation of the nerve. The combination of these factors allows one to retract the femoral nerve more safely.
- The contralateral annulus may be left intact during disc removal to protect from iatrogenic injury to contralateral structures. It may be directly released at the end of disc preparation prior to implant trialing. However, in bone-on-bone deformity, the contralateral annulus is released immediately to allow for disc space distraction.

- The width of the disc space is longer posteriorly than anteriorly, and an instrument can incorrectly appear to be contained within the disc space on the AP when working more ventrally.
- When the retractor is posterior in the disc space and removed, bleeding may be encountered. This is controlled with gel foam and pressure; bipolar cautery should be avoided to prevent injury to the femoral nerve. The surgeon can hover and use endoscopic Kittners and a sponge for pressure.
- X-Ray mastery will prevent endplate damage, limit subsidence, and improve indirect decompression of the neural elements.
- Hemostasis from segmental artery bleeding must be obtained with ligature or bipolar cautery.
- The use of angled instruments at the L1–L2 and L4–L5 levels is of significant benefit for high-angle disc spaces.
- L1–L2 and L2–L3 are often between the 11th and 12th ribs.
- In obese patients, one must correctly identify the 12th rib to avoid inadvertently entering the thoracic cavity.
- Projection of the iliac crest over the L4 pedicle prevents a lateral approach at this level.
- L5–S1 is carefully considered from a direct lateral approach due to neurovascular structures.
- Check the AP view routinely to monitor patient shifting throughout surgery.
- Longer and wider implants are more biomechanically stable. When placing an implant, one must traverse the ring apophysis, and the implant should be 1–2 mm longer than the vertebral body.

## Conclusion

When employed judiciously, the direct lateral transpsoas approach can be a useful method for safely placing a large interbody device which can be useful for indirect decompression, deformity correction, and providing a large area for fusion. In order to effectively perform this approach, it is critical to understand indications, advantages, disadvantages, surgical anatomy, patient positioning, imaging, and neuromonitoring. As this approach becomes more widespread, the neuromonitoring systems, retractors, and implants will likely become more reliable and result in improved patient safety.

## References

1. Ozgur BM, Aryan HE, Pimenta L, Taylor WR. Extreme Lateral Interbody Fusion (XLIF): a novel surgical technique for anterior lumbar interbody fusion. Spine J. 2006;6(4):435–43.
2. McAfee PC, Regan JJ, Peter Geis W, Fedder IL. Minimally invasive anterior retroperitoneal approach to the lumbar spine. Emphasis on the lateral BAK. Spine (Phila Pa 1976). 1998;23(13):1476–84. https://doi.org/10.1097/00007632-199807010-00009.

3. Pimenta L, Coutinho E, Barraza JCS, Oliveira L. Lateral XLIF fusion techniques. In: Yue JJ, Guyer R, Johnson JP, Khoo LT, Hochschuler SH, editors. Comprehensive treatment of the aging spine. Philadelphia: Elsevier; 2011. p. 408–12. https://doi.org/10.1016/B978-1-4377-0373-3.10061-2.
4. Phillips FM, Isaacs RE, Rodgers WB, et al. Adult degenerative scoliosis treated with XLIF: clinical and radiographical results of a prospective multicenter study with 24-month follow-up. Spine (Phila Pa 1976). 2013;38(21):1853–61.
5. Mobbs RJ, Phan K, Malham G, Seex K, Rao PJ. Lumbar interbody fusion: techniques, indications and comparison of interbody fusion options including PLIF, TLIF, MI-TLIF, OLIF/ATP, LLIF and ALIF. J Spine Surg. 2015;1(1):2.
6. Oliveira L, Marchi L, Coutinho E, Pimenta L. A radiographic assessment of the ability of the extreme lateral interbody fusion procedure to indirectly decompress the neural elements. Spine (Phila Pa 1976). 2010;35(26S):S331–7.
7. Elowitz EH, Yanni DS, Chwajol M, Starke RM, Perin NI. Evaluation of indirect decompression of the lumbar spinal canal following minimally invasive lateral transpsoas interbody fusion: radiographic and outcome analysis. Minim Invasive Neurosurg. 2011;54(5–6):201–6. https://doi.org/10.1055/s-0031-1286334.
8. Ahmadian A, Deukmedjian AR, Abel N, Dakwar E, Uribe JS. Analysis of lumbar plexopathies and nerve injury after lateral retroperitoneal transpsoas approach: diagnostic standardization: a review. J Neurosurg Spine. 2013;18(3):289–97.
9. Cahill KS, Martinez JL, Wang MY, Vanni S, Levi AD. Motor nerve injuries following the minimally invasive lateral transpsoas approach: clinical article. J Neurosurg Spine. 2012;17(3):227–31. https://doi.org/10.3171/2012.5.SPINE1288.

# Chapter 15
# Adjunctive Analgesia Methods

Ashley Nguyen and Trevor Myers

## Introduction

Patients undergoing complex spine surgery present many anesthetic challenges, including but not limited to opiate dependence, opioid-induced hyperalgesia, and multiple medical comorbidities. Enhanced recovery after surgery (ERAS) protocols are well established in colorectal, joint arthroplasty, and gynecologic surgery. The concept of the ERAS protocol encompassing the preoperative, intraoperative, and postoperative periods was first described in 1997 by Kehlet et al. as a multimodal approach to control and optimize postoperative pathophysiology and rehabilitation [1]. Application of ERAS to spinal surgery has been relatively recent, and consensus guidelines from the ERAS society were published in 2021 [2].

The ERAS protocol begins with preoperative optimization regarding nutrition, functional status, and management of medical comorbidities such as smoking cessation, anemia management, alcohol consumption cessation, and modification of fasting guidelines. Preemptive analgesia is accomplished with oral premedication that can include acetaminophen, gabapentinoids, and nonsteroidal anti-inflammatories when appropriate depending on the procedure and surgeon preference.

Intraoperatively, there are multiple evidence-based anesthetic considerations when implementing an ERAS protocol. The ideal regimen does not rely solely on opioids for postoperative pain management, as many spine patients have a significant history of opioid exposure from previous surgeries and chronic pain and may have opioid dependence. In addition, the extensive coverage of the national opioid epidemic has made patients understandably concerned about their exposure during and after surgery. Most concerning may be that the opioid therapeutic window is narrowed in opioid-dependent patients, making these patients vulnerable to serious

A. Nguyen (✉) · T. Myers
Dominion Anesthesia LLC, Arlington, VA, USA

© The Author(s), under exclusive license to Springer Nature Switzerland AG 2023

J. R. O'Brien et al. (eds.), *Lumbar Spine Access Surgery*,
https://doi.org/10.1007/978-3-031-48034-8_15

side effects as well as suboptimal analgesia. Anesthetic interventions specific to complex spine surgery can be divided into pharmacologic adjuncts and regional anesthesia techniques.

## Pharmacologic Adjuncts

Ketamine is a commonly used adjunct medication. It acts primarily as an N-methyl-d-aspartate antagonist with profound analgesic and dissociative properties. A large body of work in animals demonstrates that ketamine can block the development of opioid tolerance and opioid-induced hyperalgesia. Side effects include hypersalivation, hallucination, and lowering of the seizure threshold. Ketamine protocols for surgery include a bolus of up to 0.5 mg/kg prior to incision and then an infusion of 5–10 mcg/kg/min during longer procedures. These protocols may reduce cumulative opioid requirements for the first 24 to 48 h and may even reduce cumulative opioid consumption at 6 weeks [3].

Lidocaine is another useful intravenous adjunct. It is an amide local anesthetic that possesses analgesic, anti-hyperalgesic, and anti-inflammatory properties [4]. Clinical benefits in trials focus on abdominal surgery and report decreased rates of ileus, decreased visual analog scale pain scores, and lower cumulative opioid consumption 0–72 h after surgery [5]. In major spine surgery, perioperative lidocaine infusion was found to reduce pain scores and was noninferior compared with placebo. At 1 and 3 months after surgery, patients receiving lidocaine infusion reported improved quality of life as measured by the Acute Short-Form 12 Health Survey [6]. A typical lidocaine infusion is 1–2 mg/min. Although rare, lidocaine toxicity can include neurologic changes and cardiac dysrhythmias. Care should be taken to discontinue the lidocaine infusion quickly to allow prompt emergence.

Other adjuncts include magnesium 1–2 g administered as a slow bolus and muscle relaxants such as diazepam 5–10 mg or methocarbamol 500–1000 mg intravenously. Dexmedetomidine, a selective alpha-2 agonist, has mild analgesic properties and minimal respiratory depression.

## Regional Anesthesia Techniques

The incorporation of regional anesthetic techniques has been a significant addition to modern spine surgery. Regional anesthesia has long been a mainstay of postoperative pain control in extremity surgery and has become commonplace over the last two decades in thoracic and abdominal surgery as well. Intrathecal or epidural analgesia can significantly reduce opioid requirements and improve the patient experience [2]. A recently described regional technique useful in minimally invasive spine surgery is the erector spinae plane (ESP) block. This was first described in 2016 by Forero et al. as a novel technique for the treatment of a patient with thoracic neuropathic pain [7]. They described two applications of the ESP block which achieved multi-dermatomal sensory blockade. Proposed mechanisms of action include neural blockade and central inhibition through spread of local anesthetic to the paravertebral or epidural space, immunomodulatory effects of the local anesthetics, or spread via mechanosensory properties of the thoracolumbar fascia [8].

The ESP block can be performed under ultrasound preoperatively or after induction of general anesthesia. Preoperatively, the patient can be positioned sitting, lateral, or prone depending on operator preference (Fig. 15.1). If the patient is prone, a roll should be placed under the stomach to improve visualization. An ultrasound probe is used to visualize the transverse processes of the spine and the erector spinae complex at the desired level (Fig. 15.2). A linear probe can be used at both the thoracic and lumbar levels, but a curvilinear probe provides better visualization in the lumbar region due to the increased depth of the transverse process. If the block is performed after induction, the transverse process can be visualized under fluoroscopy. The needle is advanced until it touches the transverse process, and the local anesthetic is injected in 5-mL increments with intermittent aspiration to ensure there is no intravascular spread. On average, 20 mL of local anesthetic will achieve blockade of four dermatomes at the lumbar level and slightly more at the thoracic level due to the thinner ESP complex. Complications of this technique are similar to those with other nerve blocks, including, but not limited to, local anesthetic toxicity,

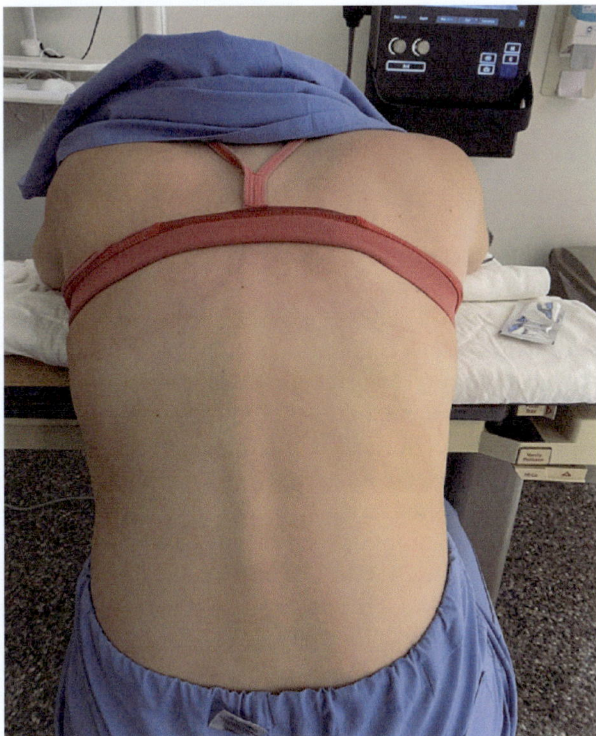

**Fig. 15.1** Patient positioned sitting for erector spinae plane block

**Fig. 15.2** Erector spinae plane complex layered over hyperechoic line of the transverse process indicated by the arrow

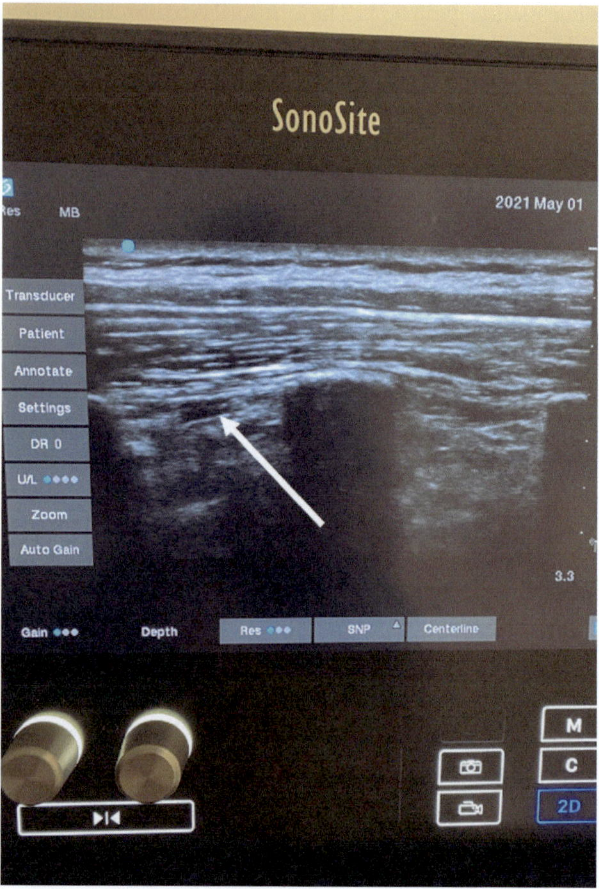


nerve injury, vascular injury, or pneumothorax if the needle is advanced too far past the transverse process.

For anterior or lateral minimally invasive spine approaches, the quadratus lumborum (QL) block is appropriate. It has been successfully used to provide analgesia for hip surgery, colorectal surgery, lower extremity amputation, breast reconstruction, radical nephrectomy, and lower extremity vascular surgery [9–14]. The QL block can be performed with the patient in the lateral position with a curvilineal probe just above the iliac crest (Fig. 15.3). Depending on the volume of local anesthetic administered, sensory blockade of the abdominal wall from T7–L2 has been described in multiple case reports. In contrast to a transverse abdominus plane (TAP) block, the QL block provides some degree of visceral analgesia in addition to somatic analgesia. The proposed mechanism of local anesthetic spread is via the fascial planes that follow the QL and psoas muscles through the medial and arcuate ligaments and aortic hiatus of the diaphragm, thus forming the endothoracic fascia [15].

**Fig. 15.3** Patient positioning for quadratus lumborum block with a curvilinear probe positioned just above iliac crest, angled caudad

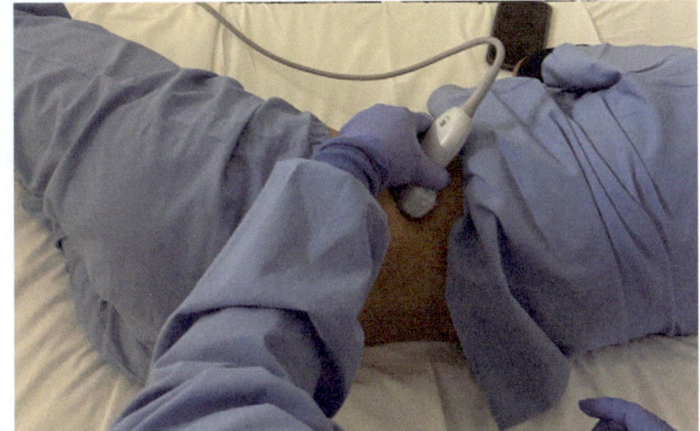

**Fig. 15.4** QL1 block with arrow indicating the plane of the transverse abdominus terminating into the QL where local anesthetic should be injected. *QL* quadratus lumborum, *EO* external oblique, *IO* internal oblique, *TA* transverse abdominus

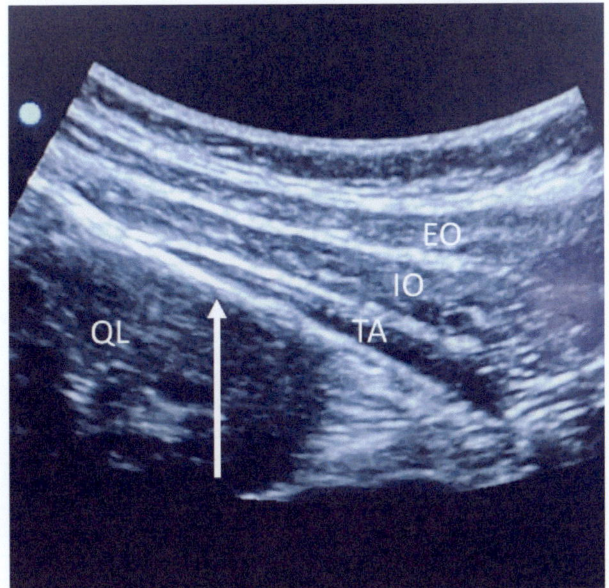


There are three subtypes of the QL block, described by Blanco et al. [16]. They include:

QL1: also known as a lateral TAP block. The local anesthetic is injected just after the termination of the transverse abdominus and internal oblique muscles adjacent to the QL, pictured below.

QL2: the local anesthetic is injected at the posterolateral aspect of the QL deep to the erector spinae complex.

QL3: also called the anterior QL block. In this approach, the local anesthetic is injected deep into the QL in the plane between QL and psoas muscles anteriorly.

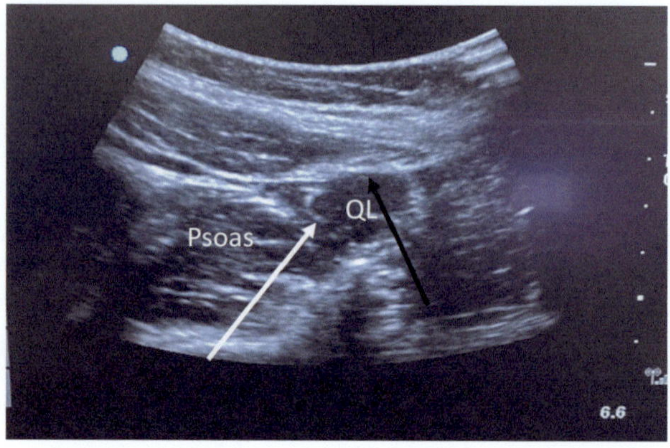


**Fig. 15.5** Black and white arrows indicate tissue planes for deposition of local anesthetic for QL2 and QL3 blocks, respectively. *QL* quadratus lumborum

There is currently insufficient evidence to recommend one approach over the other. There is, however, some risk of lower extremity weakness particularly with the QL3 block (Figs. 15.4 and 15.5) [11].

## Conclusion

Anesthesia for minimally invasive spine surgery should include preoperative oral analgesics, intravenous nonnarcotic adjuncts listed above, and the consideration of incorporating a regional anesthetic technique. The overarching goal is to provide optimal analgesia while minimizing reliance on narcotics in a challenging patient population.

## References


1. Kehlet H, et al. Multimodal approach to control postoperative pathophysiology and rehabilitation. Br J Anaesth. 1997;78:606–17.
2. Debono B, Wainwright T, Wang M, et al. Consensus statement for perioperative care in lumbar spinal fusion: enhanced recovery after surgery recommendations. Spine J. 2021;21(5):729–52.
3. Loftus RW, Yeager MP, Clark JA, Brown JR, Abdu WA, Sengupta DK, Beach ML. Intraoperative ketamine reduces perioperative opiate consumption in opiate-dependent patients with chronic back pain undergoing back surgery. Anesthesiology. 2010;113:639–46. https://doi.org/10.1097/ALN.0b013e3181e90914.
4. Baussier M, Delbos A, Maurice-Szamburski A, et al. Perioperative use of intravenous lidocaine. Drugs. 2018;78:1229–46.
5. Dunn L, Durieux ME. Perioperative use of intravenous lidocaine. Anesthesiology. 2017;126:729–37. https://doi.org/10.1097/ALN.0000000000001527.
6. Farag E, Ghobrial M, Sessler DI, Dalton JE, Liu J, Lee JH, Zaky S, Benzel E, Bingaman W, Kurz A. Effect of perioperative intravenous lidocaine administration on pain, opioid consumption, and quality of life after complex spine surgery. Anesthesiology. 2013;119:932–40.

7. Forero M, Adhikary SD, Lopez H, Tsui C, Chin KJ. The erector spinae plane block: a novel analgesic technique in thoracic neuropathic pain. Reg Anesth Pain Med. 2016;41(5):621–7.
8. Chin KJ, El-Boghdadly K. Mechanisms of action of the erector spinae plane (ESP) block: a narrative review. Can J Anaesth. 2021;68(3):387–408.
9. Shaaban M, Esa WA, Maheshwari K, Elsharkawy H, Soliman LM. Bilateral continuous quadratus lumborum block for acute postoperative abdominal pain as a rescue after opioid-induced respiratory depression. A A Case Rep. 2015;5:107–11.
10. Elsharkawy H, Salmasi V, Soliman LM, Esa WAS, Blanco R. Anterior quadratus lumborum block versus transversus abdominis plane block with liposomal bupivacaine: a case report. J Anesth Crit Care Open Access. 2016;6:1–5.
11. Ueshima H, Otake H. Lower limb amputations performed with anterior quadratus lumborum block and sciatic nerve block. J Clin Anesth. 2017;37:145.
12. Spence NZ, Olszynski P, Lehan A, Horn JL, Webb CA. Quadratus lumborum catheters for breast reconstruction requiring transverse rectus abdominis myocutaneous flaps. J Anesth. 2016;30:506–9.
13. Chakraborty A, Goswami J, Patro V. Ultrasound-guided continuous quadratus lumborum block for postoperative analgesia in a pediatric patient. A A Case Rep. 2015;4:34–6.
14. Watanabe K, Mitsuda S, Tokumine J, Lefor AK, Moriyama K, Yorozu T. Quadratus lumborum block for femoral-femoral bypass graft placement: a case report. Medicine (Baltimore). 2016;95:e4437.
15. Dam M, Moriggl B, Hansen CK, Hoermann R, Bendtsen TF, Børglum J. The pathway of injectate spread with the transmuscular quadratus lumborum block: a cadaver study. Anesth Analg. 2017;125:303–12.
16. Blanco R, Børglum J. Truncal blocks: quadratus lumborum blocks. In: Krige A, Scott MJP, editors. Analgesia in major abdominal surgery. Cham: Springer; 2018. p. 163–75.

**Part V**
**Intraoperative Complications for Lumbar
Spine Access Surgery**

# Chapter 16
# Arterial Complications

Amanda L. Chin, Jesus G. Ulloa, and Jonathan Schoeff

## Introduction

Anterior fusion of the lumbar spine has become an increasingly popular procedure to treat spinal pathology. These operations often utilize a team approach involving spine surgeons and spinal access or exposure surgeons (i.e., vascular or general surgeons) given the proximity of the spine to the abdominal vasculature. Exposure and mobilization of the iliac vein and artery, aorta, or inferior vena cava require meticulous dissection and familiarity with the retroperitoneal space.

Numerous studies describe the incidence of minor and major vascular injuries during anterior and lateral exposure of the lumbar spine. The overall rate of vascular injury is low, and venous injuries occur more commonly than arterial injuries [1]. However, arterial injuries may have devastating consequences, most of which are categorized as major vascular injuries. Arterial injury sequelae are primarily thromboembolic in nature, but direct arterial injuries, formation of arterial pseudoaneurysms, and arteriovenous fistulas have also been reported [1–3]. Exposure at the L4–L5 level has been associated with the highest incidence of vascular injury [1, 4]. Goals following arterial injury focus on durable hemostasis and restoration of distal flow following disruption of the arterial vasculature. Open and endovascular techniques have been described [1–3, 5, 6].

While arterial injuries are reported in the literature during anterior spine surgery, these injuries can and should be extremely rare. Emphasizing patient evaluation and

A. L. Chin
Perelman School of Medicine, University of Pennsylvania, Philadelphia, PA, USA

J. G. Ulloa (✉)
University of California Los Angeles, Los Angeles, CA, USA
e-mail: gro.rtcdemfscu@aollu.susej

J. Schoeff
Rocky Mountain Advanced Spine Access, Lone Tree, CO, USA

© The Author(s), under exclusive license to Springer Nature Switzerland AG 2023

J. R. O'Brien et al. (eds.), *Lumbar Spine Access Surgery*,
https://doi.org/10.1007/978-3-031-48034-8_16

procedural selection and a thorough understanding of patient specific vasculature including location, orientation, preexisting arterial disease, and prior vascular interventions, along with attention to critical intraoperative perfusion assessments and meticulous technique, should all but eliminate arterial injuries and their sequelae.

## Diagnosis and Intraoperative Monitoring

Prior to the start of any anterior spinal procedure, preoperative distal pulses should be documented. The addition of routine pulse oximetry monitoring of the left lower extremity is a useful adjunct for detection of thrombosis and embolism during spinal surgery [7]. During retraction of the left common iliac artery, the pulse oximetry waveform may be blunted or lost, and a timer may be started to measure total ischemic time. It is important to note that this is a qualitative measure, and the waveform is what guides the access surgeon. Intraoperative neuromonitoring (IOM) is often utilized by spine surgeons, and while somatosensory-evoked potentials (SSEPs) may provide insight into vascular occlusion resulting in ischemia, it is critical to understand the significant time delay required to see changes in SSEPs. Complete occlusion of the left common iliac artery, as reflected by loss of pulse oximetry waveform, does not result in a significant decrease (>50%) in SSEP amplitudes (the primary measure of ischemia) for 12–15 min. Relying on IOM may supplement, but should not supplant, the use of continuous pulse oximetry. With dampening or loss of waveform, the first maneuver should be to assess perfusion status by checking peripheral pressure via standard blood pressure cuff or arterial cannulation if available. Pharmacologically increasing the systolic blood pressure to a level 30–50 mmHg higher than the initial patient blood pressure readings may resolve dampened waveforms. This requires close and constant communication with the anesthesia team throughout the procedure. If the waveform remains dampened despite elevating the blood pressure, intermittent retractor release may be necessary. Additional maneuvers may include adjusting retractors directly on arterial vessels or the use of handheld retractors to allow for constant adjustment of retraction forces. Upon release of retraction devices, incomplete return of pulse oximetry and waveform readings suggests arterial vasospasm, injury, or thrombosis that warrants further investigation.

In contrast to thrombotic complications, arterial lacerations and avulsions are often immediately recognized intraoperatively with profuse bleeding. If clinical suspicion of arterial injury is high postoperatively, additional imaging such as duplex arterial ultrasound, computed tomography (CT), or angiography should be pursued.

## Arterial Injuries and Management

Arterial injuries have been reported to occur in 0.45% to 1.5% of cases and generally present as iliac artery thromboses [4–6]. In one study evaluating the incidence of left iliac artery thrombosis, 6 patients out of 1315 (0.45%) undergoing anterior lumbar surgery between 1997 and 2002 were identified from a prospective database [5]. All underwent exposure at the L4–L5 level. Thrombosis in five of these patients was diagnosed intraoperatively, and one was diagnosed in the post-anesthesia recovery unit. In two of the patients where thrombosis was not clinically obvious, decreased pulse oximetry levels and measurement of ankle-brachial index confirmed the diagnosis. All patients who were identified underwent attempts at mechanical thrombectomy via left femoral approach; one patient required repair of an intimal tear. In two of these patients, thrombectomy was unsuccessful and ultimately required a bypass procedure to restore flow (one femoral-femoral, one axillo-femoral). Two patients also required fasciotomies for subsequent compartment syndrome [5].

Endovascular techniques may also be employed in the management of arterial thrombosis. Percutaneous common femoral access under ultrasound guidance ipsilateral or contralateral to the thrombotic event may permit passage of a mechanical aspiration system for suction embolectomy with real-time visualization of clot extraction. On-table delivery of a thrombolytic agent via a multi-hole infusion catheter permits local thrombolysis and clot softening for mechanical aspiration. However, the risk of bleeding in the context of the index spine procedure must be weighed with the thrombolytic benefits of alteplase administration, further emphasizing the necessary partnership between the operating spine surgeon and the spinal access surgeon. It is the authors' experience and recommendation to perform mechanical or suction embolectomy but avoid the use of thrombolytics, locally and most certainly systemically, as bleeding into a fixed space such as the epidural space is likely to have devastating neurological consequences.

Arterial thromboses are hypothesized to result from arterial retraction and stretching, leading to small intimal tears that provoke thrombosis [1]. While intraoperative heparin is widely administered during the perioperative period in vascular surgery, increased risk of bleeding during concomitant spine surgery limits its use. However, a prospective study conducted by Sim et al. suggests that the administration of heparin may be safe to help prevent thrombotic events during anterior lumbar spine surgery [8]. While the overall estimated blood loss was significantly higher for the heparin study group compared to the non-heparin group, only prosthesis use and the spinal level treated were found to be related to blood loss on multivariable regression analysis. Mobilization of the left iliac artery as close as possible to the femoral canal may reduce intimal injury and stretch. This is a useful maneuver when significant traction on the iliac artery is necessary, and near immediate loss of pulse oximetry waveform is encountered even with minimal retraction; however, this is not routinely necessary and should only be utilized when indicated [5]. This avoids over-dissection in the retroperitoneum, which may result in extensive scarring, making revision surgery more difficult. Vasospasm due to arterial irritation from retraction may mimic the symptoms of acute arterial thrombosis. Papaverine or other vasodilators may be administered via the access surgeon's preferred route to distinguish spasm from thrombosis [5, 7]. Should there be a persistent loss of pulse oximetry waveform despite the release of retraction, a thrombotic complication should be further investigated and is guided by lower extremity evidence of malperfusion. With advances in imaging technology, it may be prudent to complete the primary spine procedure, close the incision, and obtain a perioperative CT angiography, which may aid in characterizing thrombotic or other arterial complications prior to directed surgical intervention. This can be achieved with the patient still intubated, allows for more detailed surgical planning specific to the arterial anatomy, and permits an endovascular approach as opposed to an open exploration of the zone of the arterial injury.

For major aortoiliac lacerations or injuries that are not amenable to direct suture repair, endovascular techniques with stenting are an effective alternative. In one study examining the long-term results of endovascular repair at a single center between 1997 and 2010, seven patients were treated for aortic or iliac artery injuries following discectomy, including lacerations, pseudoaneurysms, and arteriovenous fistulas [2]. Six of the seven reported cases involved the common iliac vessels (four left common iliac artery, two right common iliac artery). For all procedures, femoral access was established percutaneously or after surgical exposure for stent exclusion of the iliac artery injury. The use of an iliac limb, a self-expanding stent graft extension from the aorta into the external iliac artery often used in bifurcated endovascular graft devices to treat unfavorable seal zones, may also be considered. Intravascular ultrasound is a useful adjunct in the identification of arterial intimal injury, planning for stent graft implant diameter, and stent graft deployment while limiting the total dose of intravascular contrast administration. Similarly, aortic stent graft repair is also a feasible treatment option in the rare instance of aortic injury during lumbar interbody fusion [1]. In these cases, suture temporization and packing may slow the resultant hemorrhage for the patient to be repositioned and endovascular access obtained in the rare event that an aortic injury is not technically accessible through the existing incision.

Injury to the lumbar arteries is another possible complication of spinal surgery. A case report describing the formation of a left L2 lumbar artery pseudoaneurysm after lateral interbody fusion demonstrates the use of spinal angiography and embolization [3]. The patient was transferred 2 days after a lateral lumbar interbody fusion with hemorrhagic shock and a large retroperitoneal hematoma discovered on CT. Angiography demonstrated an irregular contour of the proximal left L2 lumbar artery adjacent to a fixation screw, suggesting traumatic pseudoaneurysm. This was ultimately treated with platinum coils and liquid embolization.

## Concomitant Aortoiliac Vascular Disease and Spinal Surgery

As advances in both spinal prostheses and endovascular devices for abdominal aortic aneurysm repair progress, there will be a growing cohort of patients with prior endovascular aortic repair (EVAR) who will undergo lumbar interbody fusion [9]. Preoperative vascular imaging is of increased utility in this group. It will help to better understand the aortoiliac anatomy after endograft deployment, which could contort the vessels and affect the relationship between anatomical structures, such as the level of the aortic bifurcation. While extensive aortoiliac mobilization following EVAR has been shown to be safe, careful dissection and control are necessary to avoid complications [9]. Furthermore, early postoperative follow-up imaging to confirm stent graft patency and assess for the presence of a new endoleak is recommended. Postoperative imaging with contrast-enhanced CT to confirm the absence of new endoleak or stent graft migration within 1 month following spinal exposure is recommended. Patients who have undergone prior aortoiliac revascularization via inline reconstruction (aortoiliac or aortobifemoral bypass) may represent prohibitive risk to spinal access as compared to patients who have undergone extra-anatomic reconstruction (axillobifemoral bypass) given the presence of scar tissue from prior dissection, particularly involving the artery/vein interface.

In addition to aneurysmal disease, aortoiliac occlusive disease and symptomatic degenerative disc disease may co-exist, as both affect older patients. Aortoiliac pathology and spinal conditions are treated separately. Endovascular interventions for aortoiliac occlusive disease may permit future vascular manipulation for spinal access if spinal pathology presents lifestyle-limiting symptoms following treatment of arterial disease. Routine manipulation of prior endograft-treated vessels is not recommended. Untreated aortoiliac arterial disease, which is often characterized by diffuse calcification and stenosis, may be considered in experienced hand, as there are maneuvers, mentioned previously in this chapter, to offset direct tension forces on arterial anatomy. The presence of severe aortoiliac arterial pathology should also serve as a reminder regarding the critical importance of preoperative evaluation and multidisciplinary coordination of care including close communication between spine and spinal access surgeons prior to indicating this type of approach.

## Conclusion

While arterial injuries during anterior and lateral spinal surgery are rare, they can have potentially devastating consequences if not identified and treated early by experienced surgeons familiar with vascular structures in the retroperitoneal space. Thrombosis is the most common arterial complication in the acute to subacute setting, but other arterial injuries resulting in pseudoaneurysms or arteriovenous fistulas require a high clinical suspicion postoperatively for diagnosis. Severe aortoiliac pathology should not preclude anterior spine surgery but does require critical attention to detail in the planning and procedural selection phase. In the rare event that an arterial injury does occur in the setting of anterior spine surgery, immediate recognition, followed by thorough evaluation via duplex ultrasonography and/or CT angiography to further characterize the nature of the arterial complication, with subsequent definitive intervention, is likely to achieve the best outcome. In an age with progressive advancement in surgical technology, endovascular treatment will continue to play an increasing role in the treatment of arterial injuries during spinal surgery.

## References


1. Brau SA, Delamarter RB, Schiffman ML, Williams LA, Watkins RG. Vascular injury during anterior lumbar surgery. Spine J. 2004;4(4):409–12. https://doi.org/10.1016/j.spinee.2003.12.003.
2. Canaud L, Hireche K, Joyeux F, et al. Endovascular repair of aorto-iliac artery injuries after lumbar-spine surgery. Eur J Vasc Endovasc Surg. 2011;42(2):167–71. https://doi.org/10.1016/j.ejvs.2011.04.011.
3. Santillan A, Patsalides A, Gobin YP. Endovascular embolization of iatrogenic lumbar artery pseudoaneurysm following extreme lateral interbody fusion (XLIF). Vasc Endovasc Surg. 2010;44(7):601–3. https://doi.org/10.1177/1538574410374655.
4. Hamdan AD, Malek JY, Schermerhorn ML, Aulivola B, Blattman SB, Pomposelli FB. Vascular injury during anterior exposure of the spine. J Vasc Surg. 2008;48(3):650–4. https://doi.org/10.1016/j.jvs.2008.04.028.
5. Brau SA, Delamarter RB, Schiffman ML, Williams LA, Watkins RG. Left iliac artery thrombosis during anterior lumbar surgery. Ann Vasc Surg. 2004;18(1):48–51. https://doi.org/10.1007/s10016-003-0104-0.
6. Kulkarni SS, Lowery GL, Ross RE, Ravi Sankar K, Lykomitros V. Arterial complications following anterior lumbar interbody fusion: report of eight cases. Eur Spine J. 2003;12(1):48–54. https://doi.org/10.1007/s00586-002-0460-4.
7. König MA, Leung Y, Jürgens S, MacSweeney S, Boszczyk BM. The routine intra-operative use of pulse oximetry for monitoring can prevent severe thromboembolic complications in anterior surgery. Eur Spine J. 2011;20(12):2097–102. https://doi.org/10.1007/s00586-011-1900-9.
8. Sim EM, Claydon MH, Parker RM, Malham GM. Brief intraoperative heparinization and blood loss in anterior lumbar spine surgery. J Neurosurg Spine. 2015;23(3):309–13. https://doi.org/10.3171/2014.12.SPINE14888.
9. Ullery BW, Thompson P, Mell MW. Anterior retroperitoneal spine exposure following prior endovascular aortic aneurysm repair. Ann Vasc Surg. 2016;35:207.e5–9. https://doi.org/10.1016/j.avsg.2016.01.048.

# Chapter 17
# Venous Complications

Daniel H. Newton, Natalie Wall, Jonathan Schoeff, Devin Zarkowsky, and Aparna Baheti

## Introduction

The first documented anterior exposure for spinal surgery dates back to the 1930s, with operative correction of spondylolisthesis occurring via a transperitoneal approach [1, 2]. Shortly thereafter, this was followed by a retroperitoneal approach in the surgical treatment of tuberculosis (Pott disease) [3].

As contemporary techniques have evolved, anterior spine surgery has become an accepted approach for addressing a multitude of pathologies [4, 5]. An anterior approach allows direct access to ventral spinal pathology while sparing the paraspinal anatomy. The anterior approach is also associated with improved postoperative mobility, decreased chronic muscle pain, and avoidance of posterior surgical scar [6].

However, safe anterior spinal access surgery requires detailed knowledge of both standard and anomalous anatomy, as the majority of immediate procedure-related complications are access-related. Anterior surgery puts the vascular, visceral, muscular, lymphatic, urogenital, and peripheral nervous structures at risk, rather than neural elements, dura, and vertebrae which are more likely to be injured in a posterior approach [6].

D. H. Newton · N. Wall
Division of Vascular Surgery, Virginia Commonwealth University, Richmond, VA, USA

J. Schoeff (✉)
Rocky Mountain Advanced Spine Access, Lone Tree, CO, USA
e-mail: jschoeff@rockymountainasa.com

D. Zarkowsky
Scripps Clinic, La Jolla, CA, USA

A. Baheti
Vascular and Interventional Radiologist, Tacoma, WA, USA

© The Author(s), under exclusive license to Springer Nature Switzerland AG 2023

J. R. O'Brien et al. (eds.), *Lumbar Spine Access Surgery*, https://doi.org/10.1007/978-3-031-48034-8_17

Thus, anterior spine surgery facilitates an opportunity for multispecialty collaboration among spine and spinal access surgeons including a variety of sub-specialists (including general, cardiothoracic, vascular, and urologic surgeons) for safe exposure [7]. In the United States, a two-surgeon approach has become routine; however, globally, this is not always the case. This two-surgeon approach allows for anterior access to be obtained by a surgeon well-adept to complex vascular mobilization to mitigate the risk of major vascular injury [7–9].

Vascular injury represents an infrequent but potentially catastrophic complication during anterior exposure, and it is imperative that both spinal and exposure surgeons use all available information and resources to anticipate and prevent vascular complications. Venous injuries in particular lead to most of the associated morbidity and, in some cases, mortality [10].

## Incidence and Mechanisms of Venous Injuries

Venous injury is the most common vascular complication during anterior approach spine surgery [11]. The incidence of these injuries varies widely in the literature. In an early series of 102 cases, Baker et al. reported an overall venous injury rate of 15.6%, including 11 tears of the common iliac vein, 4 tears of the inferior vena cava (IVC), and a single avulsion of the iliolumbar vein [12].

A more recent retrospective analysis of 269 anterior exposures at a single institution reported a similar incidence, with injuries to named veins occurring in 10.4% of anterior exposures. Fifty-three percent of these injuries were found to involve the left common iliac vein [10]. Furthermore, a retrospective analysis of 482 anterior exposures at a single institution found that an intraoperative vascular injury occurred in 11% of patients, with the majority of these injuries being avulsed branches or direct lacerations of the left common iliac vein [13].

A high-volume single-surgeon series of 1315 procedures by Brau et al. published in 2003 reported a markedly lower incidence of 1.4% major venous injury [11]. Finally, a review of 21 case series found that the incidence of vascular injury in anterior spine exposure ranged widely from 0.3% to 20%, with venous laceration being the most common example [14]. Venous injuries are most frequently encountered at the left common iliac vein, with injury to the IVC and iliolumbar vein occurring substantially less frequently [4, 14].

The lack of standardized definitions for major venous injury has previously hampered reliable comparison in the published literature. In 2019, the Society of Spinal Access Surgery reached a consensus definition of major and minor venous injuries (Fig. 17.1) which will allow for improved reporting and comparison.

In addition to the heterogeneity implicit in defining venous injury, the relative volume of more challenging cases also substantially affects the overall incidence of vascular injury in any series. A straightforward L5–S1 exposure below the common iliac confluence and aortic bifurcation should generally carry a very low risk of venous injury as there is access between the vessels with minimal retraction.

**Society of Spinal Access Surgery Major and Minor Venous Injuries**

| Major Injury | Minor Injury |
| --- | --- |
| One or more of the following:<br>  >300mL blood loss directly attributable to injury<br>  Need for formal repair, primary* or endovascular<br>  Alteration of initial operative plan as direct result of injury | One or more of the following:<br>  <300mL blood loss directly attributable to injury<br>  Requiring more than topical hemostatic application* for control |
| *excluding small injuries treatable by a single suture | *examples include single suture or hemoclip application |

**Fig. 17.1** Major and minor venous injuries according to the Society of Spinal Access Surgery

Exposure of the L4–L5 level, however, has been reported to carry a 2.7-fold increase of vascular injury due to the extensive rightward retraction and mobilization of the left common iliac vein that is often necessary [13, 15]. However, even the assumption that venous anatomy is constant across levels and patients can lead to miscalculation in anticipating vascular relationships relative to the spine. A more practical framework, admittedly more labor-intensive in the research setting, is to categorize exposure levels based on the targeted spine level based on its relationship to the vascular anatomy. This concept of "spinovascular" anatomic relationships will be more thoroughly discussed later in this chapter. The relative complexity of an individual practice will affect the overall incidence of vascular injury, and a higher volume of revision surgery and cases with significant inflammation adjacent to the disc space may substantially increase the incidence of venous injury [16, 17].

The mechanism of venous injury can be separated into three categories including branch avulsion (typically from the side wall and thereby technically less difficult to access and control), tears from vein adherence or over-retraction (typically from the posterior aspect of a vessel which creates a difficult, if not impossible, scenario to manage with conventional primary repair methods), and direct venous injury during spinal instrumentation (which may or may not occur in accessible locations for conventional repair). Branch avulsion can occur even in routine exposure of the spine. During standard left-sided retroperitoneal access to the spine when approaching the lateral border of the left common iliac vein for release and rotation, the left common iliac vein is often retracted to the patient's right. The iliolumbar and ascending lumbar veins, typically arising from the left common iliac vein, may be divided to allow for sufficient mobilization. Indeed, many expert access surgeons recommend routine division of these structures for typical L4–L5 exposure before attempting significant retraction of the left common iliac vein [11, 16]. Failure to divide these branches along with over-retraction may result in avulsion of the branch at its confluence with the iliac vein, ultimately leading to hemorrhage. Insufficient mobilization of a venous structure can also result in tears of the major vein itself at the point of maximum tension, which can be at a retractor blade, but may also be remote from it, especially when the vein is adherent to the underlying spine. Lastly, direct injury to the vein can occur from instruments and implants during discectomy or interbody insertion. It is not always possible to fully protect vascular structures with retractor blades without impeding the spinal portion of the procedure. However, the typical scenario for this type of injury is when aggressive use of sharp instruments such as a Cobb elevator or osteotome in conjunction with mallet use pushes the patient away from a table-mounted retractor, allowing the vein to slip under a retractor blade and become lacerated.

## Assessing the Risk for Venous Injury

One of an access surgeon's primary merits is a reduction in vascular injury incidence and blood loss [11]. Further, since any injury to the major veins involved in anterior spine exposure may result in significant hemorrhage, the primary goal of an access surgeon should be avoiding venous injury in the first place. Predicting which patients are at highest risk and which area of an exposure will pose challenges allows for optimal patient selection, alterations in the surgical technique, or particular care and attention during certain parts of the exposure.

The risk of venous injury arises from two broad patient factors. The first is the patient's native vascular anatomy and its location relative to the spine, also known as the spinovascular relationship. Because this anatomy is highly variable, understanding a patient's particular spinovascular layout is extremely useful in performing safe and expeditious access surgery. Fortunately, cross-sectional imaging with magnetic resonance imaging (MRI) is routinely obtained in most patients undergoing spine surgery. In particular, the T2-weighted sequence shows the vasculature well. This can be used to plan the mobilization and retraction strategy and stratify difficulty.

A commonly encountered example of the importance of the spinovascular relationship is in the variable position of the iliocaval junction. This confluence frequently sits significantly higher or lower than the typical position just above the L4–L5 disc space. A high iliocaval confluence may allow an approach to L4–L5 between the common iliac vessels, making the exposure similar to a standard L5–S1 level. Alternatively, a particularly low iliocaval confluence may make an L5–S1 exposure more technically challenging, requiring rightward mobilization of the lateral border of the left common iliac vein. In this case, the risk of venous injury would be similar to that of a standard L4–L5 exposure. Failing to identify these common deviations from the normal spinovascular anatomy on preoperative imaging can result in both ineffective and inefficient exposure at best and unnecessary hemorrhage at worst.

Iliocaval congenital anomalies are also frequently encountered, which can also be identified on preoperative imaging and thereafter facilitate further intraoperative planning (Fig. 17.2).

The second patient factor to consider is retroperitoneal inflammation, which is often related to the spinal pathology being treated. Prior retroperitoneal surgery, particularly laparoscopic inguinal hernia repairs, can make initial access to the

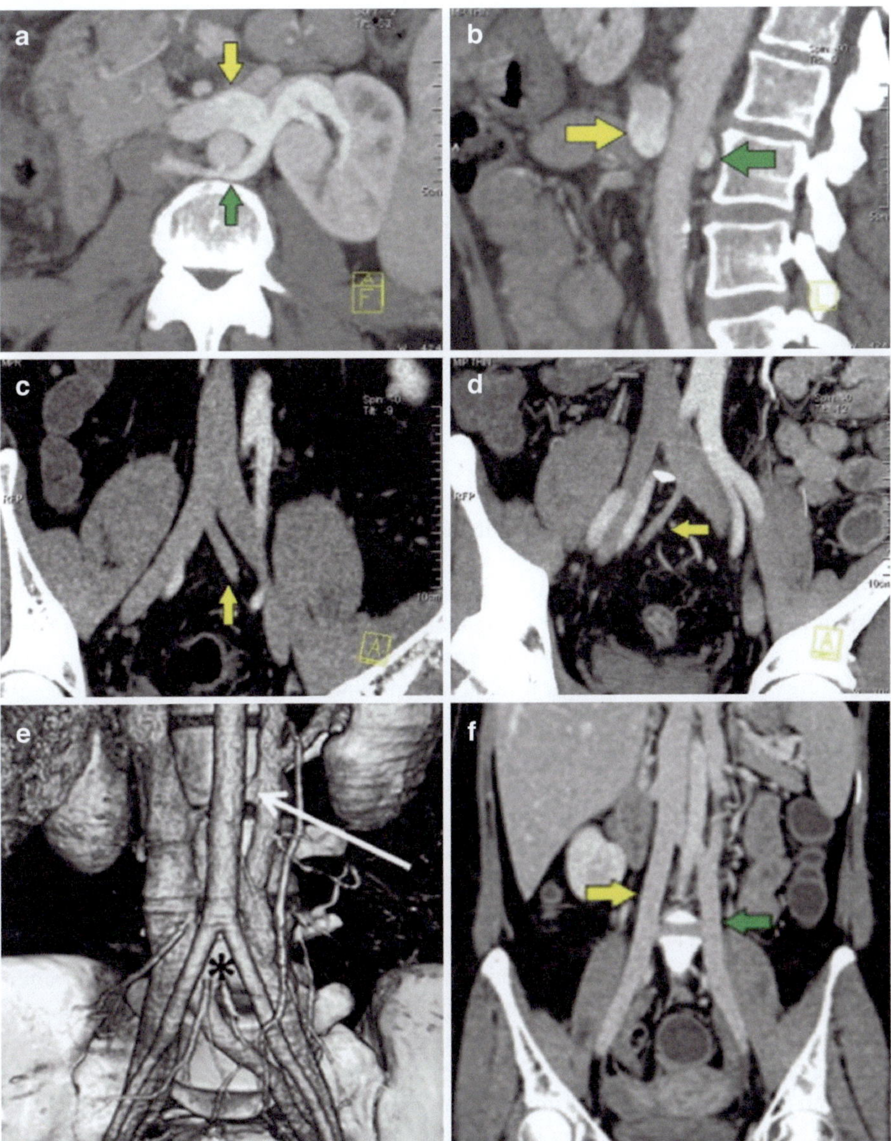

**Fig. 17.2** Congenital variants of iliocaval anatomy. (*a, b*) Retroaortic left renal vein. Encountered usually in L2–L3 exposure, this can be most easily avoided by using an oblique approach; (*c, d*) anomalous drainage of the internal iliac veins. An internal iliac vein can be ligated to facilitate anterior L5–S1 exposure when necessary; (*e, f*) duplicated IVC. There are multiple variations of the duplicated IVC, with varying drainage of the internal and external iliac veins. There are often bridging veins which may require ligation to access the desired disc space. Typically, duplicate IVC will make anterior access less difficult; (*g, h*) left-sided IVC. L4–S1 anterior access can be obtained from the right retroperitoneum. Higher levels are best accessed from an oblique approach

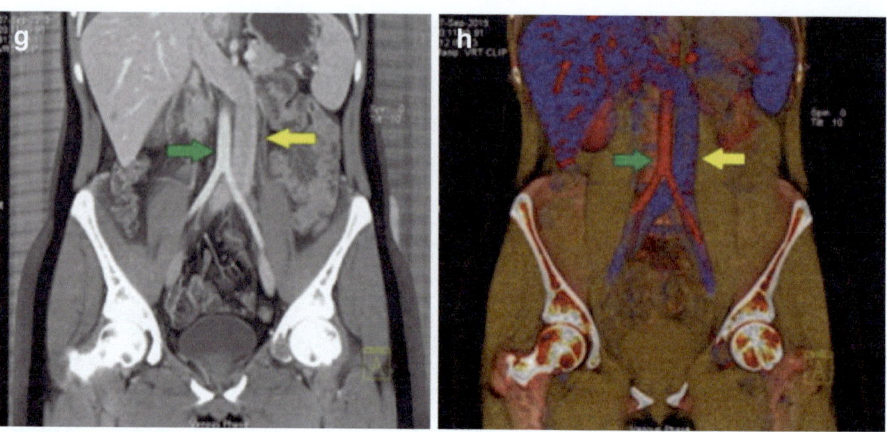

**Fig. 17.2** (continued)

correct retroperitoneal plane difficult and may impact the deep retroperitoneal dissection.

Prior retroperitoneal surgery that includes lymph node dissection can obliterate normal tissue planes and further complicate the exposure and mobilization of soft tissue (e.g., ureter) and vascular structures. Therefore, this category of prior surgical procedures should be viewed as a relative contraindication based on spinal access surgeon experience. Furthermore, pelvic and retroperitoneal radiation therapy can also obliterate normal tissue planes, make the vessel walls friable, and impede mobilization of vascular structures. The retroperitoneum can be profoundly scarred and hostile even in the absence of prior surgery. Intense inflammatory reactions affecting the retroperitoneum may be encountered in a prior history of diverticulitis (which may have been treated with nonoperative management) or pancreatitis.

A history of open or endovascular treatment of the aortoiliac junction and iliac arteries should also be considered with a great deal of trepidation. Depending on the spinal access surgeon's experience, this history is likely to be an absolute contraindication; however, primary vascular intervention may be considered a relative contraindication to anterior spine exposure if the spinal access surgeon has acquired significant experience. In the case of postsurgical arterial vasculopathy, it is imperative to have a thorough discussion with the primary spine surgeon to first determine necessity of an anterior spine procedure versus alternative approaches. A critical, in-depth review and understanding of the patient's spinovascular anatomy are also necessary, along with a detailed risk assessment and conversation with the patient. A stent or native vessel thrombosis might be easily managed under normal circumstances but would now require anticoagulation or thrombolytics in the setting of recent spine surgery which can begin a catastrophic sequence potentially leading to epidural bleeding.

While not affecting initial access to the posterior retroperitoneal space, spondylosis-related inflammation can also hinder mobilization of the vessels [4, 6]. These changes can be seen on T2-weighted sequence MRI. Effacement of the normal fat plane between the vessels and the spine indicates that this tissue plane may be obliterated by inflammatory changes [18]. This "loss of retrovascular fat plane" serves as a sign that severe vascular adherence is likely present and tedious dissection will likely be required in order to achieve successful exposure. The presence of osteophytes is not only associated with an inflammatory rind that may adhere to the vessel walls but can physically obstruct vein mobilization. Similarly, spondylolisthesis is associated with inflammatory changes and can place the veins under increased baseline tension.

Lumbar discitis and osteomyelitis present particularly challenging pathology for anterior and oblique exposures due to the intense inflammatory response. Proper timing of the operation can reduce the level of difficulty. Exposure and discectomy in the early acute phase of the infection are typically not substantially more challenging than spondylosis cases. Surgery in the late phase of the infection after a long course of antibiotics, while still challenging, can be safely performed. However, the period between the early acute phase and the chronic phase of the disease is fraught, and intervention during this period puts the patient at highest risk for significant vascular injury due to the intense inflammatory rind.

## Management of Venous Bleeding

The best way to prevent significant venous bleeding is, of course, to avoid venous injury in the first place. Veins should be mobilized in the plane directly on the annular ring or anterior longitudinal spinal ligament. This allows the vein to be moved with some protective perivenous tissue and is often the freest plane. When the vein is adherent to the spine, meticulous dissection is necessary to separate them. It is easy to put the vein under enough tension that it flattens and cannot be distinguished from the surrounding tissue. For this reason, frequent relaxing of the vein retraction allows the surgeon to visualize the vein edge and maintain safe dissection. It is necessary to remain extra vigilant for small nutrient or segmental veins during this type of dissection, as avulsion of these vessels is often what begins the cascade toward serious bleeding.

When a venotomy occurs, initial bleeding control should be obtained with direct pressure at or adjacent to the site of injury using sponge sticks or other atraumatic means. Venous injuries often appear worse than they are. The initial impetus to "do something definitive" often leads to propagation of an initially small and manageable problem. Furthermore, the nature of vein retraction in the area of injury also creates high venous pressure zones in and around the primary operative field. This phenomenon often necessitates the counterintuitive practice of relaxing or releasing retraction to relieve venous obstruction and decrease the intravenous pressure at the site of injury. This may be necessary to reduce bleeding and allow for further assessment of the injury. However, care must be taken to balance sufficient exposure to address the bleeding while also relieving focal venous hypertension near the injury. Similarly, placing the patient in Trendelenburg position decreases venous pressure and therefore bleeding. These maneuvers allow for further assessment of the injury, opportunity to organize the response, and time for anesthesia providers to replace volume [19]. If not already in use, intraoperative blood salvage should be established in anticipation of further blood loss while definitive control is established.

Small venous defects are less difficult to manage than large lacerations but can still cause significant blood loss. Attempts at clamping the vessel or direct suture repair frequently lead to tearing of an already thinned vein and worsening of the situation. Instead, control of these injuries is best achieved with topical hemostatic agents rather than direct suture repair. Ideal hemostatic agents for this purpose are not overly bulky, have structural integrity, and adhere slightly to the vein surface. Oxidized cellulose-based or collagen-based agents are cost-effective initial choices for this type of bleeding. When this fails, it is the authors' preference to use a fibrin sealant patch. This strategy can be employed reliably for lacerations up to 4 mm and sometimes larger with adjunctive maneuvers [11].

Nutrient vessel bleeding can be difficult to control when the vessels are avulsed flush from the vertebral body. Bipolar vessel sealers are a useful initial maneuver. Should this fail, liquid thrombin hemostatic agents can be forcefully injected into the nutrient foramina with the applicator. While only a small amount of material will actually enter the channel, the expanding nature of the hemostatic agent will typically seal off the hemorrhaging vessels.

When faced with major venous bleeding, the approach to repair depends on when the injury occurs in the course of the operation and injury location. Injuries that occur during the exposure portion of the case are most common. Once a linear laceration of a venous injury is sutured, one must consider the potential for further injury if the vein must be retracted again. In some cases, the vein cannot be retracted without a high likelihood of further tearing and can make proceeding with the spinal portion of the operation impossible. Therefore, suture repair of a major venous injury that occurs with initial dissection should be delayed, whenever possible, until the spine portion of the case is completed. Even significant venous injuries can usually be temporized with hemostatic agents, utilizing retractor blades, and even hand-held retractors, to maintain pressure on the injury. This allows the case to proceed and may even result in definitive hemostasis.

If a major, hemodynamically significant, venous injury occurs before initiating spinal instrumentation, it may be prudent to terminate the case after a discussion between spine and access surgeons. This decision is not taken lightly, since the patient has already undergone a surgical insult and will still be left with their spinal pathology. Abortion of an anterior spine procedure as a result of major vascular injury should be considered a major spinal access surgical complication. Injuries during spinal instrumentation and fusion can almost always be temporized until completion of this portion of the procedure with sponge stick control, packing, and use of handheld retractors.

Once the spinal portion of the procedure is complete, retractors can slowly be released and the vessels reassessed for hemostasis. Should neither hemostatic agents, direct pressure, nor time be sufficient for hemostasis, easily accessible tears (i.e., small, anterior) can be directly repaired with suture, typically 5-0 polypropylene. A minimally invasive cardiac needle driver has the necessary length and is low-profile enough to suture difficult-to-reach vessels. A traditional laparoscopic knot-pusher also facilitates suture repair in minimally invasive spine surgery exposures. Should this repair begin to fail, it is best to avoid becoming fixated on placing increasingly desperate sutures or clamps and instead consider endovascular adjuncts. Likewise, inaccessible venous injuries, such as those on the posterior wall, are best managed with endovascular repair should topical agents fail.

## Endovascular Adjuncts to Venous Bleeding

Switching from open surgery to an endovascular procedure can be awkward and time-consuming. For patients deemed elevated risk of venous injury based on pre-operative history and imaging, it may be worth obtaining preemptive venous access. At a minimum, it is the authors' practice to prep in bilateral groins for all spinal access surgical procedures. Placing 5 French sheaths in the bilateral common femoral veins and guidewires into the IVC adds negligible morbidity to the procedure and dramatically expedites endovascular control in high-risk settings. Direct hemostasis with emergent groin access can also be readily achieved. A moderately stiff wire such as a J-tipped 0.035" Amplatz wire facilitates easier passage of sheaths, balloons, and stents even in altered venous anatomy.

In the event of bleeding, 10 French, radiopaque-tipped 25-cm sheaths can be placed over the wires. These sheaths are easy to identify in a crowded surgical field, and the 10 French size provides the flexibility to deploy any of the commercially available venous stents. Contrast injection via the bilateral sheaths provides accurate visualization of the IVC bifurcation and can allow for rescue of a covered right common iliac vein from inaccurate left iliac vein deployment.

There is little evidence to support one stent over another in the situation of a bleeding iliac vein, but sizing considerations do inform stent selection. The size of the injured vein can be measured on preoperative imaging. However, in an emergency, the size can be based on normal vein anatomy. The common iliac veins are typically 14 to 16 mm, while the external iliac veins measure 12 to 14 mm [20]. The infrarenal IVC is 20 to 24 mm. Standard self-expanding covered stents are not typically large enough in diameter for the common iliac vein. Balloon-mounted stents can be secondarily expanded up to 16 mm after initial deployment, though this is a precarious maneuver for a stent that has little apposition to the vessel wall until it is post-dilated. Additionally, these balloon-expandable stents are stainless steel and can be crushed with further retraction. Nonetheless, they have been used with success [19]. Endoprostheses used for iliac limb extension in endovascular aneurysm repair have also been used successfully [21]. These endografts require excessively long coverage since most of these devices have a minimal length of about 8 cm. Additionally, they may not be readily available at all centers in useful diameters and lengths.

Bare metal stents are readily available in sizes useful for treating iliac vein injury; however, it cannot be overstressed that while there may be long-term benefits to uncovered stents, utilization of this technique must be considered and employed quite early in this management strategy as significant blood loss and ensuant coagulopathy will uniformly doom this strategy to failure. Multiple authors have noted the perhaps surprising usefulness of uncovered stents for these injuries, especially in combination with topical hemostatic agents. Because uncovered stents are less thrombogenic than covered stents, they may additionally have an advantage in long-term patency. The mechanism for their hemostatic utility is likely by two routes. First, they reduce the venous pressure at the site of bleeding by restoring the normal caliber to the vein. Second, they provide a scaffold for the externally applied hemostatic agents or tissue to provide a seal. Venous-specific stents are now available and have the advantage of appropriate sizing for iliac veins and good resistance to compression, making them safe to retract. In general, self-expanding stents should recoil back to their original shape even if compressed during retraction, but these venous-specific stents have particularly good hoop strength and resist compression (Fig 17.3).

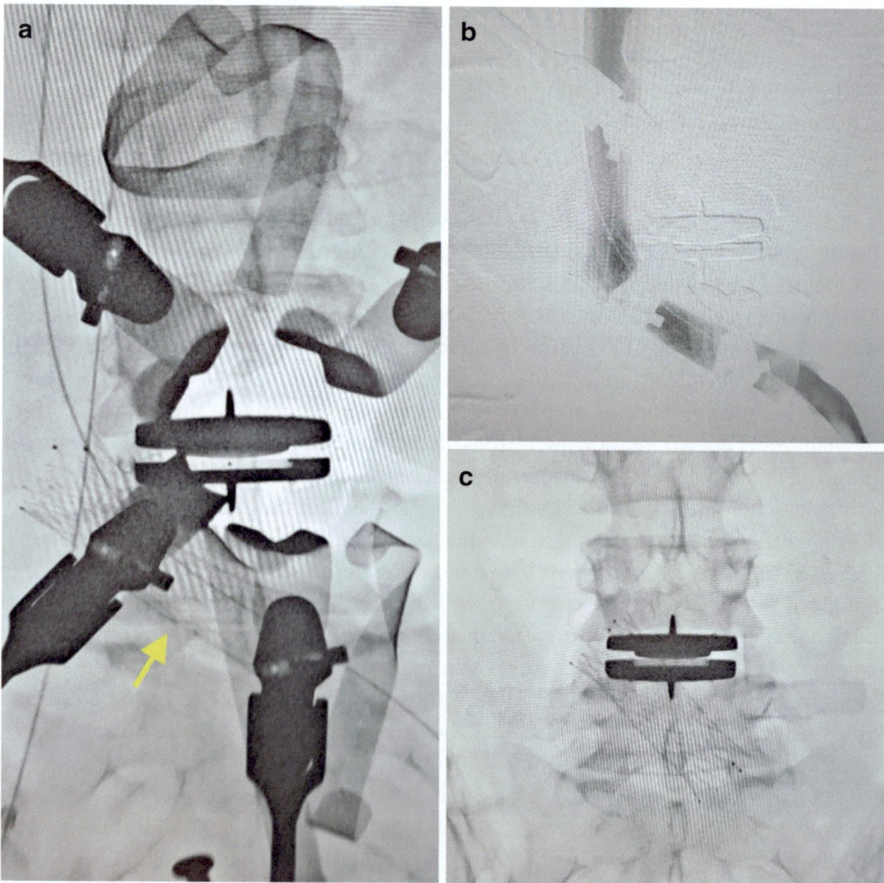

**Fig. 17.3** Anterior spine exposure performed on a patient with a pre-existing left common iliac vein stent. (**a**) Retractor blades can be placed directly on the stented left iliac vein (yellow arrow) without causing significant stent compression. (**b**) Patency of the stent under retraction is demonstrated with venography. (**c**) The self-expanding stent returned to its pre-operative shape without requiring angioplasty

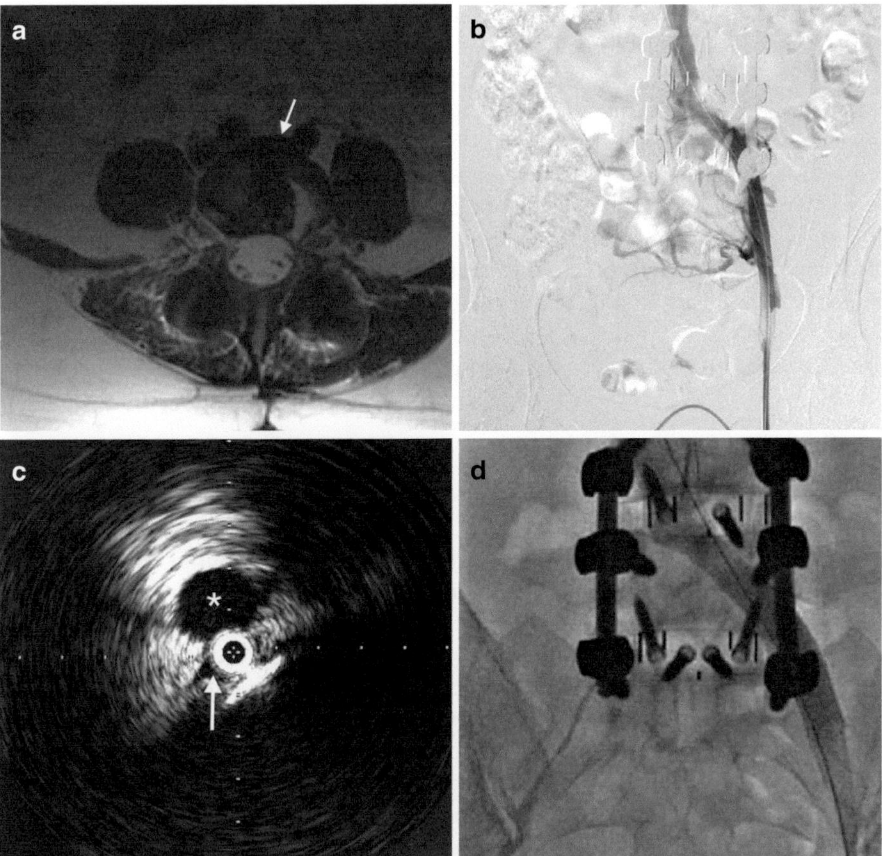

**Fig. 17.4** Case of a 42 year-old female following prior posterior instrumentation with subsequent two-level pseudoarthrosis with screw fracture. She underwent anterior exposure for L4-S1 ALIF and replacement of her posterior fixation. (**a**) The left common iliac vein was severely adherent to the L4–L5 disc (white arrow) and was lacerated during screw placement to affix the ALIF cage. The majority of blood loss (1500mL) was attributed to further exposure and direct control of the vein in order to perform suture repair. (**b**) Postoperative venography was performed based on an abnormal venous duplex. This showed cross-pelvic collaterals, though the stenosis was not directly visualized. (**c**) Intravascular ultrasound demonstrated significant stenosis of the left common iliac vein (white arrow) adjacent to the right common iliac artery (white star). (**d**) Stenosis was successfully resolved with angioplasty and stenting. This case illustrates the drawbacks to suture repair, including higher volume blood loss due to the need for more extensive exposure, as well as the high risk of late thrombosis or stenosis requiring intervention

Completion venography can be performed after visual hemostasis is obtained. A sheath may be left in place postoperatively to perform a delayed venogram, confirming no further extravasation and no thrombus formation. The appearance of significant venous collaterals suggests ongoing luminal compromise that may be further assessed with intravascular ultrasound (Fig 17.4). When ready to remove the sheath, hemostasis can be achieved at the venous access site with gentle manual pressure.

It is wise to consider an endovascular solution during the initial injury event. Long-term stent patency is significantly higher when stenting is performed in the absence of significant deep vein thrombosis; thus, preservation of lumen and restoration of normal flow should be the goal in the case of venous injury [22]. With the ability to place venous stents, ligation or oversewing of a major named vessel is largely an outdated and unnecessarily morbid conclusion to iatrogenic venous injury.

## Thrombotic Complications

Venous thromboembolism (VTE) is a well-known complication of anterior access spine surgery. Postoperative deep vein thrombosis (DVT) following anterior lumbar interbody fusion (ALIF) is reported to occur in 1–5% of patients, although this may underestimate the overall incidence since clinically occult venous thrombosis is well known to occur [23–25]. Patient risk factors for VTE include obesity, advanced age, underlying malignancy, and oral contraceptive use. Intraoperative vein retraction can cause intimal trauma from vessel stretch and stasis from compression that leads to thrombosis. Overt venous injury and subsequent repair, however, would seem to be most associated with postoperative DVT [24–26]. Not surprisingly then, typical spinovascular relationships seen at L4–L5 requiring significant medial mobilization, and more extensive exposures, are associated with increased incidence of DVT.

In addition to avoiding venous injury, surgeons can prevent DVT by employing early mobilization and intermittent pneumatic compression devices routinely. While more controversial, chemoprophylaxis may additionally lower the incidence of perioperative DVT. One of the benefits of anterior approach spine surgery in this regard is the very low risk of epidural hematomas, assuming that a minimally invasive and/or percutaneous approach to posterior fixation has been utilized. This is a critical point and requires close communication between spinal access surgeon and primary spine surgeon to individually assess not only bleeding risk but also implications of bleeding into a closed space such as the epidural space. In general, the authors recommend a more aggressive chemoprophylaxis whenever possible; however, to date, there remains no consensus on an appropriate regimen, duration, and further management. Since most patients undergoing general pelvic and abdominal surgery would receive preoperative chemoprophylaxis based on various applicable societal guidelines, it would follow that patients having anterior access spine procedures may similarly benefit. Although a modestly underpowered, non-randomized study, Vint et al. reported no major bleeding complications and no

DVT in a group of 200 patients who were given a prophylactic dose of low molecular weight heparin on the evening before ALIF [27]. The North American Spine Society gives a weak recommendation based on low-quality evidence: "These therapies should be considered carefully and on an individual case-by-case basis, as use may place patients at increased risk of bleeding complications" [28]. While many spine surgery teams do not routinely provide preoperative chemoprophylaxis, most will initiate postoperative therapy within 2–5 days depending on individualized patient risk.

Patients who have had an intraoperative venous injury are at a substantially elevated risk of venous thrombosis and may benefit from a more aggressive prophylaxis regimen. While there is no consensus on postoperative antithrombotic therapy in the management of these patients, extrapolations can be made from similar conditions such as trauma. Though there is mixed data regarding whether or not anticoagulation prevents pulmonary embolism after venous injury, many trauma studies support this practice. Frank et al. performed a multicenter retrospective study evaluating 435 trauma patients with penetrating venous injury which demonstrates withholding of VTE prophylaxis to be associated with higher rates of VTE formation and a 28% increase in incidence for each postoperative day that chemoprophylaxis is not given [29]. Therefore, it is best to initiate DVT chemoprophylaxis in the early postoperative period, especially when a venous injury occurs. These patients with venous injury likely benefit from extended prophylaxis, commonly using low-dose direct oral anticoagulants.

Currently, no consensus for postoperative DVT screening exists. Some institutions routinely screen all patients with intraoperative venous injury for lower extremity DVT prior to hospital discharge, while others evaluate patients based on clinical symptoms [24, 25]. Symptoms such as shortness of breath, hypoxia, lower extremity swelling, or tenderness should prompt vascular imaging [10]. Duplex ultrasound of the iliac veins is often impossible due to sonographic shadowing by bowel gas or retroperitoneal air following surgery. An iliac vein DVT can be subtly suggested based on abnormal duplex waveforms in the veins distal to the occlusion. These vein segments will lose their characteristic respiratory phasicity. When there is high clinical suspicion for iliac or caval thrombosis, a CT or MRI can be obtained. Shadowing from the adjacent hardware may still preclude accurate diagnosis, however. Venography is ultimately the gold standard diagnostic technique for iliocaval thrombosis.

While iliac vein thrombosis can be silent, symptomatic iliofemoral DVT is a morbid condition. It can lead to post-thrombotic syndrome in about one-third of patients, with presentation including leg swelling, venous claudication, and pain [30]. The mainstay of treatment for iliofemoral DVT remains therapeutic anticoagulation. Should the risk of bleeding be high, a careful titration of heparin can be initiated without an initial bolus. If bleeding develops, the heparin can be stopped or even reversed with protamine. If the risk of bleeding is prohibitively high, a retrievable IVC filter can be placed. As soon as the danger of bleeding has passed, standard anticoagulation should be initiated and the filter removed because of the risk of filter-associated IVC occlusion.

Catheter-directed therapies (CDT) provide an interventional alternative to standard anticoagulation [31]. These include catheter-directed thrombolysis, catheter-based mechanical thrombectomy, and pharmacomechanical thrombolysis. While some contemporary literature demonstrates CDT may be more effective in risk reduction of post-thrombotic syndrome when compared to systemic anticoagulation alone, the paucity of reproducible multicenter randomized controlled trials remains a barrier to widespread acceptance and application [32, 33]. Furthermore, since most thromboses are the result of venous injury and repair, these therapies may result in significant bleeding, and early endovascular intervention has not been commonly used. Once the patient is beyond the acute phase of a DVT, venoplasty and stenting of chronically thrombosed vein segments can be performed with good long-term outcomes [31, 34]. Considering the paucity of data surrounding these practices in the context of anterior spine surgery, conservative approaches remain the mainstay; however, it is the authors' experience that early intervention, including locally directed thrombolysis (mechanical and pharmacological) combined with venoplasty and stent, has been successful in select patients as early as 5–7 days postoperatively in the context of limb-threatening venous occlusion (i.e., phlegmasia cerulea dolens). In these cases, intervention is certainly limb-preserving, and these risky maneuvers may be justified. However, the success in these cases with limited morbidity should spark interest in the role of such maneuvers in less severe cases of postoperative DVT.

## Conclusion

Venous injuries remain the most feared and potentially devastating spine exposure-related complication. Avoiding venous injuries in the first place is the primary goal, since these injuries substantially increase the risk of morbidity from resulting post-thrombotic syndrome as well as perioperative mortality when severe hemorrhage cannot be quickly controlled. With careful planning, surgical technique, and prudent care of preventing venous injuries, significant morbidity and mortality can be minimized to 2% or less [15]. Treatment of significant injuries can often be accomplished with topical hemostatic agents alone, thus avoiding direct suture repair and further trauma. While primary sutured repair still has a role, it should largely be limited to small, accessible injuries with adequate exposure, with major vein ligation an extreme last resort.

Endovascular techniques can be used not only as salvage but also as a primary technique for venous reconstruction in the setting of anterior spine exposure. The use of endovascular treatment of venous bleeding with stents in conjunction with extravascular topical hemostatic agents may reduce morbidity and mortality and avoid the cascade of events that follows extensive DVT often seen with direct suture repair. With advances in hemostatic and endovascular therapies, future management of these injuries will likely trend further away from direct suture repair, especially as exposure techniques and spine instrumentation technology advance to allow less and less invasive surgery.

# References


 1. Capener N. Spondylolisthesis. Br J Surg. 1932;19(75):374–86.
 2. Burns BH. An operation for spondylolisthesis. Lancet. 1933;221(5728):1233. https://doi.org/10.1016/s0140-6736(00)85724-4.
 3. Ito H, Tsuchiya J, Asami G. A new radial operation for Pott's disease. J Bone Joint Surg. 1932;16(3):499–515.
 4. Czerwein JK Jr, Thakur N, Migliori SJ, et al. Complications of anterior lumbar surgery. J Am Acad Orthop Surg. 2011;19(5):251–8. https://doi.org/10.5435/00124635-201105000-00002. Erratum in: J Am Acad Orthop Surg. 2012;20(2):45a.
 5. Bateman DK, Millhouse PW, Shahi N, et al. Anterior lumbar spine surgery: a systematic review and meta-analysis of associated complications. Spine J. 2015;15(5):1118–32. https://doi.org/10.1016/j.spinee.2015.02.040.
 6. Samudrala S, Khoo LT, Rhim SC, et al. Complications during anterior surgery of the lumbar spine: an anatomically based study and review. Neurosurg Focus. 1999;7(6):e9. https://doi.org/10.3171/foc.1999.7.6.10.
 7. Ikard RW. Methods and complications of anterior exposure of the thoracic and lumbar spine. Arch Surg. 2006;141(10):1025–34. https://doi.org/10.1001/archsurg.141.10.1025.
 8. Ballard JL, Carlson G, Chen J, et al. Anterior thoracolumbar spine exposure: critical review and analysis. Ann Vasc Surg. 2014;28(2):465–9. https://doi.org/10.1016/j.avsg.2013.06.026.
 9. Asha MJ, Choksey MS, Shad A, et al. The role of the vascular surgeon in anterior lumbar spine surgery. Br J Neurosurg. 2012;26(4):499–503. https://doi.org/10.3109/02688697.2012.680629.
10. Zahradnik V, Lubelski D, Abdullah KG, et al. Vascular injuries during anterior exposure of the thoracolumbar spine. Ann Vasc Surg. 2013;27(3):306–13. https://doi.org/10.1016/j.avsg.2012.04.023.
11. Brau SA, Delamarter RB, Schiffman ML, et al. Vascular injury during anterior lumbar surgery. Spine J. 2004;4(4):409–12. https://doi.org/10.1016/j.spinee.2003.12.003.
12. Baker JK, Reardon PR, Reardon MJ, et al. Vascular injury in anterior lumbar surgery. Spine (Phila Pa 1976). 1993;18(15):2227–30. https://doi.org/10.1097/00007632-199311000-00014.
13. Hamdan AD, Malek JY, Schermerhorn ML, et al. Vascular injury during anterior exposure of the spine. J Vasc Surg. 2008;48(3):650–4. https://doi.org/10.1016/j.jvs.2008.04.028.
14. Inamasu J, Guiot BH. Vascular injury and complication in neurosurgical spine surgery. Acta Neurochir. 2006;148(4):375–87. https://doi.org/10.1007/s00701-005-0669-1.
15. Fantini GA, Pawar AY. Access related complications during anterior exposure of the lumbar spine. World J Orthop. 2013;4(1):19–23. https://doi.org/10.5312/wjo.v4.i1.19.
16. Fantini GA, Pappou IP, Girardi FP, et al. Major vascular injury during anterior lumbar spinal surgery: incidence, risk factors, and management. Spine (Phila Pa 1976). 2007;32:2751–8.
17. Wert WG Jr, Sellers W, Mariner D, et al. Identifying risk factors for complications during exposure for anterior lumbar interbody fusion. Cureus. 2021;13(7):e16792. https://doi.org/10.7759/cureus.16792.
18. Ng JP, Scott-Young M, Chan DN, et al. The feasibility of anterior spinal access: the vascular corridor at the L5–S1 level for anterior lumbar Interbody fusion. Spine (Phila Pa 1976). 2021;46(15):983–9. https://doi.org/10.1097/BRS.0000000000003948.
19. Schoeff JE, Israel TR, Green TJ, et al. Expedient endovascular hemorrhage control during anterior lumbar spinal exposure allows procedural completion in rescued patients. Ann Vasc Surg. 2022;78:377.e5–377.e10. https://doi.org/10.1016/j.avsg.2021.05.061.
20. Raju S, Buck WJ, Crim W, et al. Optimal sizing of iliac vein stents. Phlebology. 2018;33(7):451–7. https://doi.org/10.1177/0268355517718763.
21. Schneider JR, Alonzo MJ, Hahn D. Successful endovascular management of an acute iliac venous injury during lumbar discectomy and anterior spinal fusion. J Vasc Surg. 2006;44(6):1353–6. https://doi.org/10.1016/j.jvs.2006.07.049.

22. Murphy E, Gibson K, Sapoval M, et al. Pivotal study evaluating the safety and effectiveness of the abre venous self-expanding stent system in patients with symptomatic iliofemoral venous outflow obstruction. Circ Cardiovasc Interv. 2022;15(2):e010960. https://doi.org/10.1161/CIRCINTERVENTIONS.121.010960.

23. Oskouian RJ Jr, Johnson JP. Vascular complications in anterior thoracolumbar spinal reconstruction. J Neurosurg. 2002;96(1 Suppl):1–5. https://doi.org/10.3171/jns.2002.96.1.0001.

24. Ho VT, Martinez-Singh K, Colvard B, et al. Increased vertebral exposure in anterior lumbar interbody fusion associated with venous injury and deep venous thrombosis. J Vasc Surg Venous Lymphat Disord. 2021;9(2):423–7. https://doi.org/10.1016/j.jvsv.2020.08.006.

25. Garg J, Woo K, Hirsch J, et al. Vascular complications of exposure for anterior lumbar interbody fusion. J Vasc Surg. 2010;51(4):946–50.; ; discussion 950. https://doi.org/10.1016/j.jvs.2009.11.039.

26. Nourian AA, Cunningham CM, Bagheri A, et al. Effect of anatomic variability and level of approach on perioperative vascular complications with anterior lumbar interbody fusion. Spine (Phila Pa 1976). 2016;41(2):E73–7. https://doi.org/10.1097/BRS.0000000000001160.

27. Vint H, Mawdsley MJ, Coe C, et al. The incidence of venous thromboembolism in patients undergoing anterior lumbar interbody fusion: a proposed thromboprophylactic regime. Int J Spine Surg. 2021;15(2):348–52. https://doi.org/10.14444/8045.

28. Bono CM, Watters WC 3rd, Heggeness MH, et al. An evidence-based clinical guideline for the use of antithrombotic therapies in spine surgery. Spine J. 2009;9(12):1046–51. https://doi.org/10.1016/j.spinee.2009.09.005.

29. Frank B, Maher Z, Hazelton JP, et al. Venous thromboembolism after major venous injuries: competing priorities. J Trauma Acute Care Surg. 2017;83(6):1095–101. https://doi.org/10.1097/TA.0000000000001655.

30. Notten P, Ten Cate-Hoek AJ, Arnoldussen CWKP, et al. Ultrasound-accelerated catheter-directed thrombolysis versus anticoagulation for the prevention of post-thrombotic syndrome (CAVA): a single-blind, multicentre, randomised trial. Lancet Haematol. 2020;7(1):e40–9. https://doi.org/10.1016/S2352-3026(19)30209-1.

31. Sagris M, Tzoumas A, Kokkinidis DG, et al. Invasive and pharmacological treatment of deep vein thrombosis: a scoping review. Curr Pharm Des. 2022;28(10):778–86. https://doi.org/10.2174/1381612828666220418084339.

32. Enden T, Haig Y, Kløw NE, et al. Long-term outcome after additional catheter-directed thrombolysis versus standard treatment for acute iliofemoral deep vein thrombosis (the CaVenT study): a randomised controlled trial. Lancet. 2012;379(9810):31–8. https://doi.org/10.1016/S0140-6736(11)61753-4.

33. Vedantham S, Goldhaber SZ, Julian JA, et al. Pharmacomechanical catheter-directed thrombolysis for deep-vein thrombosis. N Engl J Med. 2017;377(23):2240–52. https://doi.org/10.1056/NEJMoa1615066.

34. Sharifi M, Mehdipour M, Bay C, et al. Endovenous therapy for deep venous thrombosis: the TORPEDO trial. Catheter Cardiovasc Interv. 2010;76(3):316–25. https://doi.org/10.1002/ccd.22638.

# Chapter 18
# Ureteral Injury

Daniel Mecca, Santosh Shanmuga, and Robert Mordkin

## Introduction

The ureters are retroperitoneal structures that drain urine from the renal pelvis of the kidneys to the bladder. The ureter originates at the ureteropelvic junction (UPJ), posterior to the renal artery and vein. The ureter then travels toward the pelvis along the psoas muscle. The ureter crosses over the iliac bifurcation before inserting into the trigone of the bladder. The ureter can be divided into three anatomic segments: the proximal ureter extends from the UPJ down to the sacroiliac (SI) joint, the middle ureter is the segment between the SI joint and the pelvic brim, and the distal ureter extends from the iliac vessels to the bladder [1].

Ureteral injuries, although uncommon, are a possible complication during any abdominal or pelvic surgery. Selzman et al. conducted a retrospective review of 165 ureteral injuries over a 20-year period [2]. They identified 165 injuries in 156 patients and found that upper ureteral injuries occurred in 3/165 patients (2%), middle ureteral injuries occurred in 12/165 patients (7%), and distal ureteral injuries occurred in 150/165 patients (91%) [2]. The high rate of injury to the distal ureter is not surprising considering the intimate relationship between the distal ureters and the pelvic vasculature, including the iliac vessels, uterine artery, and rectal arteries.

The blood supply to the upper third of the ureter comes from the aorta and the renal vessels and can be traced medial to the ureter. The blood supply to the bottom two-thirds of the ureter comes from the iliac, sacral, and lumbar vessels and can be traced lateral to the ureter. The location of the vascular supply to the ureter is

D. Mecca · S. Shanmuga
Walter Reed National Military Medical Center, Bethesda, MD, USA

R. Mordkin (✉)
Virginia Hospital Center, Arlington, VA, USA

© The Author(s), under exclusive license to Springer Nature Switzerland AG 2023

J. R. O'Brien et al. (eds.), *Lumbar Spine Access Surgery*,
https://doi.org/10.1007/978-3-031-48034-8_18

important to note as devascularization of the ureter is a common mechanism of injury and most often presents in a delayed fashion [1].

Ureteral injury severity can be graded on a scale from I to V. A grade I injury involves a hematoma or contusion without devascularization, a grade II injury involves less than 50% transection, a grade III injury involves more than 50% transection, a grade IV injury involves a complete transection with less than 2 cm of devascularization, and a grade V injury involves an avulsion with more than 2 cm of devascularization [3].

## Mechanism of Injury

Historically, ureteral injuries were most common during an anterior approach to the spine, as the ureter courses anterior to the psoas and just lateral to the vertebral bodies. The common iliac artery bifurcates at the L4 level, and the ureter has a more medial course while crossing over the iliac bifurcation. Ureteral injuries are much less common during a posterior approach to the spine as the ureter is anterior to the spinal column and the quadratus lumborum muscle in the retroperitoneum [4]. Minimally invasive techniques such as posterior, transforaminal, and lateral lumbar interbody fusion result in less bleeding and trauma but place the ureter in closer proximity to the dissection. The ureter is especially at risk at the L2–L3 level due to the loss of anatomic landmarks [4]. Patients who are thin, have advanced disc degeneration, or are undergoing revision with retroperitoneal scarring are at a higher risk for ureteral injuries [4].

A systematic review performed by Turgut et al. reviewed a total of 44 articles with 46 reported cases of ureteral injury during posterior or lateral spinal surgery [4]. The most common mechanism of injury was due to accidental perforation of the anterior longitudinal ligament or psoas major muscle with a rongeur-type instrument or advancing an instrument through the intertransverse space into the retroperitoneum in procedures such as discectomy or minimally invasive surgery. Most injuries were contralateral to the side of the discectomy (Fig. 18.1). Of note, out of 44 cases, only two cases were identified at the time of injury. Most of the cases had an interval of more than 1 week until time of diagnosis [4]. Thus, it is imperative that the surgeon be able to recognize the signs of a delayed ureteral injury in the postoperative patient.

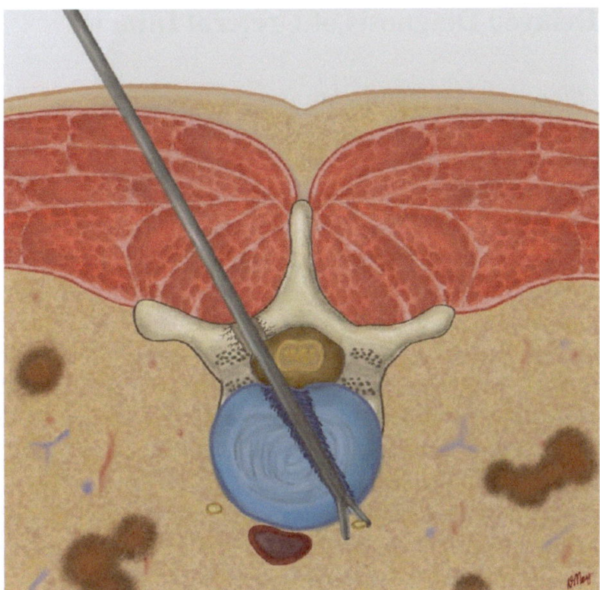

**Fig. 18.1** Mechanism of ureteral injury during posterior spinal surgery. Courtesy of Natalie May

## Early Diagnosis

Iatrogenic injury to the ureter is a feared complication of abdominal and spinal surgery. It has been postulated that prophylactic ureteral catheter or stent placement reduces the risk of ureteral injury. However, current literature suggests that ureteral catheter placement increases the rate of intraoperative diagnosis of a ureteral injury rather than preventing it [5]. An increase in intraoperative diagnosis may be useful as delayed diagnoses of ureteral injury result in significant morbidity and early detection of ureteral injuries leads to better outcomes. While placement of ureteral catheters may help increase recognition of ureteral injuries, there is no substitute for good surgical technique and care to help avoid ureteral injuries.

If ureteral injury is suspected and no prior ureteral catheters or stents were placed, a cystoscopy with retrograde pyelogram can be performed intraoperatively. A study performed by Vakili et al. demonstrated that cystoscopy with retrograde pyelogram had a 100% success rate of identifying a ureteral injury [6]. The protocol, which may differ depending on the institution, involves injecting a dye such as methylene blue, indigo carmine, or indocyanine green and evaluating for efflux of the dye into the urine. The use of intravenous dye alone had a 96% rate of diagnosing a ureteral injury [6]. Retrograde pyelogram with contrast is often performed at the time of cystoscopy to evaluate for ureteral obstruction or contrast extravasation, which is a clear indicator of ureteral injury. In summary, if ureteral injury is suspected intraoperatively, prompt urologic consultation for cystoscopy and potential retrograde pyelogram should be performed to prevent delayed diagnosis and associated complications.

## Delayed Diagnosis of Ureteral Injuries

Often, ureteral injuries are missed at the time of injury and present in a delayed fashion. This can be due to missed direct injury to the ureter, as well as thermal injury or vascular compromise of the ureter, which leads to delayed necrosis and sequelae such as urine leak or stricture formation. Most injuries are diagnosed 48–72 h after the initial procedure, with the patient exhibiting symptoms that lead to a clinical suspicion for possible ureteral injury. Clinically, the presenting symptoms may include microscopic or macroscopic hematuria, pyrexia, dysuria, abdominal pain, abdominal distention, flank pain, and signs of peritonitis. Serum studies may show leukocytosis and elevated serum creatinine levels due to resorption of extravasated urine. Some patients may even present with severe acute kidney injury or acute renal failure from an undetected ureteral injury. Of note, not all patients with ureteral injuries will exhibit hematuria, which can be absent in 15–45% of patients with ureteral injuries [7, 8].

As these clinical findings can be nonspecific, diagnostic studies are essential to make the correct diagnosis. The spectrum of diagnostic studies includes imaging procedures such as ultrasound (US), computed tomography (CT), or magnetic resonance imaging, as well as procedures such as ureteroscopy and retrograde pyelogram. At the time of ureteral injury, diagnosis is best made with intraoperative cystoscopy, ureteroscopy, and retrograde pyelogram, as detailed in the previous section. However, in the delayed postoperative setting, imaging studies are almost equally as sensitive to detecting ureteral injury and less invasive than a repeat procedure under anesthesia.

When there is concern for ureteral injury, it is important to notify the radiologist so that the right diagnostic imaging study may be performed. A triple-phase contrast-enhanced CT scan of the abdomen/pelvis with nephrogram and delayed excretory phases (performed 5–20 min after administration of contrast) is optimal to evaluate for ureteral injuries and their sequelae. The delayed excretory phase is essential for diagnosis. Urine opacification with contrast during the excretory phase will help delineate the course of the ureters, and the findings of extravasation of urine (urinoma) are highly suggestive of ureteral injury. Other radiologic findings that are concerning for ureteral injury include urinary ascites and ureteral obstruction/hydronephrosis. If any of these findings are seen on CT scan, urology should be consulted immediately for next steps in the management of the suspected ureteral injury.

Of note, urinomas can appear highly variable on CT scan and may not always opacify with contrast. Thus, urinomas are often misinterpreted as ordinary ascites, abdominal or pelvic hematomas or abscesses, seromas, cystic masses, or pancreatic pseudocysts. If a fluid collection is seen and there is still a high concern for suspected ureteral injury, the fluid collection may be percutaneously drained and the aspirate sent for a creatinine level. If the fluid creatinine is several times higher than the patient's serum creatinine, there should be a high suspicion for urine leak and thus a possible ureteral injury.

If CT scan is not available to evaluate a patient for suspected ureteral injury, renal/bladder US may be used in the interim setting. The ultrasonographic triad of hydronephrosis, ascites, and ipsilateral absent ureteral jet is suggestive for ureteral injury, though it is less sensitive than CT scan [9]. Finally, if imaging modalities are not available for evaluation or they are inconclusive, urology should be consulted to consider evaluation with direct visualization or retrograde pyelogram.

Early diagnosis of ureteral injury is paramount to avoid further complications, such as sepsis or kidney loss. The surgeon should be mindful of the potential for ureteral injury, especially if the intraoperative course was problematic, and move to establish a swift diagnosis when patients present with complications in the postoperative period.

## Short-Term Management

When ureteral injury is suspected or diagnosed, urology should be consulted immediately. From a surgical point of view, ureteral injuries can be classified as immediate if recognized at the time of injury or delayed if recognized in the postoperative period. For immediate recognition, intraoperative consultation to urology is preferred, as the urologist can come and directly assess the degree of injury. For minor or thermal injuries, initial management may consist of endoscopic double-J ureteral stent placement or percutaneous nephrostomy. If the injury is more severe, i.e., a complete transection or a large segment of injured ureter, the urologist may elect to perform a ureteral reconstruction.

It is also important to involve urology for ureteral injuries diagnosed in a delayed fashion. Management will be most likely consistent of initial urinary diversion with nephrostomy or ureteral stenting with plans for further urologic reconstruction at a later date. Additionally, if the patient has a large urinoma or large amounts of urinary ascites, percutaneous drainage may be necessary to avoid further complications or to assist with diagnosis. In the setting of severe ureteral injury, extremely delayed diagnosis, or inability to perform initial urinary diversion successfully, nephrectomy may be needed [10].

## Long-Term Management

If the patient is managed with initial urinary diversion (nephrostomy tube or ureteral stenting), they will need follow-up with urology to determine next steps of management and the potential need for further reconstruction. As above, in the setting of severe ureteral injury or extremely delayed diagnosis, nephrectomy may be unavoidable [10].

Early diagnosis, treatment, and repair provide increased renal preservation and can help avoid further complications. Additionally, early detection of ureteral injuries is associated with better operative outcomes. A meta-analysis of iatrogenic ureteral injuries among all surgical specialties revealed patients required fewer reconstructive operations (1.2 vs. 1.8, $p < 0.0006$) when the injury was identified intraoperatively versus postoperatively [2].

## Conclusion

Ureteral injury is an infrequent but severe complication of anterior and lateral lumbar spine surgery, and management of this complication is best approached by a multidisciplinary team involving the spine and access surgeons, radiology, and urology. Awareness of the possible injury and careful retroperitoneal exposure during surgery are crucial for prevention and early detection of ureteral injury. Prompt recognition of ureteral injuries with immediate diversion or repair results in the best outcomes for the patient, with fewer complications and preserved renal function.

## References


1. Haroon SA, Rahimi H, Merritt A, Baghdanian A, Baghdanian A, LeBedis CA. Computed tomography (CT) in the evaluation of bladder and ureteral trauma: indications, technique, and diagnosis. Abdom Radiol (NY). 2019;44(12):3962–77. https://doi.org/10.1007/s00261-019-02161-6.
2. Selzman AA, Spirnak JP. Iatrogenic ureteral injuries: a 20-year experience in treating 165 injuries. J Urol. 1996;155(3):878–81. https://doi.org/10.1016/s0022-5347(01)66332-8.
3. Moore EE, Cogbill TH, Jurkovich GJ, et al. Organ injury scaling. III. Chest wall, abdominal vascular, ureter, bladder, and urethra. J Trauma. 1992;33:337–9.
4. Turgut M, Turgut AT, Dogra VS. Iatrogenic ureteral injury as a complication of posterior or lateral lumbar spine surgery: a systematic review of the literature. World Neurosurg. 2020;135:280–96. https://doi.org/10.1016/j.wneu.2019.12.107.
5. Dumont S, Chys B, Meuleman C, Verbeke G, Joniau S, Van der Aa F. Prophylactic ureteral catheterization in the intraoperative diagnosis of iatrogenic ureteral injury. Acta Chir Belg. 2021;121(4):261–6. https://doi.org/10.1080/00015458.2020.1753148.
6. Vakili B, Chesson RR, Kyle BL, Shobeiri SA, Echols KT, Gist R, Zheng YT, Nolan TE. The incidence of urinary tract injury during hysterectomy: a prospective analysis based on universal cystoscopy. Am J Obstet Gynecol. 2005;192(5):1599–604. https://doi.org/10.1016/j.ajog.2004.11.016.
7. Palmer LS, Rosenbaum RR, Gershbaum MD, Kreutzer ER. Penetrating ureteral trauma at an urban trauma center: 10-year experience. Urology. 1999;54:34–6.
8. Perez-Brayfield MR, Keane TE, Krishnan A, Lafontaine P, Feliciano DV, Clarke HS. Gunshot wounds to the ureter: a 40-year experience at Grady Memorial hospital. J Urol. 2001;166:119–21.
9. Hung MJ, Huang CH, Chou MM, Liu FS, Ho ES. Ultrasonic diagnosis of ureteral injury after laparoscopic-assisted vaginal hysterectomy. Ultrasound Obstet Gynecol. 2000;16:279–83.
10. Omidi-Kashani F, Mousavi SM. Total ureteral avulsion leading to early nephrectomy as a rare complication of simple lumbar discectomy: a case report. SICOT J. 2015;1:30.

# Part VI
# Postoperative Care for Lumbar Spine Access Surgery

# Chapter 19
# Pain Management

Nirguna Thalla, Andrew Wondra, and Mehul J. Desai

## Introduction

Various pain management elements must be considered for patients undergoing lumbar spinal surgery, and despite advances in technologies, pain control after surgery remains difficult to manage adequately [1]. Achieving adequate pain control postoperatively is associated with improved patient satisfaction rates, shorter hospital stays, and lower costs [2, 3]. Although opioid-based treatment was typically used in the past for pain management because of its low cost, there is currently more evidence showing more adverse effects, hospital costs, and worse long-term outcomes with these strategies [4]. However, multimodal, nonopioid-based analgesia, which were first described by Kehlet et al. in 1993, are becoming increasingly common [5].

Factors affecting pain management may be divided into general and surgery-specific concerns. General issues include premorbid chronic pain, underlying behavioral issues, general baseline health status, appropriate selection of surgical candidates and operation, presence of acute pain following surgery, and poor pain control in the perioperative setting. Specific considerations are typically related to

N. Thalla · A. Wondra
Department of Rehabilitation Medicine, MedStar Georgetown University,
Washington, DC, USA

MedStar National Rehabilitation Hospital, Physical Medicine and Rehabilitation,
Washington, DC, USA

M. J. Desai (✉)
International Spine, Pain & Performance Center, Washington, DC, USA

School of Medicine and Health Sciences, The George Washington University,
Washington, DC, USA
e-mail: drdesai@isppcenter.com

© The Author(s), under exclusive license to Springer Nature
Switzerland AG 2023

J. R. O'Brien et al. (eds.), *Lumbar Spine Access Surgery*,
https://doi.org/10.1007/978-3-031-48034-8_19

surgical approach and may include extent of tissue trauma, adequate decompression and/or fusion, nerve root traction or injury, and lumbosacral or sympathetic plexus damage.

The general concerns listed are primarily beyond the scope of this chapter or are covered elsewhere in this text. Therefore, the focus of this chapter will be options and alternatives to provide patients with adequate analgesia in the postoperative setting as well as the approaches to specific issues that might be encountered such as nerve root or plexus injury. Furthermore, a discussion of persistent spinal pain syndrome (PSPS) will be presented.

## Persistent Pain Following Surgery

Development of chronic pain, known as chronic postsurgical pain (CPSP), is pain that persists beyond the timeframe of tissue healing. There are varying definitions that articulate the timeline for development of CPSP. The International Classification of Diseases (ICD) defines CPSP as pain developing or increasing in intensity following a surgical procedure, in the area of surgery, persisting at least 3 months and not better explained by any other causes such as the patient's presurgical pain condition [6]. An important consideration in patients who have undergone spinal surgery is this presurgical condition. Spinal surgery patients may present with complicating factors such as higher baseline opioid requirements, elevated anxiety levels, and altered presurgical pain perception [7]. This population is at higher risk for the development of CPSP. Adequate pain control in this population has far-reaching consequences including favorable outcomes for mobility and coordination, quicker recovery, lower risk of complications, and greater patient satisfaction [8].

Newly developing literature and reevaluation of chronic pain definitions following surgeries have shed light on the flaws existing in current terminology. The predominantly accepted term failed back surgery syndrome (FBSS) is misleading and may be misinterpreted [9]. The preemptive flaw with the terminology is that it ambiguously suggests the surgery failed to relieve the pain or may be the cause of the pain. It provides no differentiation of symptoms caused by surgery or those failed to be relieved by surgery. Recently, an international group of experts convened to discuss the potential of replacement terminology for utilization in the ICD-11 coding system [9]. A consensus among the panel suggested the adoption of "persistent spinal pain syndrome" (PSPS). The principle of PSPS accounts for chronic and/or recurrent symptoms after spinal surgery and other treatments and in the absence of such treatments, including surgery [9]. A proposed subclassification includes PSPS type 1 (no surgery) and PSPS type 2 (surgery) [9, 10]. The key difference is the use of "persistence" which offers context regarding a preexisting condition which then continues despite interventions, such as surgery, or altered circumstances. This newly developed terminology has yet to be formally accepted but offers a glimpse into the future direction of understanding chronic pain in the context of surgery.

There are several risk factors that are important to consider when trying to determine those at risk for the development of chronic pain. The commonly reported risk factors include psychosocial factors, female sex, younger (non-pediatric) age, genetic predisposition, and level of preexisting pain [11, 12]. However, many of these factors may simply be associations and not causative. One such factor is acute postoperative pain. Acute postoperative pain is an important predictor of chronic pain [13].

## Chronic Pain Prevention

The notion that postoperative pain control is purely a postsurgical dilemma is largely falling out of favor. Effective pain management for surgeries, regardless of the degree of invasiveness, requires a preventative approach. The methods of doing so were initially targeted at the prevention of acute pain but have now transitioned to an all-encompassing pain management model that aims to control perioperative/postoperative pain and prevent the development of CPSP.

The idea of analgesia before procedural intervention was first theorized by Woolf et al. and Wall [11, 14]. This idea of preemptive analgesia was centered around the idea that treatment before incision would decrease the intensity of postoperative pain, hyperalgesia, and prevent sensitization. This notion has since fallen out of favor due to a variety of inconclusive studies that showed no significant difference between pre-incisional and post-incisional analgesia [11, 12]. A meta-analysis conducted on 80 randomized controlled trials revealed no superiority for preemptive analgesia when compared to analgesia given after incision [15]. The idea of preemptive analgesia was simply too narrow in scope. A newer model of preventive analgesia has recently been developed that allows for a broader and more effective clinical application.

Several multimodal regimens have been described in the literature for the management of lumbar spine access surgeries and may include oral analgesics, infused analgesics, nonpharmacologic techniques, and emerging techniques (Table 19.1). A prospective trial focusing on the preventive portion of the analgesic spectrum compared the use of intravenous (IV) morphine as a single regimen versus a multimodal

**Table 19.1** Options for components of multimodal therapy for spine access surgery

| Oral analgesics | Infusion analgesics | Nonpharmacologic techniques | Emerging techniques |
| --- | --- | --- | --- |
| NSAIDs, paracetamol, gabapentinoids, opioids, antispasmodics | Lidocaine, ketamine, magnesium, dexmedetomidine | SCS, RFA, TENS | Nerve blocks (quadratus lumborum block, transversus abdominis plane block) |

*NSAIDs* nonsteroidal anti-inflammatory drugs, *SCS* spinal cord stimulation, *RFA* radiofrequency ablation, *TENS* transcutaneous electrical nerve stimulation analgesic regimen consisting of celecoxib, pregabalin, extended release oxycodone, and acetaminophen for patients undergoing posterior lumbar interbody fusion for lumbar stenosis [16]. The subjects were allocated to receive the treatment 1 h prior to surgery and twice daily following surgery until hospital discharge. Visual Analog Scale and Oswestry Disability Index (ODI) measures for pain and functional outcomes were significantly in favor of the multimodal cohort for all postoperative time points except for the ODI on postoperative day one. There were no safety concerns observed in this study [16]. A comprehensive analysis of multimodal regimens in spine surgeries was performed by Deven et al. in 2015 [17]. They evaluated various multimodal regimens based on the level of evidence available in the literature and assigned a grading system for the various agents involved. The grading system was based on the North American Spine Society Clinical Guidelines for Multidisciplinary Spine Care assigning good evidence (Grade A) based on showing level 1 studies that demonstrated consistent findings. The agents to receive this classification are gabapentinoids, acetaminophen, neuraxial blockades, and extended release local infiltrative anesthetics [17]. Additional studies have been conducted that have shown inconsistent evidence to the aforementioned study in terms of specific agents, but the idea of a multimodal regimen as an effective approach is now nearly universal. Our understanding of analgesia in the surgical world continues to evolve, specifically in spine surgery where the evidence is still lacking. There is a specific need for higher level of evidence studies for newer, advanced procedures such as anterior and lateral lumbar interbody fusions.

## Pharmacotherapy for Chronic Pain Following Spine Surgery

There is little pharmacotherapy guidance for the treatment of chronic pain following spine surgery remote to the perioperative setting. Very little data exist to support the use of any specific category of medication in these patients. Often, physicians must engage in a trial-and-error methodology to identify effective treatments in this population. Several categories of oral medications are utilized and include nonsteroidal anti-inflammatory drugs (NSAIDs), paracetamol, gabapentinoids, opioids, muscle relaxants (Table 19.2). IV medications are also considered (ketamine, lidocaine, magnesium, and dexmedetomidine) (Table 19.3).

**Table 19.2**  Oral analgesics

| | Mechanism of action | Effective for postoperative pain | Suggested starting dosage | Comments/adverse effects |
|---|---|---|---|---|
| **NSAIDs** | | | | |
| Ibuprofen | Nonselective COX inhibitor | Yes | 400 mg (NNT 2.5) | AE: gastrointestinal bleeding, oliguria, renal toxicity |
| Naproxen | Nonselective COX inhibitor | Yes | 500/550 mg (NNT 2.7) | |
| Celecoxib | COX-2 selective inhibitor | Yes | 200–400 mg (NNT 4.2–2.5) | |
| Paracetamol | Predominantly COX-2 selective inhibitor | Yes | 1000 mg (NNT 3.6) | AE: nausea, abdominal discomfort, gastrointestinal bleeding, abnormal liver function tests |
| **Gabapentinoids** | | | | |
| Gabapentin | Alpha2delta subunits of voltage-dependent $Ca^{2+}$ channels | Yes | 600–1200 mg per dose | AE: dizziness, drowsiness, fatigue, peripheral edema, hypotension, nausea, vomiting, and hallucinogens |
| Pregabalin | Alpha2delta subunits of voltage-dependent $Ca^{2+}$ channels | Yes | 150–300 mg once per day | |
| **Opioids** | Blocks calcium channels, inhibits release of substance P, glutamate | Yes | Lowest effective dose, immediate release | AE: dysphoria, euphoria, sedation, respiratory depression, constipation, endocrine suppression, cardiovascular disorders (bradycardia), convulsion, nausea, vomiting, pruritus, and miosis |
| **Antispasmodics** | | | | |

(continued)

**Table 19.2** (continued)

| | Mechanism of action | Effective for postoperative pain | Suggested starting dosage | Comments/adverse effects |
|---|---|---|---|---|
| *Benzodiazepines* | | | | |
| Alprazolam, clonazepam, diazepam, hydroxyzine | GABA-A receptor (α-2 subunit) agonist | Insufficient evidence | | Not recommended. Use with caution in patients with a history of addiction. Sudden withdrawal can cause delirium tremens. AE: lethargy, fatigue, drowsiness, dizziness, impaired motor coordination and thinking, disorientation, vertigo, slurred speech, blurry vision, mood swings, and euphoria |
| *Nonbenzodiazepines* | | | | |
| Cyclobenzaprine | Not fully understood, primarily centrally acting to reduce tonic somatic motor activity, influencing both gamma and alpha motor neurons | Insufficient evidence | 5–10 mg tid as needed or 15–30 mg ER daily | Contraindications: cardiac arrhythmias, congestive heart failure, heart block, recent myocardial infarction, hyperthyroidism AE: Xerostomia, drowsiness, dizziness, fatigue, nausea, dyspepsia |
| Tizanidine | Alpha2-adrenergic receptor agonist | Insufficient evidence | 8 mg every 6–8 h | Use caution in patients with hepatic or renal impairment |
| Methocarbamol | Currently unknown, centrally acting | Insufficient evidence | 500–1000 mg qid as needed | AE: nausea, drowsiness, blurred vision, hypotension, seizures, and coma (in overdose) |
| *Antispastics* | | | | |
| Baclofen | Not fully understood, primarily centrally acting. GABA-B analogue | Insufficient evidence | 5–10 mg tid as needed, max 80 mg daily | Use caution in patients with renal impairment. AE: drowsiness, dizziness, sedation, fatigue, seizures (with sudden withdrawal) |

*COX* cyclooxygenase, *GABA* gamma amino butyric acid, *NNT* number needed to treat, *AE* adverse effects

**Table 19.3** Intravenous analgesic

|  | Primary mechanism of action | Opioid-sparing effects | Suggested dosing | Adverse effects |
|---|---|---|---|---|
| Corticosteroids (mineralocorticoids) | Inhibits PG synthesis (blocks intracellular conversion of phospholipids to arachidonic acid) | Yes | Dexamethasone >0.1 mg/kg | Impaired healing, impaired immune function, hypertension, insomnia, increased appetite hyperglycemia |
| Ketamine | Noncompetitive, reversible NMDA inhibitor | Yes | Lacks consensus | Psychotomimetic (hallucinations, agitation, anxiety, dysphoria, and euphoria), dizziness, nausea, sedation, and tachycardia |
| Magnesium | Calcium channel blocker, noncompetitive NMDA inhibitor | Maybe beneficial | 40 mg/kg bolus + continuous 10 mg/kg/h | No significant adverse effects, low risk of toxicity |
| Dexmedetomidine | Selective a-2 adrenergic receptor agonist | Yes | 0.3–1.0 µg/kg bolus + continuous 0.2–0.6 µg/kg/h | Bradycardia, mild hypotension, sedation |

*PG* prostaglandins, *POVN* postoperative nausea or vomiting, *NMDA* N-methyl-D-aspartate, *mg* milligram, *µg* microgram, *kg* kilogram

## *Gabapentinoids*

Gabapentinoids are analogues of gamma-aminobutyric acid (GABA) which bind to and block the alpha2delta subunits of voltage-dependent $Ca^{2+}$ channels [18]. Commonly used gabapentinoids include gabapentin and pregabalin.

## *Antispasmodics*

Antispasmodics are used to decrease muscle spasm associated with painful conditions such as low back pain and can be subclassified into benzodiazepines (i.e., diazepam), nonbenzodiazepines (i.e., cyclobenzaprine, methocarbamol, tizanidine), and antispastics (i.e., baclofen). Antispasmodics have differing mechanisms of action. Benzodiazepines produce a myorelaxant effect that is primarily mediated through α2 subunit of GABA receptors in the spinal cord and motor neurons and to a lesser extent through interaction with α3 subunits [19, 20]. Nonbenzodiazepines exhibit their effects through other pathways; however, the exact mechanisms are not fully understood. Methocarbamol is thought to inhibit acetylcholinesterase in the autonomic nervous system, neuromuscular junction, and central nervous system centrally to relax muscles but does not act on the muscle or nerve motor end plate directly [21]. Cyclobenzaprine appears to act primarily at the brain stem to reduce tonic somatic motor activity, influencing both gamma and alpha motor neurons leading to a reduction in muscle spasms [22]. Baclofen is centrally acting at the spinal cord as a GABA receptor agonist, and tizanidine is a central $\alpha$2 agonist; both medications inhibit tone at the spinal cord level.

## Opioids

Opioids are commonly used to treat spine-mediated postoperative pain with good evidence supporting their use for short periods with close monitoring. Opioids bind mu, kappa, and delta opioid receptors. Presynaptically, opioids block calcium channels on nociceptive afferent nerves to inhibit the release of neurotransmitters substance P and glutamate. Postsynaptically, opioids open potassium channels and hyperpolarize cell membranes, increasing the required action potential to generate nociceptive transmission. Some opioid agents (tramadol, oxycodone, fentanyl, methadone, dextromethorphan, meperidine, codeine, and buprenorphine) can affect serotonin kinetics through weak serotonin reuptake inhibition and increase the release of intrasynaptic serotonin through inhibition of GABA. Additionally, methadone binds N-methyl-D-aspartate (NMDA) receptors antagonizing glutamate, theoretically explaining the effects on neuropathic pain [23]. Per CDC guidelines, "clinicians should consider opioid therapy only if expected benefits for both pain and function are anticipated to outweigh risks to the patient. If opioids are used, they should be combined with nonpharmacologic therapy and nonopioid pharmacologic therapy, as appropriate" [24]. With respect to acute pain, the lowest effective dose of immediate release opioids and smallest quantity for expected duration of severe pain should be prescribed [23].

Opioids are available in oral formulations, including both immediate release and extended release tablets, including methadone, oxycodone, and hydrocodone (commonly combined with acetaminophen or ibuprofen), respectively. IV formulations of opioids, including morphine, hydromorphone, and fentanyl, are frequently used for pain control in the acute inpatient setting. Fentanyl transdermal patches exist for extended absorption. Morphine can also be given epidurally for the management of acute pain, as well as intrathecally in the form of implantable pumps or the management of chronic pain and palliative care.

Adverse events include dysphoria, euphoria, sedation, respiratory depression, constipation, endocrine suppression, cardiovascular disorders (bradycardia), convulsion, nausea, vomiting, pruritus, and miosis. In the long term, opioid-induced hyperalgesia and/or allodynia can occur [25]. With respect to serotonergic opioids, serotonin syndrome is a feared complication when combined with other medications with serotonergic activity, and co-administration should be done cautiously or avoided entirely [26].

## Lidocaine

IV lidocaine may be an effective treatment in managing chronic pain of a number of etiologies, achieving both central and peripheral analgesic effects with relatively few side effects, which may be an ideal compound for managing chronic pain [27]. Specific channels play a role in subtypes of pain such as neuropathic and inflammatory pain, and our knowledge of the underlying mechanism of lidocaine has expanded considerably [28]. Van der Wal et al. concluded that IV lidocaine is effective in the management of some neuropathic pain syndromes by modulating the ectopic neuronal discharges, thus decreasing hyperalgesia and the inflammatory response. This effect is obtained through inhibition of the voltage-gated sodium channels, voltage-gated calcium channels, various potassium channels, NMDA receptors, glycine system, and G-protein pathways [29]. IV lidocaine infusions have shown promising results in managing pain related to FBSS. Investigators including Park et al. have investigated these effects with regard to neuropathic pain, the pain that occurs because of abnormal impulses originating from the dorsal root ganglion and spinal cord, as a result of nerve injury [30]. Their study demonstrated that 1 and 5 mg/kg of IV lidocaine improved chronic pain attributable to FBSS; however, 5 mg/kg was significantly more effective than 1 mg/kg [31].

## Ketamine

IV ketamine may be used in the perioperative period in subanesthetic doses. It is more frequently used as part of a multimodal postoperative analgesia regimen, sometimes as an adjuvant to opioids in painful surgical procedures, including spine surgery, or in those with opioid tolerance or dependence. Ketamine has multiple actions, primarily acting as a noncompetitive, reversible inhibitor of the NMDA receptor especially at lower doses. At higher doses, it also acts at mu-opioid receptors, dopamine $D_2$ receptors, monoaminergic receptors, and GABA receptors, but there is lack of consensus as to the appropriate bolus and infusion dosing [32, 33]. It has also been concluded that ketamine significantly reduces the postoperative IL-6 inflammatory response in surgical patients [32].

IV ketamine has been shown to significantly reduce opioid consumption in major abdominal surgery and persistent pain at 6 months postoperatively [34, 35]. A meta-analysis of randomized controlled trials showed that patients who were administered adjunctive ketamine required significantly less cumulative morphine equivalent consumption and had lower postoperative pain scores, as well as reduced postoperative nausea or vomiting within 24 h following spine surgery without statistically significant adverse events [36, 37]. The most commonly reported adverse effect of ketamine is psychotomimetic (hallucinations, agitation, anxiety, dysphoria, and euphoria), but it may also cause dizziness, nausea, sedation, and tachycardia [33].

## *Magnesium*

Magnesium (Mg) is an NMDA receptor antagonist, having direct analgesic effects, as well as central nociceptor receptor sensitization and reduction or reversal of opioid-induced hyperalgesia and a low risk of toxicity [38]. Prolonged periods of dietary restriction, operation times, and perioperative IV fluid administration may contribute to lower Mg levels. Multiple studies showed the beneficial effects of perioperative IV administration of Mg in reducing postoperative pain, analgesic consumption, but there also potential adverse effects in patients undergoing general orthopedic surgeries and spine surgery [39, 40]. A randomized, double blind, placebo-controlled study examined patients scheduled for major gastrointestinal surgery who received a bolus of 40 mg/kg of magnesium sulfate, followed by a continuous perfusion of 10 mg/kg/h for the intraoperative hours resulting in a significant reduction in postoperative ileus, severe pain, and analgesic requirements without significant side effects [41]. However, other studies have not found that IV magnesium provided a clinically significant reduction in opioid consumption or pain severity [42].

## *Alpha-2 Agonist: Dexmedetomidine*

Systemic clonidine is not routinely used as an infusion given its adverse cardiovascular effect profile (hypotension and bradycardia), but dexmedetomidine (DEX) is more frequently used as an adjunct to anesthetics, given its alpha-2 agonist causing anesthetic-sparing effect. Studies have shown various results regarding postoperative pain control and reductions in opioid requirements. Bhiken et al. found that intraoperative dexmedetomidine did not reduce postoperative opioid consumption or improve pain scores after multilevel deformity correction spine surgery [43]. However, Garg et al. found that infusion of low-dose dexmedetomidine provided good postoperative analgesia and can be used safely and effectively for postoperative pain relief in patients after spine surgery with minimal side effects [44]. A systematic review and meta-analysis showed a significant reduction of both propofol and morphine equivalent consumption both intraoperatively and postoperatively [45]. While no serious adverse effects can be directly associated with DEX, bradycardia, mild hypotension, and sedation are not uncommon.

## Interventional Options

### *Quadratus Lumborum Block*

The quadratus lumborum (QL) block is a fascial plane nerve block where local anesthetic is injected adjacent into the QL muscle with the goal of anesthetizing the thoracolumbar nerves. The QL is a posterior abdominal wall muscle that originates from the posteromedial iliac crest and inserts into the medial border of the 12th rib and the transverse processes of the first to fourth lumbar vertebrae and anterior to the erector spinae muscles (multifidus, longissimus, and iliocostalis muscles). Large systematic reviews and meta-analysis have concluded that QL block lowers postoperative opioid requirements in cesarean delivery and renal surgeries and may also be effective in abdominal and pelvic surgeries; however, the current quality of evidence is low, and there is insufficient evidence comparing QL block with other analgesia techniques such as transversus abdominal plane (TAP) block [46, 47]. Evidence is low with regard to spine surgery; however, one retrospective review showed that continuous QL blocks significantly lower opiate consumption when lumbar fusions are performed when compared to the standard opioid regimens however larger prospective randomized control design studies are warranted [48]. The main complication associated with QL block is local anesthetic toxicity.

## *Transversus Abdominis Plane Block*

The transversus abdominal plane (TAP) block involves the injection of local anesthetic solution into a plane between the internal oblique and transversus abdominis muscles targeting the thoracolumbar nerves which originate from T6 to L1 spinal roots supplying sensory input of the anterolateral abdominal wall. The local anesthetic spreads within this plane block the neural afferents ultimately providing analgesic effects to the anterolateral abdominal wall [49]. TAP blocks have been shown to improve postoperative pain outcomes in other surgical subtypes but have not been fully studied with regard to spine surgery, including anterior and lateral approaches. Extended release liposomal injections have shown good efficacy in postoperative pain relief over a period of 48 h [50].

## Interventional Approaches for Complications Related to Anterior and Lateral Approaches

Anterior and lateral interbody fusions have demonstrated improvements in patient safety outcomes compared to posterolateral approaches over the years [51]. However, several complications unique to these approaches are important to consider. For the anterior approach, injuries have been described in the literature to the lumbar sympathetic chain, ilioinguinal nerve, and iliohypogastric nerves [52]. In a majority of these cases, the patient does not suffer long-term sequelae. However, a minority of these cases do develop prolonged dysesthetic pain. Lateral approaches that have been developed to reduce the risk of vascular injury in anterior approaches have also demonstrated an appreciable risk of neural injury [53]. Multiple anatomic/cadaveric studies demonstrated how these approaches involving dissection through the psoas muscle place the sympathetic plexus, lumbar plexus, ilioinguinal,

**Table 19.4** Nonpharmacologic treatment

| | Mechanism of pain relief | Opioid-sparing | Effective for postsurgical pain |
|---|---|---|---|
| Spinal cord stimulation | Multiple theorized mechanisms; primarily thought to stimulate larger, faster fibers involved in touch and proprioception which blocks or mitigates the dysregulated, overactive pain signals produced from the slower nociceptive $A\delta$ and C fibers | Yes | Yes |
| Radiofrequency ablation | Focal delivery of thermal energy inducing thermal injury to the target nerve destroys pain-producing signals | Yes | Yes |
| Transcutaneous electrical nerve stimulation | Based on the Gate Control Theory of Pain and daily repeated application producing analgesic tolerance and increasing the toleration threshold of pain. Also results in the release of endorphins, serotonin, analgesic hormones, and reduced cytokine levels and increases blood flow to the healing muscle tissue | Yes | Yes |

iliohypogastric, genitofemoral, lateral femoral cutaneous, and subcostal nerves at risk [53]. The sequela of these injuries may include abdominal, groin, and anterior thigh sensory abnormalities. Clinical weakness such as hip flexor weakness is also a possibility. Common to all interbody fusion procedures includes the complication of pseudoarthrosis or outright failure with a return of the patient's axial, radicular, or neurogenic claudication symptoms [51]. Interventional pain physicians are uniquely equipped to deal with these surgical complications, especially as they progress to a refractory, chronic stage. Various treatment options are possible in scenarios of nerve injuries or surgical failures that include targeted nerve blocks, radiofrequency ablations, spinal cord stimulation, and peripheral nerve stimulation (Table 19.4).

Targeted peripheral nerve blocks should be considered when patients are experiencing prolonged, chronic pain signals in the distribution of a specific nerve. In most cases, these nerve blocks are a highly effective means for patients to regain their quality of life and improve their pain-limited function. These blocks are often administered with a local anesthetic such as lidocaine or bupivacaine. In cases where an inflammatory component may be contributing to pain, a combination with steroids such as dexamethasone can provide longer-lasting relief.

Radiofrequency ablation, also known as rhizotomy, is another modality used to provide long-lasting pain relief. It can be applied to peripheral nerves generating unwanted and chronic pain signals. This procedure is typically performed following a successful diagnostic nerve block. The procedure involves a focal delivery of thermal energy to induce a thermal injury to the nerve target and thereby destroy pain-producing signals [54]. The procedure is designed to provide months to even years of pain relief before the nerve regenerates. This procedure has been effectively utilized for axial and peripheral nerve pain, including in cases of pseudoarthrosis development following lumbar interbody fusions [54, 55].

Additionally, spinal cord and peripheral nerve stimulations are constantly evolving modalities that have proven to be an effective option in patients who may not be surgical candidates or those who have developed FBSS following fusions and related procedures [56]. Peripheral nerve stimulation largely remains in the early stages of research and development but has proven to be an exciting modality to individually target injured nerves with the prospects of improving both functions and reducing unwanted noxious stimulus. This option can be considered if focal neural injuries from surgical techniques do not heal adequately. There are a variety of mechanisms theorized to explain the analgesic benefit of nerve stimulation. One of the principal mechanisms of these modalities is derived from the basic idea of varying nerve fibers conducting sensory stimulus to the dorsal horn of the spinal cord [56, 57]. These modalities stimulate the larger and faster fibers involved in touch and proprioception in order to block or mitigate the dysregulated, overactive pain signals produced from the slower nociceptive A$\delta$ and C fibers [57].

## Conclusion

A variety of management strategies exist for approaching chronic pain after surgery. A multimodal approach to pain treatment at phases prior to surgery, during surgery, and after surgery has been shown to be the most effective means to achieve long-term pain relief. The very understanding of how to define the role of chronic pain before and after surgery is evolving. Newer classifications such as PSPS allow the scientific community to classify the persistent nature of symptoms more accurately. However, despite our improving understanding and earlier interventions, patients still may end up developing and experiencing persistent chronic postsurgical pain. For these patients, a variety of pharmacological or interventional options, both established and emerging in nature, may be utilized to effectively manage the pain burden. It is important for providers, both surgeons and interventionalists alike, to understand the evidence behind the variety of treatment options available and provide suitable options for their patients.

## References


1. Vadivelu N, Mitra S, Narayan D. Recent advances in postoperative pain management. Yale J Biol Med. 2010;83(1):11.
2. Berardino K, Carroll AH, Kaneb A, Civilette MD, Sherman WF, Kaye AD. An update on postoperative opioid use and alternative pain control following spine surgery. Orthop Rev (Pavia). 2021;13(2):24978.
3. Garimella V, Cellini C. Postoperative pain control. Clin Colon Rectal Surg. 2013;26(3):191.

4. Rosenblum A, Marsch LA, Joseph H, Portenoy RK. Opioids and the treatment of chronic pain: controversies, current status, and future directions. Exp Clin Psychopharmacol. 2008;16(5):405.

5. Kehlet H, Dahl JB. The value of "multimodal" or "balanced analgesia" in postoperative pain treatment. Anesth Analg. 1993;77(5):1048–56.

6. Lavand'homme P. Transition from acute to chronic pain after surgery. Pain. 2017;158(1):S50–4. https://doi.org/10.1097/j.pain.0000000000000809.

7. Singh SJ. Pain relief following spinal surgeries: a challenging task. J Spine. 2015;4:3. https://doi.org/10.4172/2165-7939.1000233.

8. Yoo JS, Ahn J, Buvanendran A, Singh K. Multimodal analgesia in pain management after spine surgery. J Spine Surg. 2019;5(Suppl 2):S154–9.

9. Simpson B, Christelis N, Russo M, Stanton-Hicks M, et al. Persistent spinal pain syndrome: a proposed replacement for failed back surgery syndrome. Br J Neurosurg. 2023;37(2):244.

10. Ounajim A, Billot M, Louis P-Y, Slaoui Y, et al. Finite mixture models based on pain intensity, functional disability and psychological distress composite assessment allow identification of two distinct classes of persistent spinal pain syndrome after surgery patients related to their quality of life. J Clin Med Res. 2021;10(20):4676. https://doi.org/10.3390/jcm10204676.

11. Wall PD. The prevention of postoperative pain. Pain. 1988;33(3):289–90. https://doi.org/10.1016/0304-3959(88)90286-2.

12. Vadivelu N, Mitra S, Schermer E, Kodumudi V, et al. Preventive analgesia for postoperative pain control: a broader concept. Local Region Anesth. 2014;7:17–22.

13. Schnabel A, Yahiaoui-Doktor M, Meissner W, Zahn PK, Pogatzki-Zahn EM. Predicting poor postoperative acute pain outcome in adults: an international, multicentre database analysis of risk factors in 50,005 patients. Pain Rep. 2020;5(4):e831.

14. Woolf CJ, Chong MS. Preemptive analgesia—treating postoperative pain by preventing the establishment of central sensitization. Anesth Analg. 1993;77(2):362–79.

15. Møiniche S, Kehlet H, Dahl JB. A qualitative and quantitative systematic review of preemptive analgesia for postoperative pain relief. Anesthesiology. 2002;96(3):725–41. https://doi.org/10.1097/00000542-200203000-00032.

16. Kim S-I, Ha K-Y, Oh I-S. Preemptive multimodal analgesia for postoperative pain management after lumbar fusion surgery: a randomized controlled trial. Eur Spine J. 2016;25(5):1614–9.

17. Devin CJ, McGirt MJ. Best evidence in multimodal pain management in spine surgery and means of assessing postoperative pain and functional outcomes. J Clin Neurosci. 2015;22(6):930–8.

18. Dooley DJ, Taylor CP, Donevan S, Feltner D. $Ca^{2+}$ channel alpha2delta ligands: novel modulators of neurotransmission. Trends Pharmacol Sci. 2007;28(2):75–82.

19. Li H, Xie W, Strong JA, Zhang J-M. Systemic antiinflammatory corticosteroid reduces mechanical pain behavior, sympathetic sprouting, and elevation of proinflammatory cytokines in a rat model of neuropathic pain. Anesthesiology. 2007;107(3):469–77.

20. Griffin CE III, Kaye AM, Bueno FR, Kaye AD. Benzodiazepine pharmacology and central nervous system–mediated effects. Ochsner J. 2013;13(2):214.

21. PubChem. Methocarbamol. n.d. https://pubchem.ncbi.nlm.nih.gov/compound/4107. Accessed 8 Oct 2021.

22. PubChem. Cyclobenzaprine. n.d. https://pubchem.ncbi.nlm.nih.gov/compound/2895. Accessed 8 Oct 2021.

23. Cohen B, Ruth LJ, Preuss CV. Opioid analgesics StatPearls. Treasure Island: StatPearls Publishing; 2021.

24. CDC guideline for prescribing opioids for chronic pain. https://www.cdc.gov/drugoverdose/pdf/guidelines_at-a-glance-a.pdf#:~:text=nonopioid%20pharmacologic%20therapy%20are%20preferred%20for%20chronic%20pain.,nonpharmacologic%20therapy%20and%20nonopioid%20pharmacologic%20therapy%2C%20as%20appropriate. Accessed 5 Oct 2021.

25. Crockett SD, Greer KB, Heidelbaugh JJ, Falck-Ytter Y, et al. American Gastroenterological Association Institute guideline on the medical management of opioid-induced constipation. Gastroenterology. 2019;156(1):218–26.

26. Smischney NJ, Pollard EM, Nookala AU, Olatoye OO. Serotonin syndrome in the perioperative setting. Am J Case Rep. 2018;19:833–5.

27. Tully J, Jung JW, Patel A, Tukan A, et al. Utilization of intravenous lidocaine infusion for the treatment of refractory chronic pain. Anesth Pain Med. 2020;10(6):e112290.

28. Anon. The role of sodium channels in neuropathic pain. Semin Cell Dev Biol. 2006;17(5):571–81.

29. van der Wal SEI, van den Heuvel SAS, Radema SA, van Berkum BFM, et al. The in vitro mechanisms and in vivo efficacy of intravenous lidocaine on the neuroinflammatory response in acute and chronic pain. Eur J Pain. 2016;20(5):655–74.

30. Park CH, Jung SH, Han CG. Effect of intravenous lidocaine on the neuropathic pain of failed back surgery syndrome. Korean J Pain. 2012;25(2):94.

31. Kandil E, Melikman E, Adinoff B. Lidocaine infusion: a promising therapeutic approach for chronic pain. J Anesth Clin Res. 2017;8(1):697.

32. Dale O, Somogyi AA, Li Y, Sullivan T, Shavit Y. Does intraoperative ketamine attenuate inflammatory reactivity following surgery? A systematic review and meta-analysis. Anesth Analg. 2012;115(4):934–43.

33. Bell RF, Kalso EA. Ketamine for pain management. Pain Rep. 2018;3(5):e674.

34. Brinck EC, Tiippana E, Heesen M, Bell RF, et al. Perioperative intravenous ketamine for acute postoperative pain in adults. Cochrane Database Syst Rev. 2018;12(12):CD012033.

35. Nielsen RV. Adjuvant analgesics for spine surgery. Dan Med J. 2018;65(3):B5468.

36. Pendi A, Field R, Farhan S-D, Eichler M, Samuel BS. Perioperative ketamine for analgesia in spine surgery: a meta-analysis of randomized controlled trials. Spine. 2018;43(5):E299.

37. Bell RF, Dahl JB, Andrew Moore R, Kalso EA. Perioperative ketamine for acute postoperative pain. Cochrane Database Syst Rev. 2006;12(1):CD004603.

38. Anon. Non-opioid analgesics: novel approaches to perioperative analgesia for major spine surgery. Best Pract Res Clin Anaesth. 2016;30(1):79–89.

39. Peng Y-N, Sung F-C, Huang M-L, Lin C-L, Kao C-H. The use of intravenous magnesium sulfate on postoperative analgesia in orthopedic surgery: a systematic review of randomized controlled trials. Medicine. 2018;97(50):e13583.

40. Yue L, Lin Z, Mu G, Sun H. Impact of intraoperative intravenous magnesium on spine surgery: a systematic review and meta-analysis of randomized controlled trials. EClinicalMedicine. 2022;43:101246.

41. Moharari RS, Motalebi M, Najafi A, Zamani MM, et al. Magnesium can decrease postoperative physiological ileus and postoperative pain in major non laparoscopic gastrointestinal surgeries: a randomized controlled trial. Anesth Pain Med. 2014;4(1):e12750.

42. Ghaffaripour S, Mahmoudi H, Eghbal H, Rahimi A. The effect of intravenous magnesium sulfate on post-operative analgesia during laminectomy. Cureus. 2016;8(6):e626.

43. Naik BI, Nemergut EC, Kazemi A, Fernández L, et al. The effect of dexmedetomidine on postoperative opioid consumption and pain after major spine surgery. Anesth Analg. 2016;122:5.

44. Garg N, Panda NB, Gandhi KA, Bhagat H, et al. Comparison of small dose ketamine and dexmedetomidine infusion for postoperative analgesia in spine surgery—a prospective randomized double-blind placebo controlled study. J Neurosurg Anesthesiol. 2016;28(1):27–31. https://doi.org/10.1097/ANA.0000000000000193.

45. Tsaousi GG, Pourzitaki C, Aloisio S, Bilotta F. Dexmedetomidine as a sedative and analgesic adjuvant in spine surgery: a systematic review and meta-analysis of randomized controlled trials. Eur J Clin Pharmacol. 2018;74(11):1377–89.

46. Anon. Single injection Quadratus Lumborum block for postoperative analgesia in adult surgical population: a systematic review and meta-analysis. J Clin Anesth. 2020;62:109715.

47. Uppal V, Retter S, Kehoe E, McKeen DM. Quadratus lumborum block for postoperative analgesia: a systematic review and meta-analysis. Can J Anesth. 2020;67(11):1557–75.

48. Wilton J, Chiu H, Codianne N, Knapp H, et al. Continuous quadratus lumborum block as post-operative strategy for pain control in spinal fusion surgery. Indian J Anaesth. 2020;64(10):869.
49. Tsai H-C, Yoshida T, Chuang T-Y, Yang S-F, et al. Transversus abdominis plane block: an updated review of anatomy and techniques. Biomed Res Int. 2017;2017:8284363.
50. Viscusi ER. Emerging techniques in the management of acute pain: epidural analgesia. Anesth Analg. 2005;101(5 Suppl):S23–9.
51. Mobbs RJ, Phan K, Malham G, Seex K, Rao PJ. Lumbar interbody fusion: techniques, indications and comparison of interbody fusion options including PLIF, TLIF, MI-TLIF, OLIF/ATP, LLIF and ALIF. J Spine Surg. 2015;1(1):2–18.
52. Choy W, Barrington N, Garcia RM, Kim RB, et al. Risk factors for medical and surgical complications following single-level ALIF. Global Spine J. 2017;7(2):141–7.
53. Epstein NE. Review of risks and complications of Extreme Lateral Interbody Fusion (XLIF). Surg Neurol Int. 2019;10:237.
54. Clarke H, Katz J, Flor H, Rietschel M, et al. Genetics of chronic post-surgical pain: a crucial step toward personal pain medicine. Can J Anaesth. 2015;62(3):294–303.
55. Liu H, Yue L, Chen SL, Hu B, et al. Anterior cervical discectomy and fusion to treat cervical spondylosis with sympathetic symptoms. Beijing Da Xue Xue Bao Yi Xue Ban. 2018;50(2):347–51.
56. Wylde V, Dennis J, Beswick AD, Bruce J, et al. Systematic review of management of chronic pain after surgery. Br J Surg. 2017;104(10):1293–306.
57. Caylor J, Reddy R, Yin S, Cui C, et al. Spinal cord stimulation in chronic pain: evidence and theory for mechanisms of action. Bioelectron Medi. 2019;5:12. https://doi.org/10.1186/s42234-019-0023-1.

# Chapter 20
# Venous Thromboembolic Issues

**Philip Parel, Bruce Seibold, Matt Walker, Ryan Smith, and Jeffrey B. Weinreb**

## Introduction

Venous thromboembolism (VTE), including deep vein thrombosis (DVT) and pulmonary embolism (PE), can be a catastrophic complication after spinal surgery and occurs in an estimated 0.06% to 18% of cases [1–4]. In patients undergoing anterior or lateral spinal surgery, VTE represents a unique entity as compared to patients undergoing posterior surgery for several important reasons. First, anterior surgery often involves some degree of mobilization and manipulation of the large anterior vessels including the inferior vena cava (IVC), aorta, and iliac vasculature, resulting in an increased risk of intraoperative and postoperative VTE [5]. This risk may be due to direct injury or prolonged retraction [6]. Second, as most anterior or lateral surgery does not involve a direct neurologic decompression, many surgeons will consider intraoperative or early postoperative chemical DVT prophylaxis, in addition to the standard mechanical prophylaxis, given the diminished risk of neurological compression from an expanding hematoma [7]. There is a lack of consensus on current recommendations, but as more research is conducted, some authors have suggested specific protocols for DVT prevention in anterior surgery [7]. The purpose of this chapter is to review the risks, perioperative prophylaxis, detection, and management of VTE in patients undergoing anterior and lateral spine surgery.

P. Parel · B. Seibold · M. Walker
School of Medicine and Health Sciences, The George Washington University,
Washington, DC, USA

R. Smith
Department of Orthopaedic Surgery, The University of Maryland, Baltimore, MD, USA

J. B. Weinreb (✉)
Department of Orthopaedic Surgery, The George Washington University,
Washington, DC, USA

Department of Orthopaedic Surgery, The University of Maryland, Baltimore, MD, USA

© The Author(s), under exclusive license to Springer Nature
Switzerland AG 2023

J. R. O'Brien et al. (eds.), *Lumbar Spine Access Surgery*,
https://doi.org/10.1007/978-3-031-48034-8_20

## Risks

One of the highest risks for postoperative VTE is an intraoperative vascular injury [8]. The most common vascular injury during an anterior lumbar interbody fusion (ALIF) is a venous laceration, typically during retraction of the great vessels [6, 9–14]. The left common iliac vein is most commonly injured during exposure due to an avulsion injury with mobilization. A significantly higher rate of injury occurs with exposure of L4–L5 compared with other levels [6, 10, 11, 14–18]. Anatomically, the bifurcation of the abdominal aorta typically occurs at the L4 vertebral body, and the confluence of the inferior vena cava is located at the L5 vertebral body [10].

These lacerations can be avoided by careful retractor manipulation and placement, appropriate structure identification, dissection, and mobilization. Preoperative imaging to assess vessel calcification can assist in operative planning [6]. When a laceration occurs, manual compression and/or primary sutures can be effective at managing the injury [9–11, 14, 17]. Other mechanisms of injury include laceration during discectomy, graft placement, and retractor frame shifting [9, 10].

As a result of prolonged retraction to the common iliac vessels, diminished flow can lead to thrombosis. This complication can be avoided by intermittently releasing retraction of the large vessels [6, 10, 13, 17]. Brau et al. recommended retractors be released if retraction time approaches 1 h in duration [6]. Intraoperative management of acute vascular injury is described in more details in Chaps. 16 and 17.

Lower extremity pulse oximetry can be used intraoperatively to monitor artery occlusion [6, 19, 20]. A preoperative baseline arterial oxygen saturation in the lower limbs can be used for comparison throughout the procedure, after the patient is turned over for a subsequent posterior procedure, and in the immediate postoperative period to detect early thrombotic occlusion [6].

One study of 204 ALIF cases compared a cohort of patients who developed DVT/PE in the postoperative period to those who did not. Patients who experienced a DVT/PE were significantly more likely to have had an intraoperative vascular injury than those who did not (36% versus 5%, $p = 0.004$) [8]. In another study of 1178 ALIF cases, there were 56 (4.75%) patients who suffered a major adverse event within a 90-day follow-up window. These included a venous injury in 13 (1.1%), arterial injury in 4 (0.34%), VTE in 20 (1.7%), myocardial infarction in 4 (0.4%), stroke in 2 (0.17%), and death in 2 (one from a stroke, the other from sudden cardiopulmonary arrest after discharge). Of the patients who developed VTE, 2/20 (10%) sustained a left iliac vein injury. Both patients underwent extensive left iliac vein reconstruction during the index procedure and were managed with anticoagulation [11].

The rate of VTE following anterior approach spine surgeries varies between 1% and 14% [3, 5, 6, 11, 13, 18, 21, 22]. During the perioperative, 30-, and 90-day periods, the odds ratio for developing VTE is between 1.5 and 3.5 in the ALIF group compared to posterior or transforaminal interbody fusion groups, after adjusting for age, sex, and patient comorbidities [5, 23–25]. In a study by Cloney et al. comparing anterior versus posterior approach lumbar fusions, anterior approach lumbar fusion increased the rate of VTE by 7.2% [24]. A propensity score-adjusted logistic regression model showed that ALIF is associated with a significantly higher odds ratio (OR) of VTE (OR = 3.49 [1.67, 7.29], $p$ = 0.001). On multivariable analysis, variables independently associated with DVT/PE within the 30-day postoperative window included anterior approach surgery (OR = 4.29 [1.98, 9.31], $p$ < 0.001), a history of VTE (OR = 8.67 [3.23, 23.22], $p$ < 0.001), age (OR = 1.53 [1.09, 2.15], $p$ = 0.014), intensive care unit admission (OR = 4.60 [1.60, 13.23], $p$ = 0.005), and length of surgery (OR = 1.16 [1.00, 1.34], $p$ = 0.044).

Patients who undergo anterior approach lumbar spine surgery are at least three times more likely to have a lower extremity duplex ultrasonography than posterior surgery patients [24]. While this introduces a degree of bias into studies that compare VTE outcomes, it also highlights the heightened awareness and concern for DVT/PE in the postoperative period for patients who undergo an anterior approach lumbar spine surgery.

## Perioperative Prophylaxis

Intraoperative and postoperative VTE prophylaxis include mechanical and chemical prophylaxis. Mechanical prophylaxis should include intermittent pneumatic calf compression and compression stockings, as well as early postoperative mobilization. All patients should be considered for intermittent pneumatic compression devices both intraoperatively and postoperatively [2, 3, 20, 26]. Chemical DVT prophylaxis during and after spine surgery, however, remains controversial. In other subspecialties, including joint replacement and trauma surgery, many elect to follow the American College of Chest Physician guidelines [27]. The *CHEST* recommended regimens include low-dose unfractionated heparin ($\leq$5000 units SC twice daily), low-molecular-weight heparin (LMWH) (such as enoxaparin 30 mg twice daily or 40 mg once daily), or fondaparinux (2.5 mg once daily) [27]. However, due to the increased risk of local hematoma and neurologic compression, these guideless are generally not recommended for low-risk patients undergoing spine surgery [28]. The most recent consensus statement from the North American Spine Society was published in 2009, with a revision currently being conducted as of 2023 [28]. To obfuscate matters further, the practice of postoperative chemical prophylaxis in patients undergoing anterior or lateral spine surgery is significantly more common due to the lack of direct exposure of the neural elements and the higher risk of VTE. Managing chemical anticoagulation for anterior spine surgeries, both intraoperatively and postoperatively, should involve an interdisciplinary approach that includes spine and vascular or approach surgeons [7]. Consulting the hospitalist or hematology services should be considered in patients with a complex medical history or a history of VTE. Placement of a preoperative IVC filter may also be an option.

In their study, Vint et al. evaluated the incidence of VTE in 200 consecutive ALIF patients that followed a specific VTE prophylaxis protocol. Subcutaneous LMWH

(4500 units of tinzaparin) was given to all patients the evening before surgery and then daily as an inpatient for the next 3 to 5 days. Patients were given 150 mg of acetylsalicylic acid and 30 mg of lansoprazole for 4 weeks following surgery. Anti-embolism stockings were worn for 6 weeks from the time of surgery. Intermittent pneumatic compression on the calves and thighs was used intraoperatively and for 24 h postoperatively, and patients were mobilized the morning after surgery. There were no intraoperative vascular injuries, symptomatic arterial occlusions, postoperative DVTs, or hematomas [7].

A prospective study by Sim et al. administered an intravenous dose of 50–75 units/kg of unfractionated heparin intraoperatively when arterial flow to the lower limbs was disrupted in patients who underwent anterior lumbar spine surgery. A pulse oximeter was placed on the patient's great toes bilaterally, and when the signal amplitude was severely diminished or completely absent (i.e., during retraction), heparin was administered. The heparin was reversed with protamine sulfate after completion of the procedure at the given level, after retraction relaxation, or upon pulse oximeter signal return. Among the 188 total patients, 72 (38.3%) received intraoperative heparin. Of the total patients, there were no intraoperative ischemic vascular complications, no complications related to the administration of heparin or protamine, and one instance of postoperative DVT. Overall blood loss was not significantly different between heparin and non-heparin groups but rather was dependent on the level and type of procedure [20].

## Detection

The clinical presentation of VTE may vary with the anatomic distribution and degree of occlusion, but specific archetypical symptoms may raise the index of suspicion. A symptomatic DVT may present with pain, numbness, erythema, muscle weakness, or significant swelling. A symptomatic PE may present with dyspnea, tachycardia, chest pain, hemoptysis, or peripheral vascular collapse [29]. The symptoms and clinical picture are relatively nonspecific, which can lead to a broad differential diagnosis including lymphedema, superficial venous thrombosis, cellulitis, improper pedicle screw positioning, and nerve root impingement. Certain preoperative factors that increase postoperative VTE risk should also raise suspicion in the postoperative period including prior VTE, polytrauma, malignancy, age greater than 60 years old, diabetes, hypertension requiring medication, a body mass index greater than 40, longer operating time/time spent anesthetized, increased time spent in sedentary state after the operation, and preoperative walking disability [30–32]. In addition to a comprehensive medical history and physical examination, standardized risk assessments can aid in stratifying patients with moderate to high risk of adverse surgical outcomes or VTE [33–35].

If postoperative DVT is suspected, ultrasonography or duplex ultrasonography (Doppler) is the primary noninvasive diagnostic study of choice [22]. Duplex ultrasonography has a high specificity (90%) but lower sensitivity for proximal and distal DVT at 62% and 48%, respectively [32, 36, 37]. In the case of a nondiagnostic study, other additional tests that can be considered include computed tomographic and magnetic resonance venography. If PE is suspected, computerized tomographic angiography (CTA) is the diagnostic imaging of choice due to its high sensitivity (83–100%) and specificity (89–96%) [38]. Although less commonly utilized recently, lung perfusion or ventilation-perfusion scans may be used to screen for PE [22].

The D-dimer laboratory test measures the levels of cross-linked fibrin clot degradation in the blood. The D-dimer is elevated in cases of VTE and can be elevated in other instances as well including the general postoperative state and cancer [32]. This leads to a high sensitivity (90%) but low specificity (55%) as these levels may be elevated in all postoperative patients to some degree [32].

These tests should be considered as part of a diagnostic algorithm as no specific test has perfect sensitivity and specificity [36]. There is no consensus on ideal length of treatment, frequency of surveillance, or screening protocols [32].

## Management

The management of postoperative VTE following anterior or lateral spine surgery, let alone spine surgery in general, is relatively limited in the literature [39]. Cain et al. reviewed nine patients treated with therapeutic heparin following PE diagnosis after undergoing spine surgery. Six patients experienced a complication including two cases of epidural hematoma requiring evacuation [40]. Schizas et al. prospectively reviewed 270 patients undergoing spinal surgery, and all patients received compression stockings and LMWH for prophylaxis. They identified six postoperative PE cases, and these patients were treated with 1 week of IVC filter followed by anticoagulation with LMWH to avoid epidural hemorrhage [41]. Postoperative DVT treatment should weigh the risks and benefits of DVT propagation/exacerbation versus hemorrhagic complications from anticoagulation. Currently, no consensus treatment has been defined [39].

## Conclusion

Postoperative VTE is thankfully uncommon in the spine surgery literature but presents a unique challenge for practitioners involved in the care of patients undergoing anterior or lateral spine surgery. In general, all patients should be treated with prophylactic mechanical compression and early mobilization. The risks and benefits of chemical prophylaxis and treatment should be weighed on an individual basis. Some studies support chemical prophylaxis in patients undergoing anterior spine surgery due to the higher VTE risk in these patients and the lack of exposure of the neural elements, which makes postoperative epidural hematoma and neurologic compromise less likely. Ultimately, the decision on how to prevent and treat VTE will differ based on institutional and individual practices as well as the unique risk profile of each patient. There remains no consensus on an ideal prophylaxis or treatment regimen.

# References


1. Inoue H, Watanabe H, Okami H, et al. The rate of venous thromboembolism before and after spine surgery as determined with indirect multidetector CT. JB JS Open Access. 2018;3:e0015.
2. Takahashi H, Yokoyama Y, Iida Y, et al. Incidence of venous thromboembolism after spine surgery. J Orthop Sci. 2012;17:114–7.
3. Piasecki DP, Poynton AR, Mintz DN, et al. Thromboembolic disease after combined anterior/posterior reconstruction for adult spinal deformity: a prospective cohort study using magnetic resonance venography. Spine. 2008;33:668–72.
4. Sansone JM, del Rio AM, Anderson PA. The prevalence of and specific risk factors for venous thromboembolic disease following elective spine surgery. J Bone Joint Surg Am. 2010;92:304–13.
5. Qureshi R, Puvanesarajah V, Jain A, et al. A comparison of anterior and posterior lumbar interbody fusions. Spine. 2017;42:1865–70.
6. Brau S. Vascular injury during anterior lumbar surgery. Spine J. 2004;4:409–12.
7. Vint H, Mawdsley MJ, Coe C, et al. The incidence of venous thromboembolism in patients undergoing anterior lumbar interbody fusion: a proposed thromboprophylactic regime. Int J Spine Surg. 2021;15:348–52.
8. Nourian AA, Cunningham CM, Bagheri A, et al. Effect of anatomic variability and level of approach on perioperative vascular complications with anterior lumbar interbody fusion. Spine. 2016;41:E73.
9. Than KD, Wang AC, Rahman SU, et al. Complication avoidance and management in anterior lumbar interbody fusion. Neurosurg Focus. 2011;31:E6.
10. Inamasu J, Kim DH, Logan L. Three-dimensional computed tomographic anatomy of the abdominal great vessels pertinent to L4-L5 anterior lumbar interbody fusion. Minim Invasive Neurosurg. 2005;48:127–31.
11. Manunga J, Alcala C, Smith J, et al. Technical approach, outcomes, and exposure-related complications in patients undergoing anterior lumbar interbody fusion. J Vasc Surg. 2021;73:992–8.
12. Brau SA. Mini-open approach to the spine for anterior lumbar interbody fusion: description of the procedure, results and complications. Spine J. 2002;2:216–23.
13. Bateman DK, Millhouse PW, Shahi N, et al. Anterior lumbar spine surgery: a systematic review and meta-analysis of associated complications. Spine J. 2015;15:1118–32.
14. Oskouian RJ, Johnson JP. Vascular complications in anterior thoracolumbar spinal reconstruction. J Neurosurg. 2002;96:1–5.
15. Chiriano J, Abou-Zamzam AM, Urayeneza O, et al. The role of the vascular surgeon in anterior retroperitoneal spine exposure: preservation of open surgical training. J Vasc Surg. 2009;50:148–51.
16. Asha MJ, Choksey MS, Shad A, et al. The role of the vascular surgeon in anterior lumbar spine surgery. Br J Neurosurg. 2012;26:499–503.
17. Hamdan AD, Malek JY, Schermerhorn ML, et al. Vascular injury during anterior exposure of the spine. J Vasc Surg. 2008;48:650–4.
18. Garg J, Woo K, Hirsch J, et al. Vascular complications of exposure for anterior lumbar interbody fusion. J Vasc Surg. 2010;51:946–50; discussion 950.
19. Kulkarni SS, Lowery GL, Ross RE, et al. Arterial complications following anterior lumbar interbody fusion: report of eight cases. Eur Spine J. 2003;12:48–54.

20. Sim EM, Claydon MH, Parker RM, et al. Brief intraoperative heparinization and blood loss in anterior lumbar spine surgery. J Neurosurg Spine. 2015;23:309–13.
21. Sebastian AS, Currier BL, Kakar S, et al. Risk factors for venous thromboembolism following thoracolumbar surgery: analysis of 43,777 patients from the American College of Surgeons National Surgical Quality Improvement Program 2005 to 2012. Global Spine J. 2016;6:738–43.
22. Dearborn JT, Hu SS, Tribus CB, et al. Thromboembolic complications after major thoracolumbar spine surgery. Spine. 1999;24:1471.
23. Shillingford JN, Laratta JL, Lombardi JM, et al. Complications following single-level interbody fusion procedures: an ACS-NSQIP study. J Spine Surg. 2018;4:17–27.
24. Cloney MB, Hopkins B, Dhillon E, et al. Anterior approach lumbar fusions cause a marked increase in thromboembolic events: causal inferences from a propensity-matched analysis of 1147 patients. Clin Neurol Neurosurg. 2022;223:107506.
25. McLynn RP, Diaz-Collado PJ, Ottesen TD, et al. Risk factors and pharmacologic prophylaxis for venous thromboembolism in elective spine surgery. Spine J. 2018;18:970–8.
26. Rokito SE, Schwartz MC, Neuwirth MG. Deep vein thrombosis after major reconstructive spinal surgery. Spine. 1996;21:853–8; discussion 859.
27. Kearon C, Akl EA, Comerota AJ, et al. Antithrombotic therapy for VTE disease: antithrombotic therapy and prevention of thrombosis, 9th ed: American College of Chest Physicians Evidence-Based Clinical Practice Guidelines. Chest. 2012;141:e419S–96S.
28. Bono CM, Watters WC III, Heggeness MH, et al. An evidence-based clinical guideline for the use of antithrombotic therapies in spine surgery. Spine J. 2009;9:1046–51.
29. Reddy D, Mikhael MM, Shapiro GS, et al. Extensive deep venous thrombosis resulting from anterior lumbar spine surgery in a patient with iliac vein compression syndrome: a case report and literature review. Global Spine J. 2015;5:22–7.
30. Schairer WW, Pedtke AC, Hu SS. Venous thromboembolism after spine surgery. Spine. 2014;39:911–8.
31. Zhang L, Cao H, Chen Y, et al. Risk factors for venous thromboembolism following spinal surgery: a meta-analysis. Medicine (Baltimore). 2020;99:e20954.
32. Lee SI, Allen RT, Garfin S. Venous thromboembolism in spine surgery: review of the current literature and future directions. Semin Spine Surg. 2019;31:100757.
33. Eskildsen SM, Moll S, Lim MR. An algorithmic approach to venous thromboembolism prophylaxis in spine surgery. J Spinal Disord Tech. 2015;28:275–81.
34. Rocha AT, Paiva EF, Lichtenstein A, et al. Risk-assessment algorithm and recommendations for venous thromboembolism prophylaxis in medical patients. Vasc Health Risk Manag. 2007;3:533–53.
35. Goz V, McCarthy I, Weinreb JH, et al. Venous thromboembolic events after spinal fusion: which patients are at high risk? JBJS. 2014;96:936–42.
36. Wells P, Anderson D. The diagnosis and treatment of venous thromboembolism. Hematology Am Soc Hematol Educ Program. 2013;2013:457–63.
37. Furlan JC, Fehlings MG. Role of screening tests for deep venous thrombosis in asymptomatic adults with acute spinal cord injury: an evidence-based analysis. Spine. 2007;32:1908–16.
38. Doğan H, de Roos A, Geleijins J, et al. The role of computed tomography in the diagnosis of acute and chronic pulmonary embolism. Diagn Interv Radiol. 2015;21:307.
39. Zelenty WD, Sama AA. Venous thromboembolism and pulmonary embolism in spine surgery: incidence, prevention, and management. Semin Spine Surg. 2022;34:100923.
40. Cain JE Jr, Major MR, Lauerman WC, et al. The morbidity of heparin therapy after development of pulmonary embolus in patients undergoing thoracolumbar or lumbar spinal fusion. Spine. 1995;20:1600–3.
41. Schizas C, Neumayer F, Kosmopoulos V. Incidence and management of pulmonary embolism following spinal surgery occurring while under chemical thromboprophylaxis. Eur Spine J. 2008;17:970–4.

# Chapter 21
# Wound Complications

Ama J. Winland and Paul W. White

## Introduction

Exposures for anterior lumbar interbody fusion (ALIF) are typically performed through either Pfannenstiel, midline, or paramedian incisions (Figs. 21.1 and 21.2). The exposures for oblique lumbar interbody fusion (OLIF) and lateral lumbar interbody fusion (LLIF) are performed through incisions on the lateral abdominal wall or flank. Wound complications associated with these incisions include dehiscence, incisional hernia, wound infection, and others. Dehiscence and wound infections typically occur in the immediate postoperative period, while hernias occur more remotely from surgery. Wound complications have been found to occur in about 2.63–6.5% of cases [1–3]. This chapter will describe specific complications, highlight techniques and strategies to mitigate risk, and describe management when a complication does occur. To provide a more thorough understanding of wound complications in general, some of the data presented are representative of all midline laparotomy incisions rather than anterior lumbar-specific approaches. Data specific to ALIF approaches will be identified as such.

A. J. Winland (✉)
Walter Reed Military Medical Center, Department of Surgery, Bethesda, MD, USA

P. W. White
Inova Heart and Vascular Institute, Falls Church, VA, USA

© The Author(s), under exclusive license to Springer Nature
Switzerland AG 2023
J. R. O'Brien et al. (eds.), *Lumbar Spine Access Surgery*,
https://doi.org/10.1007/978-3-031-48034-8_21

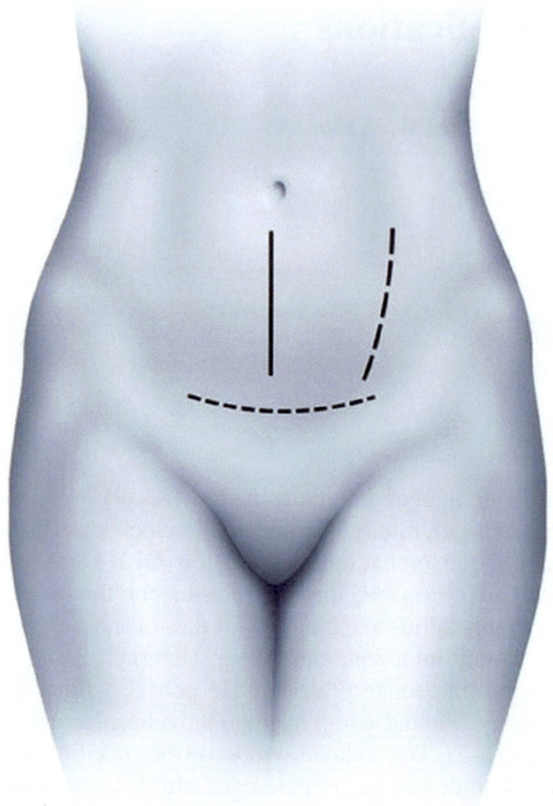

**Fig. 21.1** Examples of Pfannenstiel, midline, and paramedian ALIF incisions. Aryan, H.E., Berven, S.H., Ames, C.P. (2009). Anterior Lumbar Interbody Fusion (ALIF). In: Ozgur, B., Benzel, E., Garfin, S. (eds) Minimally Invasive Spine Surgery. Springer, New York, NY. https://doi. org/10.1007/978-0-387-89831-5_17

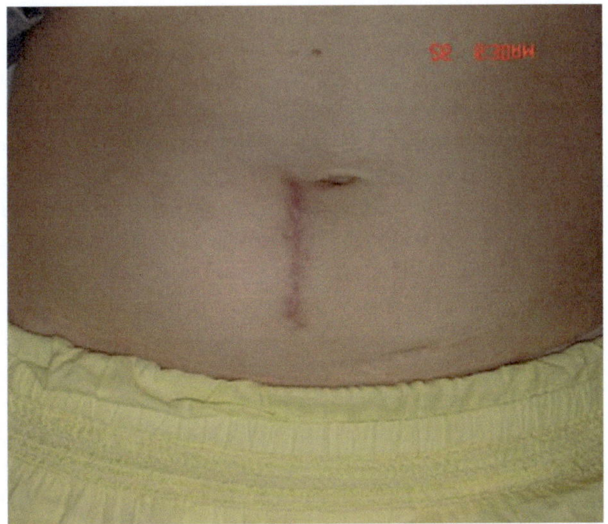

**Fig. 21.2** Paramedian incision. http://www.ijssurgery.com/content/4/3/87

# Complications

## *Dehiscence*

The rates of surgical wound dehiscence for typical midline laparotomy incisions range from 0.2 to 6% [4]. This is slightly higher than the rates of dehiscence cited in the literature for ALIF exposures, which range from as low as 0.11 to 1.8% [2, 5]. There is a paucity of literature comparing Pfannenstiel, midline, and paramedian incisions, and these incisions are often grouped together to garner more powerful analyses.

Risk factors for dehiscence for ALIF exposures are similar to those of traditional midline laparotomy incisions. Obesity is one of the most significant risk factors for dehiscence, and body mass index (BMI) of greater than 30 has been reported to have rate of dehiscence of 3.8% when compared to 0.5% for nonobese patients [2]. A study utilizing the American College of Surgeons National Surgical Quality Improvement Program (NSQIP) database found a BMI greater than 35 increased the risk of wound disruption by an odds ratio of 2.8 [6]. It is not surprising that obese patients are at an increased risk of all wound complications (including infection, hernia, and dehiscence) with rates of 11.4% versus 3.4% [3]. Other risk factors for dehiscence include male gender, postoperative surgical site infection (SSI), use of glucocorticoids, hypoalbunemia, anemia, and emergency operations [3].

Multiple studies have evaluated wound dehiscence risk reduction strategies without much success. However, preoperative antibiotics have been shown to decrease the rate of dehiscence significantly due to their ability to decrease the rate of postoperative surgical site infection (SSI) [7]. Superficial skin breakdown is mitigated by subcuticular suturing, decreasing the rate of breakdown by 90% [8]. Otherwise, no suture type (braided versus monofilament, absorbable versus nonabsorbable, looped versus non-looped) or suture method has been shown to significantly affect the rate of dehiscence [3, 8, 9]. Similarly, the amount of suture and wound length have also not been shown to significantly affect the rates of dehiscence [3]. Though there is some evidence negative pressure wound therapy (NPWT) decreases the rate of SSI, there is no evidence that it affects the rate of dehiscence or superficial skin breakdown [10].

There are multiple options for the treatment of abdominal wall dehiscence. If primary closure is possible, as is often the case with spine exposure, the patient may be taken back to the operating room for debridement and repeat primary fascial closure. Evidence of evisceration is a surgical emergency. A moist dressing should be placed over the wound or exposed bowel at the bedside for protection. The patient should then be taken emergently to the operating room for wound exploration and attempt at abdominal wall closure.

If there are no signs of infection, the wound may be loosely primarily closed, or NPWT may be placed if there is any concern for infection or otherwise left open. If primary closure of the fascial defect is not possible, NPWT can be initiated directly over the area of dehiscence. The resulting soft tissue defect is then addressed with either skin flap mobilization or split thickness skin grafting later once the enough granulation tissue has formed. A multidisciplinary approach with plastic surgery consultation or an experienced abdominal wall surgeon is highly encouraged.

## *Hernias*

The rate of incisional hernias for abdominal incisions varies widely and can be anywhere from 10% to 23% [11]. The rate of incisional hernia after ALIF is much lower in the literature, ranging anywhere from 0.5 to 3.2%. One study with either a mini-Pfannenstiel or vertical midline incision quoted a rate of 1.3% versus a separate study that utilized a paramedian approach resulting in incisional hernias in 0.5% of patients [1, 12]. There were no studies that directly compared the surgical approach to the rate of incisional hernias. OLIF and LLIF have a very low rate of hernias. Fujibayashi et al. reported only three hernias in a series of nearly 3000 patients [13].

The risk factors for incisional hernias are similar to those for dehiscence. In the setting of ALIF, Safaee et al. demonstrated a 5.3% risk of hernia in those with BMI greater than 30 versus 2% for those with BMI less than 30 ($p = 0.0007$) [2]. Preoperative patient counseling becomes important for patients with increased BMI as patients with BMI greater than 30 may benefit from weight loss prior to their elective surgery to reduce their risk of wound complications. It was also noted by Safaee et al. that, regardless of BMI, suture length and suture technique for fascial closure did not affect the rate of incisional hernias in their study [2].

While there were no trials that specifically addressed ways to prevent incisional hernias, there is a large body of literature for abdominal surgical incisions. A trial done by Deerenberg et al. (2015), called the STITCH trial, demonstrated that a running technique with long-lasting monofilament suture, such as polydioxanone

(PDS), decreased incisional hernia rates significantly [11]. Patel et al. demonstrated that monofilament suture decreased the rate of incisional hernia [RR 0.76 95% CI 0.59, 0.98] [14]. Zucker et al. showed that both nylon and PDS demonstrated a reduction in incisional hernias when compared to other popular sutures used for closure (regardless of braided versus monofilament or absorbable versus permanent) [9]. Patel et al. also suggested that there was no significant difference for absorbable versus nonabsorbable, mass versus layered closure, continuous versus interrupted suture, and fast absorbable versus slow absorbable suture [14].

With regard to the more nuanced components of fascial closure, the STITCH trial was a large randomized controlled trial for elective abdominal midline laparotomy fascial closure in patients 18 years and older. The study examined incisional hernia rates with sutures placed 5 mm deep and 5 mm apart with 2-0 PDS (small bite group) and sutures placed 1 cm deep and 1 cm apart with looped #1 PDS (large bite group) [11]. They found that the large bites group had a 21% rate of incisional hernia versus 13% for the smaller bites group ($p = 0.0220$, covariate adjusted odds ratio 0.52, 95% CI 0.31–0.87; $p = 0.0131$) [11]. Because both the needle size and the depth and spacing of the bites differed in both groups, it is difficult to say what matters more: smaller bites or a smaller needle. It is possible that both contribute to a superior fascial closure, which is why for elective laparotomy cases the STITCH trial has now become standard of care. A specific technique, deemed the continuous double-layer closure (CDLC) technique, should *not* be used. Not only did it not result in fewer wound complications, but those in the CDLC group were found to have increased pulmonary complications and increased mortality, thought to be secondary to loss of abdominal compliance from the tightness of the closure [7].

All incisional hernias should be repaired, with the type of repair being dependent on surgeon preference (Fig. 21.3). Strangulation is a surgical emergency and should be treated as such, with immediate repair. Incarceration should be addressed urgently. Reducible hernias can be repaired on an elective, outpatient basis, but these patients should still be referred to a general surgeon for repair, either laparoscopic or open.

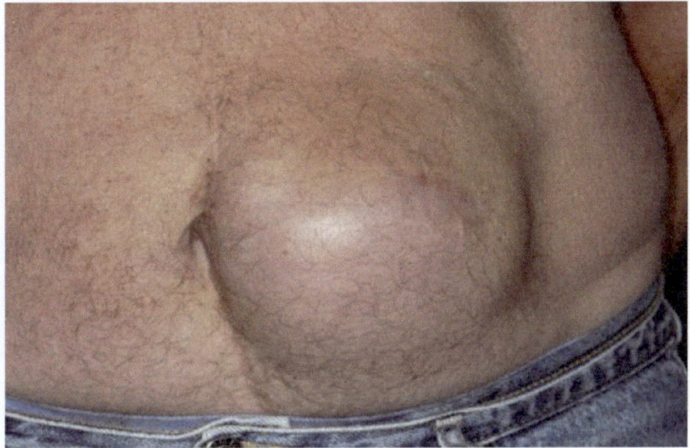

**Fig. 21.3** Incisional hernia. Merck manual photo library

## *Surgical Site Infections*

The current rate of SSI ranges anywhere from 1 to 5% for all-comers who have had abdominal surgery versus 1.1–4.3% for those undergoing ALIF [2, 5, 15, 16]. The rate of superficial SSI for ALIF ranges anywhere from 1 to 2.2% with deep surgical site infections being much less prevalent at 0.08% (Fig. 21.4) [5, 12]. There were no data to suggest atypical organisms or more virulent infections after ALIF when compared to other abdominal surgeries. Therefore, prevention of infections in those who have undergone ALIF is comparable to anyone undergoing abdominal surgery. The rate of SSI for OLIF and LLIF also is very low [13, 17]. Shillingford et al. discovered no difference in infection rates between ALIF/OLIF/LLIF and posterior approaches for one-level spinal fusion in a study that looked at over 7500 patients from NSQIP [18].

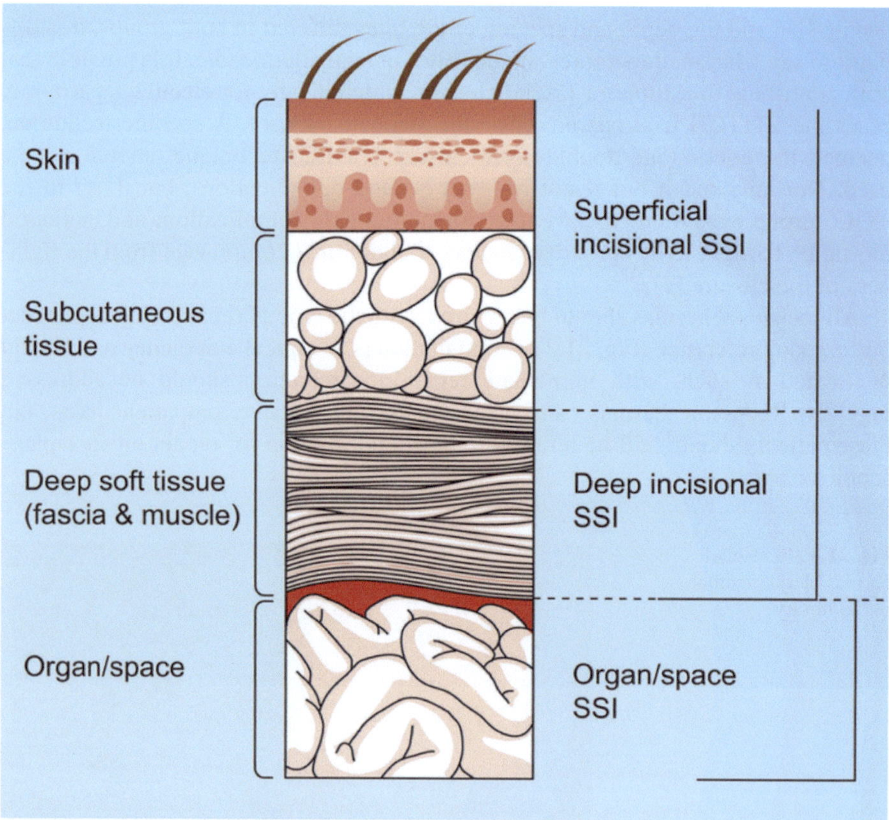


Classification of surgical site infections according to CDC National Nosocomial Surveillance System SSI: Surgical site infection. Reproduced from [14].

**Fig. 21.4**  Classification of SSI according to depth

The type of suture and fascial/skin closure methods have been studied extensively with regard to prevention of dehiscence, hernia, and SSI. There is no evidence that continuous versus interrupted skin closure or mass versus layered closure significantly affects SSI, though most opt for a continuous closure of the abdominal wall as it has been shown to decrease the rate of incisional hernia in the elective general surgery population [8, 14]. Furthermore, the STITCH trial showed that there was no difference in SSI for small (5 mm) versus large (1 cm) bites or small (2-0 PDS) versus large (#1 PDS) suture and needle [19]. It has also been shown that there is no difference in the rate of SSI for absorbable versus nonabsorbable suture or fast absorbable versus slow absorbable suture [5]. Monofilament versus multifilament also demonstrated no significant difference in SSI rates. It is important to note that the use of monofilament, slow absorbable, continuous suture to close the abdominal wall is regarded as the standard as it has been shown to significantly decrease the risk of incisional hernia, but that trend does not apply to SSI.

Other factors that have been investigated include the use of prophylactic antibiotics, use of irrigation, use of NPWT, and patient factors that could potentially increase the risk of SSI. Prophylactic intravenous antibiotics prior to skin incision are standard of care and have been shown to decrease SSI for almost all operations. Topical antibiotics have been shown to be statistically better than applying nothing to an incision for preventing SSI, regardless of type, with no increased incidence of contact dermatitis (RR 0.61, CI 0.42–0.87) [20]. While there is no high-certainty evidence regarding irrigation and prevention of SSI, there is low-certainty evidence that pulsatile irrigation compared to non-pulsatile irrigation may prevent infection as well as antibacterial irrigation being superior to nonbacterial irrigation [21]. There is moderate-certainty evidence that NPWT decreases risk of surgical site infection generally speaking, though cost-effectiveness has been questioned in the setting of ALIF [10]. For those undergoing ALIF, obesity has been shown to significantly increase the SSI rate, with those with a BMI greater than 30 having an infection rate of 3.2% versus 1.1% ($p = 0.022$) [22]. Miller et al. demonstrated an increased risk of SSI for patients with a BMI over 35 [6].

The treatment of surgical site infections after ALIF does not differ from standard treatment of all surgical site infections. Antibiotics should be prescribed for at least 7–10 days with appropriate antibiotic coverage depending on whether the infection is superficial or deep. All abscesses should be drained for source control.

## Other Complications

The following are less common or less significant complications than those addressed above; however, they still merit mention.

## Seromas and Hematomas

The rate of superficial hematomas and seromas is not well characterized in the literature, as most studies did not separate incisional hematomas/seromas from retroperitoneal seromas/hematomas in their analyses. Most only reported hematomas/seromas that required a return to the operating room or other interventions. Bateman et al. reported an incidence of 0.53% [5]. A separate chapter will discuss postoperative fluid collections and their management. Drainage of a hematoma or seroma is required if they are symptomatic, large, or infected.

## Hypertrophic Scarring and Keloid Formation

Hypertrophic scarring and keloid formation are not unique to abdominal or even surgical incisions. They can occur anywhere and are thought to be driven by an inappropriate response to the typical inflammatory response of wound healing. In addition to being a cosmetic concern, they can also be quite painful. Specific risk factors include: increased BMI; non-Caucasian background or dark skin; early postoperative incisional pain and itching; younger age (11–30 years of age); individuals with significant allergies, skin bacterial colonization, and skin tension [22, 23]. Conversely, multiple factors have also been found to be protective and include antihypertensive agents, chemotherapy, smoking, and erythropoiesis-inducing substances (proton pump inhibitors and erythropoietin) [22, 23]. Of note, there was no association between the type and the amount of suture used [23]. Typically, hypertrophic scarring and keloids are treated primarily with corticosteroid injections, while re-excision is reserved for recalcitrant cases. However, there is always the risk of forming another hypertrophic scar or keloid at the revision site, especially if prior risk factors persist.

## Rectus Muscle Atrophy/Changes in Cutaneous Sensation

Rectus muscle atrophy is typically associated with thoracotomy incisions or abdominal incisions that are off midline and close to the costal margin (chevron incision, open nephrectomy/adrenalectomy), thereby implicating intercostal and subcostal nerves as the site of injury. However, a small retrospective study showed all 12 patients in the study with a paramedian incision for a retroperitoneal approach had significant left-sided rectus muscle atrophy as evidenced by computed tomographic imaging postoperatively (Fig. 21.5) [12]. Furthermore, the rate of an abdominal bulge after an extraperitoneal approach, thought to be due to abdominal wall musculature denervation, is 11–23% [24]. This can lead to significant morbidity as there is no operative solution to denervation of the abdominal wall. While it may improve over time, the deficits are likely permanent, leading to cosmetic and functional issues for the patient for the rest of their lives (Fig. 21.6).

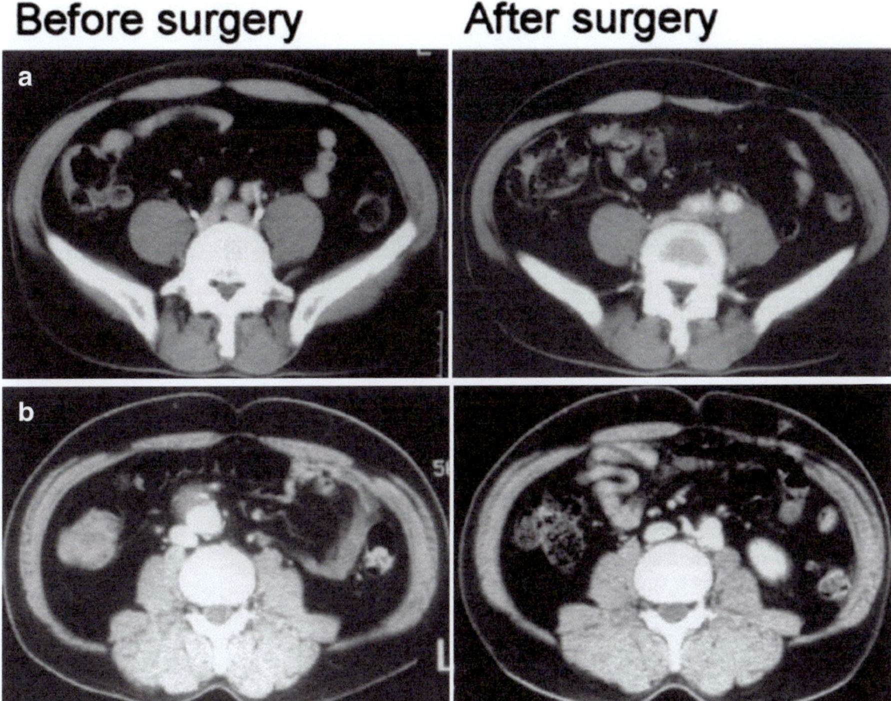


**Fig. 21.5** Computed tomographic findings of abdominal wall rectus muscle atrophy following anterior lumbar interbody fusion. (**a**) Note muscle atrophy in rectus abdominis muscle only 2 months after surgery, but thickness of lateral abdominal muscles did not change. (**b**) Note remarkable atrophy only in rectus abdominis muscle 24 months after surgery

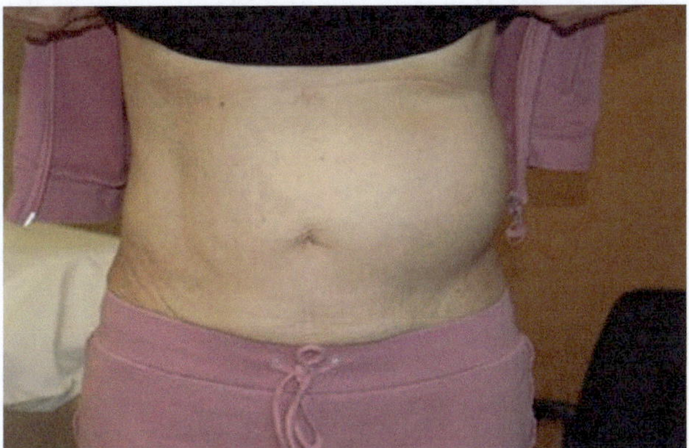

**Fig. 21.6** Dakwar, Elias, Tien V. Le, Ali A. Baaj, Anh X. Le, William D. Smith, Behrooz A. Akbarnia, and Juan S. Uribe. "Abdominal wall paresis as a complication of minimally invasive lateral transpsoas interbody fusion", Neurosurgical Focus FOC 31, 4 (2011): E18, doi: https://doi.org/10.3171/2011.7.FOCUS11164

## Conclusion

Practitioners who are involved in either anterior or lateral approaches to the spine should be aware of potential wound-related complications that may occur postoperatively. Expeditious recognition of potentially catastrophic complications like herniation with strangulation or evisceration can help minimize patient morbidity. Optimizing controllable patient factors and meticulous surgical technique can minimize the risk of wound issues. A close working relationship with any approach surgeon and other members of the surgical team can help lead to optimal patient outcomes and reduce the risk of unplanned return to the operating room and infection.

## References


1. Manunga J, Alcala C, Smith J, Mirza A, Titus J, Skeik N, et al. Technical approach, outcomes, and exposure-related complications in patients undergoing anterior lumbar interbody fusion. J Vasc Surg. 2021;73(3):992–8.
2. Safaee MM, Tenorio A, Osorio JA, Choy W, Amara D, Lai L, et al. The impact of obesity on perioperative complications in patients undergoing anterior lumbar interbody fusion. J Neurosurg Spine. 2020;33(3):332–41.
3. Walming S, Angenete E, Block M, Bock D, Gessler B, Haglind E. Retrospective review of risk factors for surgical wound dehiscence and incisional hernia. BMC Surg. 2017;17(1):19.
4. Aksamija G, Mulabdic A, Rasic I, Aksamija L. Evaluation of risk factors of surgical wound dehiscence in adults after laparotomy. Med Arch. 2016;70(5):369–72.
5. Bateman DK, Millhouse PW, Shahi N, Kadam AB, Maltenfort MG, Koerner JD, et al. Anterior lumbar spine surgery: a systematic review and meta-analysis of associated complications. Spine J. 2015;15(5):1118–32.
6. Miller EM, McAllister BD. Increased risk of postoperative wound complications among obesity classes II & III after ALIF in 10-year ACS-NSQIP analysis of 10,934 cases. Spine J. 2022;22(4):587–94.
7. Niggebrugge AH, Trimbos JB, Hermans J, Steup WH, Van De Velde CJ. Influence of abdominal-wound closure technique on complications after surgery: a randomised study. Lancet. 1999;353(9164):1563–7.
8. Gurusamy KS, Toon CD, Allen VB, Davidson BR. Continuous versus interrupted skin sutures for non-obstetric surgery. Cochrane Database of Syst Rev. 2014;14:CD010365. https://doi.org/10.1002/14651858.CD010365.pub2.
9. Zucker B, Simillis C, Tekkis P, Kontovounisios C. Suture choice to reduce occurrence of surgical site infection, hernia, wound dehiscence and sinus/fistula: a network meta-analysis. Ann R Coll Surg Engl. 2019;101(3):150–61.
10. Norman G, Goh EL, Dumville JC, Shi C, Liu Z, Chiverton L, et al. Negative pressure wound therapy for surgical wounds healing by primary closure. Cochrane Database Syst Rev. 2020;6:CD009261. https://doi.org/10.1002/14651858.CD009261.pub5.
11. Deerenberg EB, Harlaar JJ, Steyerberg EW, Lont HE, van Doorn HC, Heisterkamp J, et al. Small bites versus large bites for closure of abdominal midline incisions (STITCH): a double-blind, multicentre, randomised controlled trial. Lancet. 2015;386(10000):1254–60.
12. Mobbs RJ, Phan K, Daly D, Rao PJ, Lennox A. Approach-related complications of anterior lumbar interbody fusion: results of a combined spine and vascular surgical team. Global Spine J. 2016;6(2):147–54.

13. Fujibayashi S, Kawakami N, Asazuma T, Ito M, Mizutani J, Nagashima H, et al. Complications associated with lateral interbody fusion: Nationwide survey of 2998 cases during the first 2 years of its use in Japan. Spine (Phila Pa 1976). 2017 Oct 1;42(19):1478–84.
14. Patel SV, Paskar DD, Nelson RL, Vedula SS, Steele SR. Closure methods for laparotomy incisions for preventing incisional hernias and other wound complications. Cochrane Database Syst Rev. 2017;11:CD005661. https://doi.org/10.1002/14651858.CD005661.pub2.
15. Quraishi NA, Konig M, Booker SJ, Shafafy M, Boszczyk BM, Grevitt MP, et al. Access related complications in anterior lumbar surgery performed by spinal surgeons. Eur Spine J. 2013;22(S1):16–20.
16. Liu Z, Dumville JC, Norman G, Westby MJ, Blazeby J, McFarlane E, et al. Intraoperative interventions for preventing surgical site infection: an overview of Cochrane reviews. Cochrane Database Syst Rev. 2018;2018(2):CD012653. https://doi.org/10.1002/14651858.CD012653.pub2.
17. Ricciardi L, Piazza A, Capobianco M, Della Pepa GM, Miscusi M, Raco A, et al. Lumbar interbody fusion using oblique (OLIF) and lateral (LLIF) approaches for degenerative spine disorders: a meta-analysis of the comparative studies. Eur J Orthop Surg Traumatol. 2021;33:1. https://doi.org/10.1007/s00590-021-03172-0.
18. Shillingford JN, Laratta JL, Lombardi JM, Mueller JD, Cerpa M, Reddy HP, et al. Complications following single-level interbody fusion procedures: an ACS-NSQIP study. J Spine Surg. 2018;4(1):17–27.
19. Momin AA, Barksdale EM, Lone Z, Enders JJ, Nowacki AS, Winkelman RD, et al. Exploring perioperative complications of anterior lumber interbody fusion in patients with a history of prior abdominal surgery: a retrospective cohort study. Spine J. 2020;20(7):1037–43.
20. Heal CF, Banks JL, Lepper PD, Kontopantelis E, van Driel ML. Topical antibiotics for preventing surgical site infection in wounds healing by primary intention. Cochrane Database Syst Rev. 2016;11:CD011426. https://doi.org/10.1002/14651858.CD011426.pub2.
21. Norman G, Atkinson RA, Smith TA, Rowlands C, Rithalia AD, Crosbie EJ, et al. Intracavity lavage and wound irrigation for prevention of surgical site infection. Cochrane Database Syst Rev. 2017;2017(10):CD012234. https://doi.org/10.1002/14651858.CD012234.pub2.
22. Butzelaar L, Ulrich MMW, Mink van der Molen AB, Niessen FB, Beelen RHJ. Currently known risk factors for hypertrophic skin scarring: a review. J Plast Reconstr Aesthet Surg. 2016;69(2):163–9.
23. Butzelaar L, Soykan EA, Galindo Garre F, Beelen RHJ, Ulrich MM, Niessen FB, et al. Going into surgery: risk factors for hypertrophic scarring. Wound Repair Regen. 2015;23(4):531–7.
24. Yamada M, Maruta K, Shiojiri Y, Takeuchi S, Matsuo Y, Takaba T. Atrophy of the abdominal wall muscles after extraperitoneal approach to the aorta. J Vasc Surg. 2003;38(2):346–53.

# Chapter 22
# Fluid Collections

**Conor P. Lynch, Elliot D. K. Cha, and Jonathan A. Myers**

## Introduction

Postoperative complications are uncommon following anterior lumbar interbody fusion (ALIF) and lateral lumbar interbody fusion (LLIF) procedures, especially with the collaboration of an access surgeon [1]. However, reported occurrences include vascular or neurologic injury, urological or gastrointestinal (GI) complications, implant failure, and infection. An intra-abdominal or retroperitoneal fluid collection is a rarer but potentially clinically significant complication and generally represents a hematoma or seroma.

Although the true prevalence of this complication is hard to determine, prior studies have suggested hematomas/seromas occur at a rate of approximately 0.53%, which may be reduced by more than 50% with the inclusion of a dedicated access surgeon [2]. However, the true incidence may further vary based on whether or not asymptomatic accumulations are recognized, making this complication an important consideration during and after an anterior retroperitoneal approach to the spine. Given the relatively low prevalence among anterior and lateral spinal procedures, treatment algorithms should be optimized based on the type of fluid accumulation, which can include, but is not limited to, cerebrospinal fluid (CSF), hematoma, urinoma, lymphocele/seroma, and abscess. In this chapter, we describe the diagnosis, treatment, and consideration of the various types of postoperative fluid accumulations associated with the anterior and lateral approaches to the spine.


C. P. Lynch · E. D. K. Cha
Department of Orthopaedic Surgery, Rush University Medical Center, Chicago, IL, USA

J. A. Myers (✉)
Department of Surgery, Rush University Medical Center, Chicago, IL, USA



© The Author(s), under exclusive license to Springer Nature Switzerland AG 2023

J. R. O'Brien et al. (eds.), *Lumbar Spine Access Surgery*, https://doi.org/10.1007/978-3-031-48034-8_22

## Diagnosis

Although symptomatic fluid accumulations are uncommon following anterior or lateral spinal surgery, a number of cases have been reported in the literature [2]. Symptoms vary based on the etiology leading to the collection, as well as patient-specific characteristics. More broadly, fluid accumulations can lead to generalized abdominal symptoms related to intra-abdominal mass effect and pressure, such as abdominal distention, pain, and nausea or vomiting [3]. In some cases, the abdomen is appreciably distended with fluid accumulation palpable upon physical examination [4].

When fluid accumulation is suspected, computed tomography (CT) or ultrasound of the abdomen and pelvis should be obtained for confirmation. In fact, many intra-abdominal or retroperitoneal fluid collections present asymptomatically but are initially recognized incidentally on imaging performed for other purposes. For example, CT is a regular part of postoperative follow-up for some surgeons following spinal fusion procedures, and a fluid collection may be identified on these images. Once identified, it is important to determine the depth and location of the fluid accumulation. Depending on the nature and origin of the fluid, accumulations may be relatively superficial or located deep within the pelvic space.

Following recognition and localization of a fluid collection on imaging, percutaneous aspiration under ultrasound or CT guidance may be considered to obtain a fluid sample when the location is accessible and further diagnosis is indicated. For smaller fluid collections, percutaneous aspiration may prove to be therapeutic as well as diagnostic. Accumulations that are especially deep or intimately associated with vulnerable structures will require return to the operating room for surgical exploration to pursue definitive diagnosis and management. In addition to patient symptoms and clinical presentation, chemical and histological analyses of aspirated fluid are often key to diagnosing the specific etiology of an abdominal or retroperitoneal fluid collection. Characteristic findings are discussed in association with each potential etiology of fluid collection in the following sections.

## Lymphocele and Lymphatic Leak

Among the various causes of postoperative fluid collection, a lymphatic leak resulting in a lymphocele is one of the most common. Incidence has previously been estimated around 1.0% [5]; however, there is a paucity of high-quality epidemiological data on this phenomenon. Some surgeons have speculated that the relatively low lymphatic pressure after preoperative fasting may contribute to the rarity of this complication. However, if a lymphatic injury does occur, low lymphatic pressure may also translate to a low likelihood of intraoperative recognition or diagnosis [3].

After obtaining a fluid sample, cytology will be key in confirming the diagnosis of a lymphatic leak. Analysis of lymphatic fluid will characteristically demonstrate a high white blood cell count with lymphocytic predominance (>95%). Additional analysis includes culture, staining with Sudan III, demonstrating elevated specific gravity, and determining levels of amylase, lipase, creatinine, protein, and triglycerides [3].

For relatively mild or asymptomatic cases, observation versus management with needle aspiration followed by sclerosis with doxycycline or povidone iodine will typically be sufficient [6, 7]. However, these nonoperative strategies are associated with relatively high rates of lymphocele recurrence, which requires additional intervention. If more definitive management is required, the next step will be to determine the location of the lymphatic leak. There are several methods that can be employed to localize the defect. A lymphangiogram can localize the trajectory of the leakage within the lymphatic system. Specifically, contrast is injected into a lymph node proximal (based on flow) to the site of fluid accumulation and is followed under radiographic imaging to locate the leak. If more precise localization of the defect is needed, injection of methylene blue dye into the lymph node will allow for direct visualization as it leaks from the defect. Once located in this manner, the defect should then be ligated with sutures, taking care not to damage underlying structures, such as the iliac vasculature or ureter.

Management of the fluid accumulation itself will largely depend upon the volume of fluid as well as patient-specific symptoms. Smaller collections may spontaneously reabsorb, while larger symptomatic accumulations may necessitate further intervention. One such option is transabdominal laparoscopic fenestration of a retroperitoneal collection to allow the fluid to drain into the peritoneal cavity where it may be more readily absorbed. However, a very large accumulation may exceed the absorptive capacity of the peritoneum which may require surgical exploration and external drainage.

## Hematoma

Rates of retroperitoneal hematoma have been reported as 0.76–0.9% following anterior lumbar spinal surgery [8, 9]. Following lateral approach spinal surgery, rates of psoas hematoma have been reported at 0.18% [10]. More superficial hematomas localized to the abdominal wall have also been reported [11]. The specific mechanism of injury leading to hematoma formation is not clear [8, 9]; however, some surgeons speculate that injury to segmental arteries may be a potential cause of hematoma specific to the transpsoas approach and suggest identification of these vessels on preoperative imaging [10].

Hematomas are visualized on CT or magnetic resonance imaging (MRI) but in some cases will need to be differentiated from an abscess, which can present with a similar appearance on imaging. If a postoperative hematoma is asymptomatic and sterile, it will likely resolve spontaneously with no further intervention. However, a number of cases of intra-abdominal or retroperitoneal hematomas which required reoperation for surgical evacuation have previously been reported [8, 9]. Additionally, psoas hematomas may present with significant pain as well as neurological deficit in the form of hip or lower extremity weakness secondary to lumbar plexus compression [10]. Several reported cases of neurological deficit persisted following surgical evacuation [10]. In the event that a hematoma is discovered to be the cause of new-onset postoperative pain or neurological deficit, prompt surgical evacuation should be performed.

## Cerebral Spinal Fluid Leak

Most causes of abdominal and retroperitoneal fluid accumulation are related to the surgical approach. However, a CSF leak may be secondary to intraoperative durotomy due to spinal instrumentation. Dural tears are relatively uncommon in association with anterior spine surgery, though reports do exist in the literature [2]. While most of the complications described in this chapter are best addressed by a dedicated access surgeon, the relation and proximity of a dural injury to the spinal instrumentation operation itself is typically better addressed by an orthopedic or neurological spine surgeon. As management of intraoperative durotomy is extensively described in other literature, this discussion will be limited to the identification of dural tears as a cause of a postoperative fluid accumulation.

Dural tears may present with symptoms including postural headaches as well as nausea and vomiting [12]. CSF accumulation secondary to anterior or lateral approach spine surgery will typically be found at a relatively deep location; therefore, significant fluctuance or fluid mass is unlikely to be appreciable upon physical examination. Furthermore, given the relatively low overall volume of CSF compared with other potential sources, fluid accumulations secondary to a dural tear are likely to be relatively small. While CSF accumulation is visible on CT imaging, MRI should be considered for identification of a dural fistula if a CSF leak is suspected. On histochemical examination, clear fluid with minimal leukocytes, low protein, and presence of glucose (40–80 mg/dL) is indicative of CSF [13].

## Urinoma/Urine Leak

Ureteral injury with subsequent presence of urine in a fluid collection in the retroperitoneum is rare [14–18]. After a fluid accumulation is identified on CT or other forms of imaging, the location of fluid may provide insight as to the site of injury. Additionally, intravenous (IV) contrast can be used to confirm a urinoma, whereby the fluid collection will become opacified on delayed CT imaging [15, 19, 20]. Percutaneous drainage and testing for creatinine will confirm the presence of a urinoma.

Difficulty in diagnosing a urinoma is magnified by nonspecific presentation of symptoms, including abdominal pain, nausea, vomiting, and fever. Patients may also have a delayed presentation (days to months) which can further complicate management. After recognition, interventional radiology can perform retroperitoneal urinoma drainage and percutaneous catheter placement. After consultation with urology, cystoscopy and a retrograde pyelogram should be performed to accurately localize the site of injury. Once identified, low-grade ureteral injuries are generally managed with cystoscopy and retrograde ureteral stenting. In instances of unsuccessful stenting by an inferior approach, a superior approach via percutaneous nephrostomy and antegrade stent placement should be performed by interventional radiology. If a complete avulsion of the ureter is discovered, surgical intervention will be necessary. Depending on the timing of diagnosis, delayed surgical repair should be considered to allow the inflammatory response to resolve after a period of nephrostomy diversion.

## Abscess

Infections and abscesses after anterior spine surgery can occur at either a superficial or a deep level. A systematic review of complications related to anterior retroperitoneal approaches to lumbar fusion surgery detailed an incidence of 0.05% for deep infections and 0.73% for superficial infections among studies involving an access surgeon [1]. As with other forms of abscesses, initial diagnosis is reliant upon drainage and confirmation of purulent fluid. Clinical findings such as a positive psoas sign also reinforce a diagnosis of retroperitoneal abscess.

Patients can demonstrate clinical presentations and laboratory values indicative of an infection (erythema and/or induration, fever, diaphoresis, leukocytosis); however, latent infections are of greater concern as they can develop over a period of time ranging from days to weeks or even several years [21]. Once an abscess is confirmed, treatment should include drainage and subsequent culture of the purulent fluid. Drainage can be performed under the guidance of ultrasound or CT imaging or using an open approach. Common pathogens include methicillin-resistant *S. aureus*, which is associated with nosocomial infections. Once the abscess has been drained, wound debridement and administration of IV antibiotics should be considered. Further management of abscesses associated with spinal instrumentation should be deferred to the spine surgeon.

## Bowel Injury

Although injury to the GI tract is a rare complication following anterior lumbar fusion, it can occur due to manipulation of the rectosigmoid portion of the intestine during access to the lumbosacral disk space [22]. Reports of GI complications associated with the exposure stage of ALIF procedures include intraoperative small bowel and large bowel enterotomy or other injuries and rectal perforation [22–24].

Patients present with clinical signs and symptoms such as abdominal pain, fever, and potentially grossly bloody stools or occult fecal blood. Perforation of the bowel also places patients at risk for infection and abscess formation, which is described in a previous section. Diagnosis will involve the use of CT imaging with oral/rectal contrast or a lower GI study to locate the site of perforation. Depending on the level and extent of the injury and subsequent infection, drainage of the area with subsequent repair and possible diverting ostomy may be required [24].

## Bone Morphogenic Protein Reaction

The use of bone morphogenic protein (BMP) is common among lumbar fusion procedures. While its use can promote bone growth and potentially improve fusion rates, a number of associated postoperative complications have been reported. Currently, there is little evidence to suggest that this biologic agent places patients at increased risk for postoperative fluid accumulation. However, it is suggested that the use of BMP in thoracolumbar fusion may promote serous inflammation of the fusion site [25]. Informal surveys among access surgeons suggested that surgeons should be aware of the potential complication of a painful seroma following rhBMP-2 use in minimally invasive lumbar spine surgery, but its incidence still requires additional study [26]. Though there is a lack of consensus on development of inflammatory responses and subsequent fluid accumulation in lumbar fusion procedures, a similar approach to the diagnosis (imaging and drainage) and treatment should be considered.

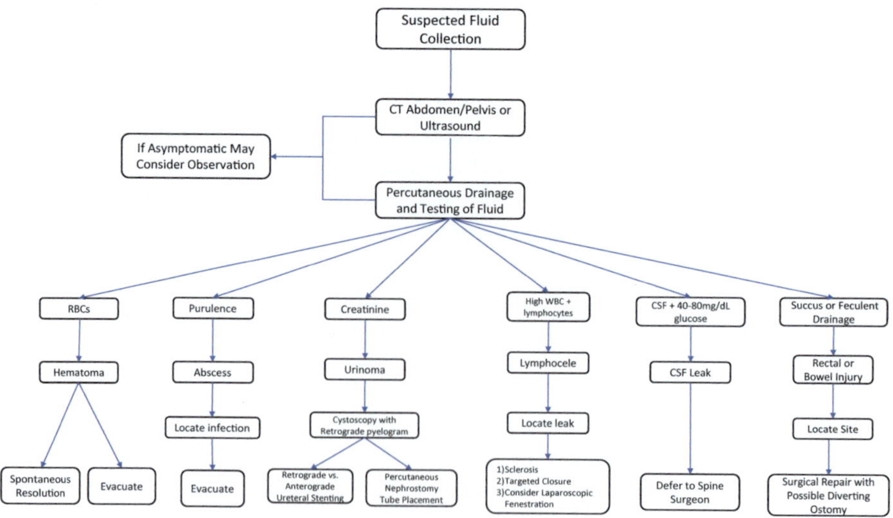


**Fig. 22.1** Diagnosis and management algorithm

# Conclusion

When a fluid collection is identified and the level of urgency has been established, management can be determined based on the patient presentation (symptomatic versus asymptomatic) and fluid type (Fig. 22.1). While postoperative fluid collections are relatively uncommon following anterior and lateral lumbar spine surgery, the underlying etiologies can vary greatly in terms of the risk they present and the complexity of their management. Therefore, prompt and accurate diagnosis is key to successful management. To this end, it is important for any surgeon navigating the anterior or lateral approaches to the spine to understand the typical presentations and standard treatment protocols for common causes of postoperative fluid collection.

# References


1. Phan K, Xu J, Scherman DB, Rao PJ, Mobbs RJ. Anterior lumbar interbody fusion with and without an "access surgeon": a systematic review and meta-analysis. Spine. 2017;42(10):E592–601.
2. Bateman DK, Millhouse PW, Shahi N, et al. Anterior lumbar spine surgery: a systematic review and meta-analysis of associated complications. Spine J. 2015;15(5):1118–32.
3. Patel AA, Spiker WR, Daubs MD, Brodke DS, Cheng I, Glasgow RE. Retroperitoneal lymphocele after anterior spinal surgery. Spine. 2008;33(18):E648–52.
4. Thaler M, Achatz W, Liebensteiner M, Nehoda H, Bach CM. Retroperitoneal lymphatic cyst formation after anterior lumbar interbody fusion: a report of 3 cases. J Spinal Disord Tech. 2010;23(2):146–50.
5. Hussain NS, Hanscom D, Oskouian RJ Jr. Chyloretroperitoneum following anterior spinal surgery. J Neurosurg Spine. 2012;17(5):415–21.
6. Levi AD. Treatment of a retroperitoneal lymphocele after lumbar fusion surgery with intralesional povidone iodine: technical case report. Neurosurgery. 1999;45(3):658–60; discussion 660-661.
7. Jagannathan J, Anton T, Baweja H, Kleiner DE, Peeler B, Arlet V. Evaluation and management of abdominal lymphoceles after anterior lumbar spine surgery. Spine. 2008;33(22):E852–7.
8. Manunga J, Alcala C, Smith J, et al. Technical approach, outcomes, and exposure-related complications in patients undergoing anterior lumbar interbody fusion. J Vasc Surg. 2021;73(3):992–8.
9. Mobbs RJ, Phan K, Daly D, Rao PJ, Lennox A. Approach-related complications of anterior lumbar interbody fusion: results of a combined spine and vascular surgical team. Global Spine J. 2016;6(2):147–54.
10. Beckman JM, Vincent B, Park MS, et al. Contralateral psoas hematoma after minimally invasive, lateral retroperitoneal transpsoas lumbar interbody fusion: a multicenter review of 3950 lumbar levels. J Neurosurg Spine. 2017;26(1):50–4.
11. Momin AA, Barksdale EM 3rd, Lone Z, et al. Exploring perioperative complications of anterior lumber interbody fusion in patients with a history of prior abdominal surgery: a retrospective cohort study. Spine J. 2020;20(7):1037–43.
12. A review article on the diagnosis and treatment of cerebrospinal fluid fistulas and dural tears occurring during spinal surgery—surgical Neurology International. 2015. https://surgicalneurologyint.com/surgicalint-articles/a-review-article-on-the-diagnosis-and-treatment-of-

cerebrospinal-fluid-fistulas-and-dural-tears-occurring-during-spinal-surgery/. Accessed May 29 2021.
13. Jurado R, Walker HK. Cerebrospinal fluid. In: Walker HK, Hall WD, Hurst JW, eds. Clinical methods: the history, physical, and laboratory examinations. Butterworths; Oxford 2011.
14. Guingrich JA, McDermott JC. Ureteral injury during laparoscopy-assisted anterior lumbar fusion. Spine. 2000;25(12):1586–8.
15. Gayer G, Zissin R, Apter S, et al. Urinomas caused by ureteral injuries: CT appearance. Abdom Imaging. 2002;27(1):88–92.
16. Van Valkenburg S, Trussell JC, Lavelle WF. Retroperitoneal fluid collection following anterior spine surgery—differential and management. Can J Urol. 2016;23(2):8243–6.
17. Isiklar ZU, Lindsey RW, Coburn M. Ureteral injury after anterior lumbar interbody fusion. A case report. Spine. 1996;21(20):2379–82.
18. Wymenga LF, Buijs GA, Ypma AF, Werkman DM. Ureteral injury associated with anterior lumbosacral arthrodesis in a patient who had crossed renal ectopia, malrotation, and fusion of the kidneys. A case report. J Bone Joint Surg Am. 1996;78(5):772–4.
19. Gayer G, Caspi I, Garniek A, Hertz M, Apter S. Perirectal urinoma from ureteral injury incurred during spinal surgery mimicking rectal perforation on computed tomography scan. Spine. 2002;27(20):E451–3.
20. Ghali AM, El Malik EM, Ibrahim AI, Ismail G, Rashid M. Ureteric injuries: diagnosis, management, and outcome. J Trauma. 1999;46(1):150–8.
21. Hresko MT, Hall JE. Latent psoas abscess after anterior spinal fusion. Spine. 1992;17(5):590–3.
22. Bianchi C, Ballard JL, Abou-Zamzam AM, Teruya TH, Abu-Assal ML. Anterior retroperitoneal lumbosacral spine exposure: operative technique and results. Ann Vasc Surg. 2003;17(2):137–42.
23. Rajaraman V, Vingan R, Roth P, Heary RF, Conklin L, Jacobs GB. Visceral and vascular complications resulting from anterior lumbar interbody fusion. J Neurosurg. 1999;91(1 Suppl):60–4.
24. Bohinski RJ, Jain VV, Tobler WD. Presacral retroperitoneal approach to axial lumbar interbody fusion: a new, minimally invasive technique at L5-S1: clinical outcomes, complications, and fusion rates in 50 patients at 1-year follow-up. SAS J. 2010;4(2):54–62.
25. Saulle D, Fu K-MG, Shaffrey CI, Smith JS. Multiple-day drainage when using bone morphogenic protein for long-segment thoracolumbar fusions is associated with low rates of wound complications. World Neurosurg. 2013;80(1-2):204–7.
26. Benglis D, Wang MY, Levi AD. A comprehensive review of the safety profile of bone morphogenetic protein in spine surgery. Neurosurgery. 2008;62(5 Suppl 2):ONS423–31. discussion ONS431.

# Chapter 23
# Ileus Prevention and Management

J. R. Salameh

## Introduction

Postoperative ileus (POI) is a major cause of morbidity in patients undergoing elective spine surgery. An ileus is a functional motility impairment of the gastrointestinal (GI) tract, especially the small intestine, marked by the absence of peristalsis leading to intestinal dilatation and accumulation of fluid and gas within the bowel lumen. A consensus conference in 2006 proposed a definition of POI as a "transient cessation of coordinated bowel motility after surgical intervention, which prevents effective transit of intestinal contents or tolerance of oral intake" [1].

Patients typically present with nausea, vomiting, and abdominal distention as well as absence of flatus. As opposed to mechanical small bowel obstruction, patients with POI have abdominal discomfort related to distension, but not colicky abdominal pain. POI is a temporary disorder that spontaneously resolves over time, particularly as inciting factors are corrected.

A retrospective study of 220,522 patients who underwent lumbar fusion found an overall incidence of POI in 2.6% of patients undergoing a posterior approach, 7.5% of patients undergoing an anterior approach, and 8.4% of patients undergoing both anterior and posterior approaches [2]. Other studies looking at lateral access spine surgery also showed an incidence of ileus between 3.9% and 7% [3, 4]. Invariably across all studies, patients with POI demonstrate greater length of stay and increased costs.

J. R. Salameh (✉)
Surgery, Georgetown University School of Medicine, VHC Health, Washington, DC, USA
e-mail: jrs2574@virginiahospitalcenter.com

© The Author(s), under exclusive license to Springer Nature Switzerland AG 2023
J. R. O'Brien et al. (eds.), *Lumbar Spine Access Surgery*,
https://doi.org/10.1007/978-3-031-48034-8_23

## Pathophysiology of POI

Following most abdominal and retroperitoneal surgeries, the motility of the GI tract is transiently impaired. Among the proposed mechanisms responsible for this dysmotility are surgical stress-induced sympathetic reflexes, inflammatory mediator release, and anesthetic/analgesic side effects, each of which can inhibit intestinal motility. The return of normal motility generally follows a characteristic temporal sequence, with small intestinal motility returning to normal within the first 24 h after surgery, gastric motility returning to normal by 48 h, and colonic motility normalizing in 2 to 5 days [5]. Functional evidence of coordinated GI motility in the form of passing flatus or bowel movement is the most useful indicator of return of normal bowel function.

Risk factors for POI include male gender, three or more levels fused, alcohol abuse, anemia, fluid/electrolyte disorders, and weight loss [2]. In another study of oblique lateral interbody fusion, multivariate analysis identified inadvertent end-plate fracture and the amount of intraoperative opioid use as independent risk factors for the development of POI [6].

In some situations, POI is caused or exacerbated by specific factors that impair local neuromuscular function and activate neurogenic inhibitory pathways, resulting in impaired contractility, motility, relative hypoxemia, and bowel edema. Such inciting factors include electrolyte abnormalities, such as hypokalemia, hyponatremia, hypomagnesemia, and hypermagnesemia; pharmacologic agents, most commonly opiates, such as morphine or meperidine and other drugs including anticholinergics, autonomic blockers, antihistamines, calcium channel blockers; and various psychotropic agents, such as haloperidol and tricyclic antidepressants. Other factors include pneumonia, intra-abdominal abscess/peritonitis, generalized sepsis from a non-abdominal source, and retroperitoneal hematoma.

## Workup of POI

POI is often defined as two or more of the following at 72 h postoperatively: (1) ongoing nausea or vomiting, (2) absence of flatus over last 24-h period, (3) inability to tolerate an oral diet over last 24-h period, (4) ongoing abdominal distention postoperatively, and (5) radiological confirmation [5]. Radiologic diagnosis is often established on plain abdominal X-rays, flat and upright (if the latter is not possible, cross-table lateral views can be obtained), which show distended small bowel loops with air-fluid levels and presence of gas in the colon.

If the clinical picture and plain radiography provide an inconclusive diagnosis, a contrast radiography study or a computed tomography (CT) scan can be obtained. In a contrast study, diatrizoate given orally should reach the cecum in 4 h in cases of adynamic ileus; a stationary column for 4 h indicates complete obstruction. A CT scan of the abdomen and pelvis with intravenous (IV) and oral contrast can also be considered and is usually a better test, not only to confirm an ileus and rule out mechanical small bowel obstruction but also to rule out other postoperative complications that may be presenting as an ileus, such as a retroperitoneal hematoma, an unrecognized bowel injury, an internal hernia secondary to violation of the peritoneum, or a lower lobe pneumonia.

Imaging is also important to rule out pseudo-obstruction of the colon or Ogilvie's syndrome, which is another more severe and potentially life-threatening form of impaired bowel motility. It is characterized by acute colonic dilatation in the absence of mechanical obstruction. Massive colonic distention is noted on plain abdominal films, especially in the ascending colon and cecum, which can reach a diameter of more than 12 cm and lead to perforation. A water-soluble contrast enema or, more frequently, a CT scan of the abdomen and pelvis can reliably distinguish between a mechanical colonic obstruction and pseudo-obstruction.

## Treatment of POI

The treatment of POI is purely supportive along with correction of any contributing factors. Proper resuscitation is critical in these patients; isotonic crystalloids and potassium should be substituted via IV in equivalent volume to losses to maintain euvolemia [7]. Any electrolyte abnormalities should be corrected.

Opioids should be discontinued if possible and replaced with non-opioid analgesics such as IV nonsteroidal anti-inflammatory (NSAID) drugs and acetaminophen. Nutritional status should be regularly assessed and total parenteral nutrition started if the patient has been unable to tolerate adequate oral intake by 7 days postoperatively or even sooner based on the patient's frailty and baseline condition.

Nasogastric (NG) decompression should be considered if the patient is having nausea or vomiting or if the abdominal distention is significant and causing discomfort or compromising respiratory function. Clinicians should ensure that an NG tube is always in working order to decrease the risk of aspiration.

There are currently no effective pharmacologic agents to treat POI. Drugs that block sympathetic input or stimulate parasympathetic activity and prokinetic agents such as metoclopramide, erythromycin, or cisapride do not appear to alter adynamic ileus [8]. IV lidocaine, neostigmine, and alvimopan, a peripheral mu-receptor antagonist, might show a potential effect but remain investigational [8, 9]. The therapeutic use of hyperosmotic, orally administered, water-soluble contrast media such as diatrizoate has been studied, as it theoretically mitigates bowel wall edema, but it has not been found to be clinically useful in shortening POI duration [10].

In the case of Ogilvie's syndrome, initial management is the same supportive care employed in POI. In addition, rectal tube placement for decompression may be helpful. Close clinical monitoring with serial abdominal exams and regular daily abdominal X-rays are needed as further colonic dilation, ischemia, and perforation are feared complications. In cases that do not improve with supportive care or in those with a cecal diameter greater than 12 cm but no evidence of ischemia or perforation, pharmacologic decompression with the acetylcholinesterase inhibitor neostigmine in a monitored setting or colonoscopic decompression is the treatment of choice and has a high success rate. Patients who do not respond to all these treatment modalities or develop systemic toxicity, ischemia, or perforation require surgical intervention. Surgical options range from a cecostomy to a total abdominal colectomy and ileostomy based on the condition of the patient and the status of the colon.

## Prevention of POI

Various measures have been investigated aimed at accelerating postoperative intestinal recovery and preventing POI after various abdominal surgeries including spine surgery. These measures have variable quality of evidence supporting their efficacy, but many of them have been incorporated in multimodal enhanced recovery after surgery (ERAS) or fast-track protocols (Table 23.1).

### *Mechanical Bowel Preparation*

Mechanical bowel preparation includes the use of oral laxatives and dietary restriction to only clear liquids 24 h prior to surgery. It has been liberally used in the past before most transperitoneal and retroperitoneal abdominal surgeries. However, numerous studies have failed to demonstrate any improved outcomes of bowel preparation in transabdominal gynecologic, urologic, and even colorectal surgeries. In addition, bowel preparation leads to patient discomfort, insomnia, electrolyte disturbances, and dehydration.

In anterior and lateral spine surgery, bowel preparation was believed to improve peritoneal mobilization and the quality of surgical field exposure. In retrospective

**Table 23.1** Measures to reduce postoperative ileus in spine surgery

| Measures to reduce POI in spine surgery |
| --- |
| • Avoid mechanical bowel preparation |
| • Balance intraoperative and postoperative IV fluid administration |
| • Correct electrolyte abnormalities |
| • Use opioid-sparing multimodal analgesia |
| • Avoid nasogastric tubes |
| • Early enteral feeding |
| • Gum chewing |
| • Early ambulation |

*POI* postoperative ileus, *IV* intravenous

studies and randomized trials, however, bowel preparation did not improve surgical performance, intraoperative complications, or postoperative bowel function in spine fusion [11, 12]. Given the lack of benefits and presence of adverse effects, the routine use of mechanical bowel preparation in spine surgery should be avoided.

## Fluid and Electrolyte Management

Although IV fluid administration is intended to compensate for intraoperative fluid losses and maintain circulating blood volume, there is no consensus on the optimal fluid management strategy. In a multivariate analysis of risk factors associated with POI following anterior lumbar interbody fusion, patients with perioperative fluid and electrolyte imbalances were four times more likely to experience POI [13]. Generally, there are three fluid replacement regimens: restrictive, liberal, and goal-directed volume therapies. Liberal fluid therapy might lead to intestinal wall edema and subsequent POI and has been correlated with an increased length of hospital stay and an increased time to bowel movement by 2 days [14, 15]. Liberal protocols have generally been abandoned and replaced by restrictive or goal-directed regimens. Whether goal-directed therapy is superior to a restrictive fluid strategy remains uncertain [15].

## Early Ambulation

Immobilization or bed rest may result in delayed functional recovery, slower pain relief, and increased risk of postoperative complications [16]. In a study of 23,295 lumbar surgery patients, patients that ambulated postoperatively on the day of surgery had a significantly decreased length of stay and ileus rate, as compared to those who did not [17]. Early ambulation using nursing or physical therapy protocols should be encouraged in all patients undergoing lumbar surgery.

## Opioid-Sparing Analgesia

Pain control following spine surgery is a prerequisite to promoting early ambulation and postoperative functional recovery. Given the detrimental influence of opioids on POI, opioid-sparing or multimodal analgesic regimens have been employed. Such regimens use a combination of various systemic and regional analgesic therapies to reduce overall opioid consumption and have been implemented in surgeries across most disciplines.

Preoperative or intraoperative acetaminophen and NSAIDs or cyclooxygenase-2-specific inhibitors are recommended as part of a multimodal pain regimen and should be continued postoperatively [18]. Short-term use of low-dose NSAIDs around the time of surgery is safe and has not been shown increase the rate of pseudoarthrosis and does not increase the risk of bleeding [18]. Intraoperative ketamine infusion is effective in reducing perioperative opiate consumption due to its significant opioid-sparing effect, especially in opiate-dependent chronic pain patients, but should not be continued in the postoperative period [18–20].

The use of epidural analgesia with local anesthetic, with or without opioids, using a catheter placed under direct visualization by the surgeon at the end of surgery is an effective component of multimodal analgesia, but its use should be individualized [18]. Because of concerns about loss of sensory function and motor weakness and the possibility of delayed diagnosis of neurological complications, low concentrations of local anesthetics should be used.

Intramuscular local anesthetic infiltration at closure has also been shown to reduce postoperative analgesic requirements and delay the time to first postoperative analgesic requests for patients undergoing lumbar spine surgery [21]. Pre-incisional transverse abdominis plane block has been used in abdominal surgery and may also be effective as an adjunct in anterior and lateral approaches to spine surgery [22, 23].

## Chewing Gum

The practice of gum chewing is hypothesized to reduce POI by stimulating early recovery of GI function through cephalo-vagal stimulation [24]. A 2015 Cochrane review showed that gum chewing resulted in a significant reduction in time to first postoperative flatus and bowel movement, but most research focused primarily on caesarean section and colorectal surgery and largely consisted of small, poor-quality trials [24]. In posterior lumbar spine surgery, chewing gum has been shown to promote bowel function recovery based on a small retrospective study, although no difference in length of hospital stay or postoperative complications was shown [25]. Although there are no studies specifically examining the effect of chewing gum on POI prevention in anterior or lateral approaches to the lumbar spine, it can be considered as it is safe and inexpensive. Current postoperative protocols after lumbar surgery allow for early oral intake, which in turn has been shown to be associated with significantly less ileus in various GI surgeries, which may obviate the need for gum chewing [26, 27].

## Enhanced Recovery After Surgery Pathways

Fast-track programs through variable ERAS pathways have been extensively examined in other surgical disciplines and have gained popularity in spine surgery in recent years. They aim at combining various preoperative, perioperative, and postoperative multimodal interventions to optimize the postsurgical recovery process. They typically include many of the interventions discussed in this chapter.

When spine surgery ERAS protocols are examined, the most common interventions are patient education (72.7%), assessment of patient health and comorbidities (45.5%), carbohydrate loading (40.9%), and a modified preoperative fasting regimen (31.8%) [28]. Common perioperative elements include perioperative multimodal analgesia (68.2%), infection prophylaxis (54.5%), "preemptive" analgesia (50%), catheter and surgical drain-sparing (50%), and minimally invasive surgery (40.9%) [28]. Common postoperative ERAS elements include postoperative multimodal analgesia (81.8%), early mobilization/rehabilitation (77.3%), and early nutrition (54.5%) [28]. Systemic analysis of available initial studies demonstrate the potential of spine surgery-specific ERAS protocols to reduce complications, accelerate return of function, minimize postoperative pain and opioid use, shorten length of stay, and reduce hospital readmissions [28, 29].

## Conclusion

POI can complicate anterior and lateral approaches to the lumbar spine and remains a significant clinical and economic burden. The management of POI is purely supportive, and the surgeon should look for any complications or correctable factors. There are several multimodal strategies that have been proven effective in reducing the overall incidence of POI, and surgeons should look at incorporating such evidence-based measures in ERAS protocols with continuous quality monitoring to assess outcomes at the local level.

## References

1. Augestad KM, Delaney CP. Postoperative ileus: impact of pharmacological treatment, laparoscopic surgery and enhanced recovery pathways. World J Gastroenterol. 2010;16(17):2067–74.
2. Fineberg SJ, Nandyala SV, Kurd MF, Marquez-Lara A, Noureldin M, Sankaranarayanan S, Patel AA, Oglesby M, Singh K. Incidence and risk factors for postoperative ileus following anterior, posterior, and circumferential lumbar fusion. Spine J. 2014;14(8):1680–5.
3. Al Maaieh MA, Du JY, Aichmair A, Huang RC, Hughes AP, Cammisa FP, Girardi FP, Sama AA. Multivariate analysis on risk factors for postoperative ileus after lateral lumbar interbody fusion. Spine (Phila Pa 1976). 2014;39(8):688–94.
4. Park SC. Risk factors for postoperative ileus after oblique lateral interbody fusion: a multivariate analysis. Spine J. 2021;21(3):438–45.
5. Tavakkoli A, Ashley SW, Zinner MJ. Small intestine. Schwartz's principle of surgery. 11th ed. New York: McGraw Hill Professional; 2010. p. 1219–57.
6. Park SC, Chang SY, Mok S, Kim H, Chang BS, Lee CK. Risk factors for postoperative ileus after oblique lateral interbody fusion: a multivariate analysis. Spine J. 2021;21(3):438–45.
7. Vather R, Bissett I. Management of prolonged post-operative ileus: evidence-based recommendations. ANZ J Surg. 2013;83(5):319–24.

8. Traut U, Brügger L, Kunz R, Pauli-Magnus C, Haug K, Bucher HC, Koller MT. Systemic prokinetic pharmacologic treatment for postoperative adynamic ileus following abdominal surgery in adults. Cochrane Database Syst Rev. 2008;1:Cd004930.

9. Chamie K, Golla V, Lenis AT, Lec PM, Rahman S, Viscusi ER. Peripherally acting μ-opioid receptor antagonists in the management of postoperative ileus: a clinical review. J Gastrointest Surg. 2021;25(1):293–302.

10. Vather R, Josephson R, Jaung R, Kahokehr A, Sammour T, Bissett I. Gastrografin in prolonged postoperative ileus: a double-blinded randomized controlled trial. Ann Surg. 2015;262(1):23–30.

11. Olsen U, Brox JI, Bjørk IT. Preoperative bowel preparation versus no preparation before spinal surgery: a randomised clinical trial. Int J Orthop Trauma Nurs. 2016;23:3–13.

12. Jeon CH, Lee HD, Chung NS. Does mechanical bowel preparation ameliorate surgical performance in anterior lumbar interbody fusion? Global Spine J. 2019;9(7):692–6.

13. Horowitz JA, Jain A, Puvanesarajah V, Qureshi R, Hassanzadeh H. Risk factors, additional length of stay, and cost associated with postoperative ileus following anterior lumbar interbody fusion in elderly patients. World Neurosurg. 2018;115:e185–9.

14. Sommer NP, Schneider R, Wehner S, Kalff JC, Vilz TO. State-of-the-art colorectal disease: postoperative ileus. Int J Color Dis. 2021;36(9):2017–25.

15. Corcoran T, Rhodes JE, Clarke S, Myles PS, Ho KM. Perioperative fluid management strategies in major surgery: a stratified meta-analysis. Anesth Analg. 2012;114(3):640–51.

16. Huang J, Shi Z, Duan FF, Fan MX, Yan S, Wei Y, Han B, Lu XM, Tian W. Benefits of early ambulation in elderly patients undergoing lumbar decompression and fusion surgery: a prospective cohort study. Orthop Surg. 2021;13(4):1319–26.

17. Zakaria HM, Bazydlo M, Schultz L, Abdulhak M, Nerenz DR, Chang V, Schwalb JM. Ambulation on postoperative day #0 is associated with decreased morbidity and adverse events after elective lumbar spine surgery: analysis from the Michigan spine surgery improvement collaborative (MSSIC). Neurosurgery. 2020;87(2):320–8.

18. Waelkens P, Alsabbagh E, Sauter A, Joshi GP, Beloeil H. Prospect working group of the European Society of Regional Anaesthesia and Pain therapy (ESRA). Pain management after complex spine surgery: a systematic review and procedure-specific postoperative pain management recommendations. Eur J Anaesthesiol. 2021;38(9):985–94.

19. Loftus RW, Yeager MP, Clark JA, Brown JR, Abdu WA, Sengupta DK, Beach ML. Intraoperative ketamine reduces perioperative opiate consumption in opiate-dependent patients with chronic back pain undergoing back surgery. Anesthesiology. 2010;113(3):639–46.

20. Garg N, Panda NB, Gandhi KA, Bhagat H, Batra YK, Grover VK, Chhabra R. Comparison of small dose ketamine and dexmedetomidine infusion for postoperative analgesia in spine surgery—a prospective randomized double-blind placebo controlled study. J Neurosurg Anesthesiol. 2016;28(1):27–31.

21. Perera AP, Chari A, Kostusiak M, Khan AA, Luoma AM, Casey ATH. Intramuscular local anesthetic infiltration at closure for postoperative analgesia in lumbar spine surgery: a systematic review and meta-analysis. Spine (Phila Pa 1976). 2017;42(14):1088–95.

22. Soffin EM, Freeman C, Hughes AP, Wetmo Re DS, Memtsoudis SG, Girardi FP, Zhong H, Beckman JD. Effects of a multimodal analgesic pathway with transversus abdominis plane block for lumbar spine fusion: a prospective feasibility trial. Eur Spine J. 2019;28(9):2077–86.

23. Ogura Y, Gum JL, Steele P, Crawford CH 3rd, Djurasovic M, Owens RK 2nd, Laratta JL, Davis E, Brown M, Daniels C, Dimar JR 2nd, Glassman SD, Carreon LY. Multi-modal pain control regimen for anterior lumbar fusion drastically reduces in-hospital opioid consumption. J Spine Surg. 2020;6(4):681–7.

24. Short V, Herbert G, Perry R, Atkinson C, Ness AR, Penfold C, Thomas S, Andersen HK, Lewis SJ. Chewing gum for postoperative recovery of gastrointestinal function. Cochrane Database Syst Rev. 2015;2015(2):CD006506.

25. Du X, Ou Y, Jiang G, Luo W, Jiang D. Chewing gum promotes bowel function recovery in elderly patients after lumbar spinal surgery: a retrospective single-center cohort study. Ann Palliat Med. 2021;10(2):1216–23.
26. Barlow R, Price P, Reid TD, Hunt S, Clark GW, Havard TJ, Puntis MC, Lewis WG. Prospective multicentre randomised controlled trial of early enteral nutrition for patients undergoing major upper gastrointestinal surgical resection. Clin Nutr. 2011;30(5):560–6.
27. Boelens PG, Heesakkers FF, Luyer MD, van Barneveld KW, de Hingh IH, Nieuwenhuijzen GA, Roos AN, Rutten HJ. Reduction of postoperative ileus by early enteral nutrition in patients undergoing major rectal surgery: prospective, randomized, controlled trial. Ann Surg. 2014;259(4):649–55.
28. Tong Y, Fernandez L, Bendo JA, Spivak JM. Enhanced recovery after surgery trends in adult spine surgery: a systematic review. Int J Spine Surg. 2020;14(4):623–40.
29. Pennington Z, Cottrill E, Lubelski D, Ehresman J, Theodore N, Sciubba DM. Systematic review and meta-analysis of the clinical utility of enhanced recovery after surgery pathways in adult spine surgery. J Neurosurg Spine. 2020;6:1–23.

# Part VII
# Additional Considerations for Lumbar Spine Access Surgery

# Chapter 24
# Revision Anterior and Lateral Spinal Access Surgery

R. Mark Hoyle

## Introduction

Anterior or lateral exposure of the lumbar spine can be safe and efficient with minimal blood loss [1]. However, even when conducted by an experienced spinal access surgeon, revision spinal access surgery presents unique risks, including ureter injury, vascular injury requiring repair, venous and arterial thrombosis, sympathetic chain injury, and retrograde ejaculation [2–5]. The highest rate of vascular injury occurs at the L4–L5 level in both primary and revision surgeries followed by the L5–S1 level [1]. There is a paucity of literature concerning revision due to the potential for vascular injuries.

When considering anterior or lateral spine surgery, the spine surgeon should work closely with the access surgeon, especially in revision cases. Prior to deciding on an anterior or lateral approach, alternative approaches may be considered including interbody cages placed from a posterior approach. Due to associated scar tissue formation or altered anatomy, many access surgeons will not attempt an anterior revision at a previously exposed level. Additionally, access to levels adjacent to previous surgical levels may present similar risks due to scar tissue formation or an inflammatory rind encasing the vasculature. The surgeon should also consider other prior anterior surgical procedures, such as a caesarian section or open hysterectomy. Other factors, such as discitis or a previous interbody device, may also lead to abnormal scarring or altered anatomy and can complicate an anterior or lateral approach.

R. M. Hoyle (✉)
Methodist Hospital for Surgery in Addison, Addison, TX, USA

© The Author(s), under exclusive license to Springer Nature Switzerland AG 2023
J. R. O'Brien et al. (eds.), *Lumbar Spine Access Surgery*,
https://doi.org/10.1007/978-3-031-48034-8_24

## Anterior Approach Selection

### *Anterior Retroperitoneal Approach*

Most access surgeons perform ipsilateral revision, which is usually a left-sided retroperitoneal approach. This approach is fraught with problems from scar tissue which may predispose injury to the major vessels or the ureters and may prevent adequate exposure [2, 5]. The left-sided approach is performed through the same incision and the same planes as the original, taking great care to identify the ureter which is often stuck to the psoas muscle. If adherent, the ureter is left attached to the psoas and not mobilized. The vessels are mobilized in a similar fashion to the index procedure, although sharp rather than blunt dissection is often necessary. A right-sided retroperitoneal approach for revisions and for adjacent-level disease from L2–L3 to L5–S1 may be utilized due to virgin tissue planes and minimal to no scarring of the right ureter or great vessels. The inferior vena cava (IVC) and the iliac veins are easily circumferentially dissected and easier to control with vascular clamps or sponge stick compression. The approach to L5–S1 is the same anatomically via the left or right side. Some surgeons think all initial L5–S1 anterior fusions should be approached via the right side to preserve the left side for adjacent-level disease. When approaching the upper anterior lumbar spine from the right side, the IVC must be adequately visualized and mobilized. With adequate mobilization, especially in the craniocaudal plane, the IVC easily crosses the spine without undue tension and is held in place with Wylie vein retractors. The initial steps after entering the right retroperitoneal space are to sharply dissect the lateral aspect of the IVC with Metzenbaum scissors, or a number 15 scalpel blade if significant scar exists, and to establish a plane where the IVC is then bluntly mobilized to the left of the spine with Kittner sponges and Wylie retractors. The iliolumbar (or ascending lumbar) vein is encircled with a right-angle clamp and doubly or triply clipped. The use of suture ligation of this vessel is limited as the structure is deep and easily torn so clips may be used. The right iliolumbar vein is much shorter with a steeper takeoff angle than the left. If the vessel is injured or retracts under the psoas before being ligated, packing with hemostatic matrix followed by a cellulose polymer hemostatic agent with gentle pressure for a minimum of 3 min will usually achieve hemostasis. Bleeding that is controlled with this technique is considered definitive, and further attempts at repair (suture, clips, etc.) often restart the bleeding. Small venous branches of the IVC (less than 1–2 mm) are clipped, as are any lumbar venous or arterial branches. Once the surgeon has dissected down to the anterior lateral aspect of the spine, a rind of scar is encountered and is incised with a number 15 scalpel blade near the vasculature in a craniocaudal fashion while applying left-sided pressure with Kittners or Wylie vein retractors to the vessel being mobilized. Oftentimes, a nerve root retractor can be placed under the vessel before enough room is established to place a Wylie vein retractor and is invaluable in dissection initiation. The dissection proceeds to the left of the spine using sharp and blunt dissection as needed. Down-biting curettes (blunt on the vessel side and sharp on the spine side) are used to undermine the scar and push the vessels and scar to the left. This dissection proceeds slowly in 1-mm increments in case vessel injury occurs. This same technique is used in revision left-sided exposures at L2–L3 and L3–L4. In this case, the IVC is kept to the right of the spine, and the aorta is dissected to the left of the spine. At the L4–L5 level, both the IVC and aorta are mobilized to the left of the spine. However, depending on the amount and extent of the scar tissue, both major vessels can be mobilized to the left from L2–L3 to L4–L5. Interestingly, this does not seem to interfere with right heart venous return, and anesthesia providers almost never note blood pressure instability despite total IVC occlusion with retraction at these levels. The IVC will have multiple small venous branches along its lateral and medial border that will need to be ligated with small clips, and at the L2–L3 levels the testicular vein emptying into the anterior aspect of the IVC will occasionally need to be ligated to facilitate mobilization.

## *Anterior Transperitoneal Approach*

Occasionally, retroperitoneal scarring will be so significant that the surgeon may have to abandon the approach and perform transperitoneal access. In performing a transperitoneal approach, the small bowel is packed to the right upper quadrant with wet laparotomy pads. The ligament of Treitz is taken down sharply, and the mesentery is opened in a vertical fashion with electrocautery. Then, the mesentery is bluntly dissected with Kittners to the level of the spine. At higher levels (L2–L3 and L3–L4), the aorta is typically dissected to the left of the spine and the IVC to the right; however, the aorta can be mobilized to either side using a combination of blunt and sharp dissection. At L4–L5, the mesentery is opened over the aortic bifurcation, and the left iliac artery and vein are usually mobilized to the left of the spine. At L5–S1, the mesentery is opened vertically over the sacral promontory, and the left iliac vessels are mobilized to the left of the spine. When performing transperitoneal exposure (primary or revision), the location of the inferior mesenteric artery (IMA) must be noted to avoid avulsion due to aortic retraction over the disc space. The IMA is usually at the L3–L4 level but can be higher and must be identified. At that level, the aorta should not be pulled to the patients' right as the IMA can be easily avulsed. If the IMA is avulsed, most of the time it can be ligated, but if the colon becomes ischemic, it is reimplanted. A small IMA can usually be ligated while the larger ones are usually reimplanted. With transperitoneal revisions, the ureter is usually very close to the spine, stuck to the psoas muscle, or in between the psoas and the spine. It should be identified and avoided. Ureteral stenting may be useful in this regard as previously mentioned. Dissection of the vessels proceeds with the use of number 15 scalpel blades, Kittners, down-biting curettes, nerve root retractors, and Wylie vein retractors as previously detailed.

## Additional Considerations

### *Lumbar Disc Replacement*

Artificial lumbar disc replacements, while less common, present a special situation. In most cases, when an anteriorly placed artificial disc has failed, a posterior fusion can be performed and alleviate the patient's symptoms while leaving the artificial disc in place [6]. However, many spine surgeons prefer to have them removed anteriorly and an anterior interbody fusion performed. At L2–L3 and L3–L4, this is not technically difficult, but most artificial discs are placed at L4–L5 and or L5–S1 where the revision exposure is a major undertaking with wider than normal exposure performed for implantation and extraction. Vascular complications are increased compared with revision exposures for anterior fusions [3–5, 7].

### *Scar Tissue Prevention*

There are several patches used to cover spinal implants and placed under the vessels to prevent scarring in case future revision is necessary [7]. A polytetrafluoroethylene (PTFE) patch has been shown to be effective at reducing scar, and the vessels seem to easily mobilize once the patch has been reached during the dissection [7]. The PTFE patch can be sewn in place or simply held in place with forceps, while the peritoneal sac and vessels are released and observed to ensure they cover the patch and that the patch stays in a good position.

## Anterior Revision Complications

### *Ureter Injury*

Ureteral injury is a feared complication of revision anterior surgery, and some surgeons stent the ureters when revisions are performed [3]. This requires urologic coordination and is time-consuming. Typically, ureteral injuries are caused by traction (blunt ischemic injury) in both primary and revision exposures and present as a urinoma with left-sided flank pain 1 to 3 weeks postoperatively. A sharp injury to the ureter results in an immediate urinoma. Urological consultation with retrograde ureteroscopy and stenting with percutaneous drainage of the urinoma should be considered. If retrograde stenting is not technically possible, immediate exploration with attempted repair of the ureter, as opposed to percutaneous nephrostomy and delayed repair, should be considered.

## Vascular Injury

Venous tears during the revision procedure are handled with either hemostatic matrix and cellulose polymer hemostatic agent application or suture repair with 5-0 polypropylene on a small vascular needle. Many times, hemostatic agent application followed by gentle retraction with a Wylie vein retractor will control the bleeding while the dissection is continued.

On occasion, blood loss from the right-sided approach necessitates converting to a transperitoneal approach, while the bleeding is packed with hemostatic agents and a few gauze sponges. In most instances, the sponges can be removed at the end of the procedure when the bleeding has stopped while leaving the hemostatic agents in place without revisualizing the previous bleeding site. In cases where packing does not control the bleeding, the IVC and right common iliac vein can easily be clamped or controlled with sponge stick occlusion while a suture repair is performed. Other hemostatic agents, such as fibrin sealant patches, can also be applied. These agents are best used at the end of the procedure as further dissection may cause additional bleeding.

Some spinal access surgeons advocate putting in IVC or iliac venous stents a few months before the revision procedure to make the vein easier to find and dissect. However, a stent in an artery or vein may increase inflammation in the vessel and surrounding soft tissue as well as additional complications including thrombosis, migration, or perforation. The stented vessel is also more difficult to move across the disc space.

It may be beneficial to prepare bilateral inguinal creases in the field in case guidewires and venous stenting are necessary due to massive venous bleeding or injury [3]. This can be useful if the access surgeon has endovascular capability or if that capability is available on standby during the procedure.

## Sympathetic Chain Injury

Ipsilateral revision approaches may injure the sympathetic chain where contralateral approaches may not. In either case, the clinical sequelae are negligible as transection of the sympathetic chain in one location seldom results in a clinical sympathectomy. A minimum of three sympathetic ganglia removed are usually required to achieve a sympathectomy on one side.

## Thromboembolic Events

Arterial thrombosis during revision or primary access surgery is usually due to atherosclerotic disease with fracturing of plaque during retraction causing a dissection. Standard vascular techniques including thromboembolectomy, endarterectomy, or bypass with PTFE graft can be performed. Thrombosis typically occurs at the aortoiliac bifurcation or proximal external iliac artery, and if an embolectomy fails to restore flow, a short segment bypass usually through the same incision can be performed. Bypass to the femoral artery in the groin is occasionally necessary. On rarer occasions, clots can extend into the popliteal or trifurcating vessels, and a below knee embolectomy of all three vessels is required with or without fasciotomy as indicated. Equipment that must be available to deal with arterial thrombosis include a full set of vascular clamps, suture, needle holders, embolectomy catheters (#3,4 and 5), and 6- and 8-mm PTFE grafts. Limb loss is a devastating complication and is usually the result of delayed vascular intervention or if the thrombosis occurs postoperatively and the diagnosis is delayed. During initial and revision procedures, ipsilateral toe pulse oximetry as well neuromonitoring can alert the surgeon to arterial ischemia of the lower limbs. At L4–L5, the iliac artery may be occluded during the procedure, and the retraction of the vessels is frequently released as dictated by the pulse oximetry to allow intermittent blood flow to the leg. However, if the pulse oximetry shows no decrease in blood flow, the vessels are held over with Wylie vein retractors without release. Frequent release and retraction in the presence of arterial plaque may contribute to plaque fracturing and thrombosis.

Vena cava or iliac clot can be lysed or mechanically removed and a stent placed across the injured venous segment. Not all iliofemoral deep venous thromboses must be treated in this fashion, and many do well on long-term anticoagulation. However, with massive leg swelling, clot removal with stenting is the preferred treatment option. Venous injuries that are repaired with no vein narrowing are at a low risk of thrombosis postoperatively. A subset of patients with no venous injury will experience a deep venous thrombosis after initial or revision anterior access surgery. These patients need a full hypercoagulable workup postoperatively to evaluate for a hypercoagulable state and often need long-term anticoagulation with hematology consultation and follow-up. If the spine surgeon decompresses the nerves posteriorly, anticoagulation medication cannot be used due to the risk of epidural hematoma, and therefore only sequential compression devices on the feet or legs are used postoperatively.

## Retrograde Ejaculation

Retrograde ejaculation is also a concern and has been reported to occur at higher rates in the revision setting [8]. Retrograde ejaculation is most commonly seen following revision at the L5–S1 level and has been theorized to be related to the inability to do a "gentle sweep" of the tissues in front of L5–S1 [8]. For men who are considering having children in the future, a serious consideration of preoperative sperm banking should be discussed.

## *Preoperative Planning*

Given the complex nature of planning for revision anterior access surgery, Gumbs et al. have proposed a preoperative checklist consisting of repeat history and physical, obtaining old operative reports, repeat spine films, consideration of ureteral stents, angiogram and venogram for revisions below the L3–L4 level, and preoperative sperm banking in appropriate male patients [9].

## Lateral Revision Access

If the previous anteriorly placed interbody cage does not have screws placed through it, an alternative approach to removal and revision fusion is a pure lateral approach going under the major vessels (requiring no mobilization) at L2–L5. An oblique lateral interbody fusion can be performed at L5–S1 as an initial procedure, but for a revision, a direct anterior right-sided or transperitoneal approach is strongly advised to avoid vascular injury. In the lateral position, a transverse incision is made over the disc space marked on the skin by fluoroscopy localization, the psoas muscle is mobilized on its anterior medial surface and retracted posteriorly, and the disc space entered underneath the major vessels where the unfused cage is removed by standard orthopedic techniques and a revision fusion is performed. This is especially useful for L4–L5 revision procedures to avoid vascular injury.

Laterally placed interbody cages occasionally require removal and revision after nonunion. These cages are best removed from an anterior approach. However, if a screw was placed laterally through the cage, a lateral approach may be required. When extracting these laterally placed cages anteriorly, the opposite side is chosen to avoid scar. The cage can be flipped out of the disc space with an angled curette, and the remaining anterior disc is removed. Typically, these laterally placed cages do not inflame the disc space and surrounding tissues as much as anteriorly placed cages, but occasionally the inflammation and scar are extensive and just as difficult as an anterior revision surgery.

## Proximal Revision Approaches

Revision exposures at L1 are extremely rare and are approached laterally dissecting either in front or through the psoas muscle. Initial L1–L2 exposures can be done transperitoneally as long as the renal arteries are at or above the L1–L2 disc space as seen on magnetic resonance imaging or computed tomography scans. If the renal arteries are below the disc space, the procedure can still be done but requires extensive mobilization of the renal arteries as well as ligation of the adrenal branch of the left renal vein and is a difficult procedure and best done via a left lateral retroperitoneal approach. Exposures above L1–L2 require a lateral thoracic approach. Small thoracic incisions with or without partial rib removal can expose thoracic levels T12–L1 all the way up to T2–T3. A contralateral thoracic approach for revisions is preferred if feasible.

## Conclusion

Revision access to the anterior or lateral lumbar spine presents a unique set of challenges which can result in devastating intraoperative and postoperative complications. However, with close coordination with an access surgeon and careful preoperative planning, the approach can be done in a safe and effective manner. The decisions of which side to approach a revision procedure and whether to pursue a retroperitoneal, transperitoneal, or lateral exposure require a thorough understanding of normal anatomy, prior procedures a patient may have undergone, surgical goals, and when to change or abort an approach in the face of unamenable anatomy.

## References

1. O'Brien MF, Hoyle MR, Kirby RP, Hostin RA. Anterior access to the thoracic and lumbar spine. In: Dubousset J, Challier V, Farcy JP, Schwab FJ, Lafage, editors. Global spinal alignment: principles, pathologies, and procedures. St. Louis, MO: Quality Medical Publishing; 2015. p. 499–509.
2. Brau SA, Delamarter RB, Kropf MA, Watkins RG III, Williams LA, Schiffman ML, Bae HW. Access strategies for revision in anterior lumbar surgery. Spine. 2008;33(15):1662–7.
3. McAffee PC, Gonz M. Lumbar TDR revision strategies. In: Cheng B, editor. Handbook of spine technology. Cham: Springer; 2019. https://doi.org/10.1007/978-3-319-33037-2_78-1.
4. Wagner WH, Regan JJ, Leary SP, et al. Access strategies for revision of the spine for removal of lumbar devices and implants. Spine. 2006;31:2449–53.
5. Wagner WH, Regan JJ, Leary SP, Lanman TH, Johnson JP, Rao RK, Cossman DV. Access strategies for revision or explantation of the Charite lumbar artificial disc replacement. J Vasc Surg. 2006;44(6):1266–72.
6. Freeman BJ, Davenport J. Total disc replacement in the lumbar spine: a systematic review of the literature. Eur Spine J. 2006;15(3):439–47.

7. Yue JJ, Sumpio B. Use of spinal vessel protection to facilitate anterior revision surgery. New Haven, CT: Yale University School of Medicine White Paper; 2009.
8. Schwender JD, Casnellie MT, Perra JH, Transfeldt EE, Pinto MR, Denis F, et al. Perioperative complications in revision anterior lumbar spine surgery: incidence and risk factors. Spine. 2009;34(1):87–90.
9. Gumbs AA, Hanan S, Yue JJ, Shah RV, Sumpio B. Revision open anterior approaches for spine procedures. Spine J. 2007;7(3):280–5.

# Chapter 25
# Anterior Lumbar Spine Access Surgery in Ambulatory Surgery Centers and Outpatient Settings

Harvinder Bhatti, Navraj S. Sagoo, and Willis Wagner

## Introduction

Healthcare costs have risen dramatically in the United States over the past several decades and are projected to grow at an average annual rate of 5.4%, reaching up to $6.2 trillion by 2028 [1, 2]. A significant portion of this cost has been attributed to inpatient hospital care, particularly for orthopedic and spine procedures [3]. The desire for cost control, improved quality of care, and advancements in minimally invasive technology have led to a shift from procedures performed in inpatient settings to outpatient and ambulatory surgical centers (ASCs). When compared with standard inpatient experiences, benefits of ASCs include shorter length of stay (LOS), lesser exposure to nosocomial infections, and improved patient experiences by allowing an early, at-home recovery.

Several studies have reported favorable outcomes following outpatient transforaminal lumbar interbody fusion (TLIF), posterior lumbar interbody fusion (PLIF), posterior lumbar laminectomy and discectomy, lateral lumbar interbody fusion (LLIF), cervical disc arthroplasty (CDA), and anterior cervical discectomy and fusion (ACDF) [4–7]. These procedures have repeatedly been shown to result in fewer complications and hospital readmissions, along with equivalent long-term clinical efficacy when compared with inpatient procedures. The cost-effectiveness of these outpatient procedures has also been shown in numerous studies, with significantly decreased costs compared with inpatient procedures [5, 8, 9].

H. Bhatti (✉)
Atlanta Spine, Atlanta, GA, USA
e-mail: bhatti@atlantaspineclinic.com

N. S. Sagoo
Department of Orthopaedic Surgery, UT Southwestern Medical Center, Dallas, TX, USA

W. Wagner
Department of Orthopaedic Surgery, Cedars-Sinai Medical Center, Los Angeles, CA, USA

© The Author(s), under exclusive license to Springer Nature Switzerland AG 2023

J. R. O'Brien et al. (eds.), *Lumbar Spine Access Surgery*,
https://doi.org/10.1007/978-3-031-48034-8_25

However, there is a relative paucity of literature investigating the indications, outcomes, and safety of anterior lumbar spine access surgery performed in ASCs. One of the primary concerns with the anterior approach is related to the complexities involved in attaining retroperitoneal access, especially at the caudal levels, due to the aortic bifurcation and its associated vasculature which require extensive mobilization and protection. Accordingly, this procedure requires a vascular access surgeon with significant experience with the anterior retroperitoneal approach to the lumbar spine. A mini-open approach utilizing a small incision, blunt muscular dissection, and direct visualization has been developed with the potential to decrease the morbidity of anterior lumbar approaches, demonstrating the increased feasibility of this procedure in the ASC setting. However, complications associated with the anterior approach are still prevalent and include intraoperative vascular, neurologic, and visceral injury, adjacent segment degeneration, subsidence, and retrograde ejaculation [10, 11].

This chapter will review anterior lumbar spine access surgery as it is performed in ASCs. We will consider preoperative factors such as appropriate patient selection thresholds. Furthermore, this chapter will investigate intraoperative considerations such as anesthesia protocol and surgical technique. Finally, postoperative considerations including multimodal analgesic medication regimens, clinical outcomes, and potential complications will be discussed.

## Preoperative Considerations

### *Patient Selection*

It is necessary to carefully select patients for anterior lumbar spine access surgery in an outpatient facility, where there is limited availability of multidisciplinary medical support and emergency services. The increased number of outpatient spine surgeries performed over the past decade has prompted the need for standardized guidelines to select patients, and there are no currently established selection criteria for anterior lumbar spine surgery in ASCs. Suggested thresholds for patient selection in anterior lumbar surgery at an ASC include American Society of Anesthesiologists (ASA) class 1 or 2, age less than 65 years old, and operation on one- or two- level lumbar pathology. The ASA categorizes patients based on comorbidities and allows surgeons to weigh risks and could be a helpful predictor of both complications and outcomes in anterior lumbar surgery [12, 13].

Obstructive sleep apnea (OSA) is an important risk factor when considering patients for surgery. Patients with OSA have a significantly higher chance of developing intraoperative complications which may lead to difficult intubation and ventilation, the requirement for supplemental oxygen, and the need for vasoactive medications to correct hemodynamic abnormalities. The body mass index of the patient is also a particularly important indicator which must be evaluated in conjunction with the body habitus of the patient when selecting patients for outpatient anterior lumbar access surgery. Patients with centripetal obesity exhibit a higher risk of sustaining a vascular injury, and vascular repair is often more difficult in this subset of patients [5]. Furthermore, patients who have high-risk cardiovascular (New York Heart Association Grades III–IV) disease or metabolic disease are generally contraindicated from receiving surgery in the outpatient setting [5, 14]. Other contraindications also include support services that are necessary but are not available in the ASC setting such as dialysis, the potential requirement for intensive care, and a blood bank for possible transfusion.

Patients who are chronic opioid users and active substance abusers are also discouraged from receiving anterior lumbar surgery in ASCs. Increased opioid consumption preoperatively is correlated with adverse postoperative patient outcomes in elective spine surgery [15, 16]. Villavicencio et al. evaluated whether preoperative opioid use predicted poor clinical outcomes in patients undergoing TLIF and noted that the use of opioids preoperatively correlated with significantly worse clinical outcome scores at 1 year follow-up [17]. Thus, it is prudent to establish an opioid-weaning scheme for patients ahead of their scheduled surgery with the intention of safely decreasing opioid dosage. Pain management consultation may be required for patients on high-dose opioids in whom weaning is expected to be challenging. Suggested indications for anterior lumbar surgery in ASCs are further outlined in Table 25.1. The ideal patient for anterior lumbar surgery in ASCs would be

**Table 25.1** Suggestions for patient selection for anterior lumbar access surgery in ASCs

| Relative indications for anterior lumbar surgery in ASCs |
| --- |
| One- or two-level pathology |
| Young patients (<65 years) |
| Body mass index <30 kg/m2 |
| Has fundamental skills required for independent living |
| Has safe home environment with responsible caretaker |
| No history of chronic opioid use or active substance abuse |
| Low comorbidity index |
| No variant abdominal or vascular anatomy |
| No history of major acute trauma or spinal deformity |
| Low risk for urinary retention |
| No history of previous lumbar surgery |
| No history of previous retroperitoneal surgery |
| Low to moderate anesthesia risk (ASA scores 1–3) |

a younger patient requiring one-level surgery without significant spinal deformity, with minimal comorbidities and appropriate retroperitoneal anatomy without anatomical variants. To improve the safety of an anterior surgical approach, preoperative vascular imaging studies of the pelvis may be obtained to identify any anatomic anomalies.

Some patients may also be anxious about receiving anterior lumbar surgery at an ASC. Clear disclosure can help establish rapport and alleviate any anxiety they may experience. However, in the event where a patient maintains anxiety regarding the procedure, this should be considered a contraindication to anterior lumbar surgery in the ASC setting. Kuo et al. retrospectively reviewed 166 patients who underwent ALIF at an ASC and aimed to determine which risk factors correlated with prolonged LOS [18]. On multivariate logistic analysis, age greater than 65 years, preoperative benzodiazepine use, 12-item Short Form Mental Component Score (FS-12 MCS), estimated blood loss, time to mobilization, and total operative time were independent predictors for extended LOS. Accordingly, subjective impairment from mood-related issues as determined by SF-12 MCS might make patients suboptimal candidates for outpatient ALIF. Patients with lower scores may be more likely to have an extended recovery course because of perceptions of increased pain and disability.

Furthermore, when considering a patient for anterior lumbar surgery at an ASC, it is important to determine that the patient has a safe home environment with a responsible caretaker who can provide basic care and supervision for at least 24 h following surgery. Additionally, patient household proximity to the ASC and an appropriate emergency room should be considered. Those patients without family support and cognitive limitations for self-care would complicate outpatient discharge. Surgeons should consider home care needs and family support in the context of the anticipated postoperative activity limitations. Finally, a surgeon's familiarity and experience with the procedure should also be factored into the decision-making process. Prevention of complications and achievement of optimal outcomes in anterior lumbar surgery in outpatient settings primarily rest on the proficiency of both the spine and vascular access surgeons. Taking note of objective surgical outcomes and patient-reported outcomes further aids in improving surgical proficiency in an outpatient setting and allows surgeons to compare their results to published standards. With such data, outcomes can be better predicted and improved upon, allowing for an excellent physician and patient experience.

A rigorous approach to quality assessment and monitoring is important as greater numbers of anterior lumbar spine access surgeries are being performed at ASCs. ASCs are often smaller and more specialized, with fewer staff who are less transient and who are familiar with the specifics of the procedures performed, therefore optimizing efficiency. Patients value an open dialogue with the medical staff, nurses, and surgeons concerning the procedure, which leads to a comfortable, transparent, and successful patient experience.

# Intraoperative Considerations

## *Anesthesia*

Anesthetic management during anterior lumbar spine access surgery at ASCs should aim to sustain patient immobility, provide safe and rapid emergence, minimize postoperative complications, and facilitate neurophysiologic monitoring. To successfully achieve these goals, rapid onset and offset of anesthesia, quick recovery of protective reflexes, mobility and micturition, and adequate control of postoperative analgesia and nausea are integral in obtaining successful outcomes. Such approaches in the ambulatory setting not only decrease morbidity and mortality but also save hospital costs and operative time.

Anesthesia in ASCs can employ general and regional anesthesia, local anesthesia, monitored anesthesia care, or a combination of these methods. Specifically for anterior lumbar spine access surgery, general anesthesia is employed typically via induction with intravenous (IV) propofol and maintained with an inhaled anesthetic via endotracheal intubation. Non-opioid intraoperative adjuncts, such as ketamine, may be utilized during general anesthesia and have been shown to reduce perioperative opioid consumptions in opioid-dependent patients undergoing lumbar spine surgery [19]. Standard monitors (blood pressure monitoring, electrocardiogram, pulse oximetry, end expired carbon dioxide, and temperature) are used for all patients undergoing general anesthesia. Pulse oximetry of the left foot is useful for monitoring oxygen saturation while the iliac vasculature is compressed by the retractors. Often, oxygen saturation may drop to zero when the iliac vessels are retracted from left to right but returns to preoperative levels following the release of retraction. A preoperative or postoperative local anesthetic injection using a long-acting agent, such as Marcaine or a bupivacaine liposomal injectable suspension, may be administered prior to incision or at the end of the operation following closure. This often achieves more than 24 h of complete or near complete peri-incisional and abdominal pain relief.

## *Anterior Spine Exposure Technique*

For L5-S1 exposures, a transverse skin incision is typically made, approximately one-third the distance between the pubis and the umbilicus. For levels above L5-S1, longitudinal paramedian or oblique midline skin incisions may be used. Access is typically performed via a left retroperitoneal approach to achieve better visualization of the retroperitoneal vessels. A right-sided approach is only utilized in the event that the index level is L5-S1 and/or if there is a high likelihood of requirement of future anterior spine exposure. For operations on L5-S1, the middle sacral levels can be taken between clips, ligatures, or cautery. For exposure at L4–L5 and usually at L3–L4, the iliolumbar veins are typically ligated and cut as they may prevent mobilization of the iliac vein away from the anterior portion of the spine, thus preventing adequate exposure. Lymphatic-bearing tissue crossing the iliac vessels and lateral to the aorta may be divided between clips for prevention of postoperative lymphatic collections. Upon completion, sequential removal of the retractor blades is typically done, leaving the right-sided blade for last. Following thorough checks on the integrity of the vasculature for signs of arterial thrombosis, the lap sponge is removed, allowing the tissues to fall back together anatomically. The individual fascial layers are closed separately with running absorbable sutures, making sure that the anterior rectus sheath is well approximated.

## Blood Loss Control

In most studies, the incidence of major vascular injury during open anterior lumbar spinal surgery is reported at less than 5% [7, 20, 21]. In the event of a vascular injury at an ASC, intraoperative blood salvage technology must be available to transfuse the patient with autologous blood. This is not only a cost-effective approach, but it helps mitigate potential adverse events from allogeneic transfusions and has been a critical component to the success of ASC facilities. In addition, the use of topical hemostatic agents can further reduce the requirement for blood transfusions and consequently decrease operative time and reduce the cost of surgery. These absorbable hemostatic products are a cost-effective option to bleeding during spinal surgery, in an attempt to avoid transfusions. Willner et al. discussed the effectiveness of tranexamic acid (TXA) therapy as having a 49% reduction in blood loss and requiring fewer blood transfusions, all without significant side effects [22]. TXA has been found to effectively reduce intraoperative blood loss without the risks of venous thromboembolism. Dorenkamp et al. retrospectively reviewed blood product utilization in 50 patients undergoing lumbar total disc arthroplasty at a single ASC [20]. In this study, there was no need for transfusion of allogeneic packed red blood cells, and 4 of the 50 patients had enough blood salvage output for autologous transfusion. Thus, a combination of modern blood salvage technology and hemostatic agents can enable less blood loss and thus efficient resource utilization during surgery.

## Transfer Options

It is recommended that ASCs exhibit a 23-h stay capability with adjacent recovery suites. Importantly, a protocol for rapid transfer to a nearby acute care hospital must be in place in the instance that this becomes necessary.

# Postoperative Considerations

## *Postoperative Pain Control*

The ideal postoperative course is one that enables patients to rapidly recover, allowing for a same-day discharge. However, such outcomes are only feasible when utilizing an appropriate anesthetic and analgesic plan. As such, both surgeons and anesthesiologists should discuss the preoperative evaluation, anesthetic technique, postoperative analgesia, and special considerations prior to the day of surgery. Postoperative analgesia is particularly challenging in the ASC setting. For example, in the inpatient setting, opioid patient-controlled analgesia (PCA) devices are often utilized following spine surgery during the immediate postoperative period. However, when similar surgeries are performed on an outpatient basis, PCA is not an option. Additionally, inpatient IV opioids, which are commonly used for breakthrough postoperative pain, may lead to complications such as respiratory compromise or oversedation. To this end, a multimodal pain management protocol is imperative to achieving successful outcomes following outpatient anterior lumbar spine surgery. Several variations of analgesia protocols have been shown to be effective, which typically include a mixture of local, systemic, short-acting, and long-acting medications with varying mechanisms of action. Protocols typically consist of a combination of gabapentinoids, antispasmodics, low-affinity opioids, nonsteroidal anti-inflammatories, acetaminophen, and topical lidocaine. Overall, the patient should be educated that different methods of analgesia will be implemented postoperatively, but that zero pain is not possible.

## *Nausea and Vomiting*

Nausea and vomiting (N/V) often affect early discharge following anterior lumbar spine surgery. Risk factors associated with N/V include patients greater than 50 years of age, female gender, nonsmokers, and a history of N/V or motion sickness. Preoperative screening is imperative to determine the risk of developing N/V, and a transdermal scopolamine patch can be applied preoperatively which may prevent N/V. Opioid medications may also contribute to N/V, and decreasing or weaning narcotics prior to surgery can decrease postoperative requirements. Moreover, non-opiate medications may be added, significantly reducing the risk of N/V. Other recommendations for reducing N/V include administration of first-line antiemetics such as 5-hydroxytryptamine receptor antagonists and/or steroid medications along with aggressive hydration on arrival. In patients who have persistent N/V, metoclopramide may also be utilized as a rescue therapy.

## *Urinary Retention*

Urinary retention is another potential complication that may arise following anterior lumbar surgery and may lead to morbidity and an increased LOS. Isolated urinary retention often resolves without serious sequelae. Distention of the bladder, removal of a catheter and inability to void with a residual bladder volume greater than 600 mL, and failure to void within 8 h of surgery are all typical signs of urinary retention [23]. Patients who fail to spontaneously void prior to discharge should be admitted overnight for inpatient observation. In addition, urology consultation and potential home discharge with an indwelling catheter may be indicated in refractory cases. Altschul et al. reported a 2.1% postoperative rate of urinary retention in patients following anterior lumbar surgery [23]. Risk factors identified for urinary retention include medications such as phenylephrine and neostigmine. In addition, benign prostatic hypertrophy, chronic constipation, prior urinary retention, and the use of PCA have also been reported as risk factors [18, 23, 24]. A rare cause of urinary retention may be attributed to cauda equina syndrome due to epidural hematoma or abscess. Awareness of the risk factors for the development of postoperative urinary retention may potentially reduce the rate of this complication. Limitation of intraoperative IV fluids, opioid dosage, and decreasing surgical time may decrease the incidence of urinary retention.

## *Follow-Up*

General discharge criteria following anterior lumbar surgery often include adequate pain control, toleration of oral intake, urine voiding, stable vital signs, and a stable neurological exam. With appropriate preoperative and intraoperative planning and execution, these goals can be achieved within a few hours following the procedure. It is important that the patient has a home caretaker who can supervise and monitor medication use to prevent early overuse. The surgeon may also consider an adjustable lumbosacral orthosis for the first few weeks to restrict motion and enable soft tissue healing. During the first week, early mobilization, soft tissue rest, and wound care are priorities. At 2 weeks, physical therapy can be initiated.

## *Complications, Readmissions, and Other Outcomes*

Most of the literature in the past 5 years has focused on the feasibility of performing outpatient spine surgery, specifically ensuring that it can be done safely and that clinical outcomes are non-inferior to hospital-based historical standards. Few studies have examined clinical outcomes and safety of anterior lumbar spine access surgery in ASCs. Snowden et al. reported on 62 patients who underwent single-level ALIF at

L5-S1 in the ASC ($n = 29$) or inpatient ($n = 33$) setting [25]. A postoperative complication rate of 10.3% was observed in the ASC group compared to 15.1% in the hospital group. No significant difference in patient reported outcomes was observed between inpatient and outpatient groups. Cuellar et al. reported on 51 patients (34 artificial disc replacements, 29 ALIFs) at an ASC [14]. In the 30-day postoperative period, there was an observed major complication rate of 0% and hospital readmission rate of 2% (1/51). Cuellar et al. published a retrospective comparative study on 226 anterior lumbar surgeries performed at an ASC ($n = 124$) or in the inpatient setting ($n = 102$) [5]. In the 90-day postoperative period, fewer complications (0.9% versus 5.6%), reoperations (0% versus 0.8%), and readmissions (1.9% versus 1.6%) were observed in the ASC cohort versus the inpatient cohort, respectively.

Given the concerns for postoperative ileus or vascular and visceral injury, there has been a slow transition to performing anterior lumbar surgeries in ACSs. To address these concerns, Parrish et al. retrospectively reviewed 111 patients who underwent single-level ALIF and sought to identify factors associated with stay >24 h [26]. Their findings suggested that coexisting degenerative disc disease with foraminal stenosis, operation at the L4–L5 level, and a herniated nucleus pulposus increased the likelihood of inpatient admission.

## Conclusion

Outpatient anterior lumbar access surgery has been reported to demonstrate similar clinical and functional outcomes, complication rates, and readmission rates in carefully selected patients compared to surgery performed in the inpatient setting. Although the available data suggests the clinical and economic benefits of anterior lumbar surgery, particular attention must be paid to the selection of surgical candidates, anterior lumbar access techniques, preoperative anesthesia protocols, postoperative pain control, and avoidance of postoperative complications. Anterior lumbar spine surgery will continue to shift toward the outpatient setting as both spine surgeons and patients become more comfortable with the process and higher-quality studies continue to demonstrate promising outcomes, low complications, and economic cost-effectiveness.

## References


1. Keehan SP, Cuckler GA, Poisal JA, et al. National Health Expenditure Projections, 2019-28: expected rebound in prices drives rising spending growth. Health Aff (Millwood). 2020;39(4):704–14.
2. Orszag PR, Ellis P. Addressing rising health care costs—a view from the Congressional Budget Office. N Engl J Med. 2007;357(19):1885–7.

3. Koltsov JCB, Sambare TD, Alamin TF, Wood KB, Cheng I, Hu SS. Healthcare resource utilization and costs 2 years pre- and post-lumbar spine surgery for stenosis: a national claims cohort study of 22,182 cases. Spine J. 2022;22(6):965–74.
4. Chin KR, Pencle FJ, Coombs AV, et al. Lateral lumbar interbody fusion in ambulatory surgery centers: patient selection and outcome measures compared with an in hospital cohort. Spine (Phila Pa 1976). 2016;41(8):686–92.
5. Cuellar JM, Nomoto E, Saadat E, et al. Outpatient versus inpatient anterior lumbar spine surgery: a multisite, comparative analysis of patient safety measures. Int J Spine Surg. 2021;15(5):937–44.
6. DelSole EM, Makanji HS, Kurd MF. Current trends in ambulatory spine surgery: a systematic review. J Spine Surg. 2019;5(Suppl 2):S124–s132.
7. Pendharkar AV, Shahin MN, Ho AL, et al. Outpatient spine surgery: defining the outcomes, value, and barriers to implementation. Neurosurg Focus. 2018;44(5):E11.
8. Parrish JM, Jenkins NW, Brundage TS, et al. Outpatient minimally invasive lumbar fusion using multimodal analgesic Management in the Ambulatory Surgery Setting. Int J Spine Surg. 2020;14(6):970–81.
9. Sivaganesan A, Hirsch B, Phillips FM, McGirt MJ. Spine surgery in the ambulatory surgery center setting: value-based advancement or safety liability? Neurosurgery. 2018;83(2):159–65.
10. Burkus JK, Dryer RF, Peloza JH. Retrograde ejaculation following single-level anterior lumbar surgery with or without recombinant human bone morphogenetic protein–2 in 5 randomized controlled trials: clinical article. J Neurosurg Spine. 2013;18(2):112–21.
11. Udby PM, Bech-Azeddine R. Clinical outcome of stand-alone ALIF compared to posterior instrumentation for degenerative disc disease: a pilot study and a literature review. Clin Neurol Neurosurg. 2015;133:64–9.
12. Basil GW, Wang MY. Trends in outpatient minimally invasive spine surgery. J Spine Surg. 2019;5(Suppl 1):S108–s114.
13. Basques BA, Ferguson J, Kunze KN, Phillips FM. Lumbar spinal fusion in the outpatient setting: an update on management, surgical approaches and planning. J Spine Surg. 2019;5(Suppl 2):S174–s180.
14. CuÉllar JM, Wagner W, Rasouli A. Low complication rate of anterior lumbar spine surgery in an ambulatory surgery center. Int J Spine Surg. 2020;14(5):687–93.
15. Kurd MF, Kreitz T, Schroeder G, Vaccaro AR. The role of multimodal analgesia in spine surgery. J Am Acad Orthop Surg. 2017;25(4):260–8.
16. Lui B, Weinberg R, Milewski AR, et al. Impact of preoperative opioid use disorder on outcomes following lumbar-spine surgery. Clin Neurol Neurosurg. 2021;208:106865.
17. Villavicencio AT, Nelson EL, Kantha V, Burneikiene S. Prediction based on preoperative opioid use of clinical outcomes after transforaminal lumbar interbody fusions. J Neurosurg Spine. 2017;26(2):144–9.
18. Kuo CC, Hess RM, Khan A, Pollina J, Mullin JP. Factors affecting postoperative length of stay in patients undergoing anterior lumbar interbody fusion. World Neurosurg. 2021;155:e538–47.
19. Loftus RW, Yeager MP, Clark JA, et al. Intraoperative ketamine reduces perioperative opiate consumption in opiate-dependent patients with chronic back pain undergoing back surgery. Anesthesiology. 2010;113(3):639–46.
20. Dorenkamp BC, Janssen MK, Janssen ME. Improving blood product utilization at an ambulatory surgery center: a retrospective cohort study on 50 patients with lumbar disc replacement. Patient Saf Surg. 2019;13:45.
21. Sheha ED, Derman PB. Complication avoidance and management in ambulatory spine surgery. J Spine Surg. 2019;5(Suppl 2):S181–s190.
22. Willner D, Spennati V, Stohl S, Tosti G, Aloisio S, Bilotta F. Spine surgery and blood loss: systematic review of clinical evidence. Anesth Analg. 2016;123(5):1307–15.
23. Altschul D, Kobets A, Nakhla J, et al. Postoperative urinary retention in patients undergoing elective spinal surgery. J Neurosurg Spine. 2017;26(2):229–34.

24. Wert WG Jr, Sellers W, Mariner D, et al. Identifying risk factors for complications during exposure for anterior lumbar interbody fusion. Cureus. 2021;13(7):e16792.
25. Snowden R, Fischer D, Kraemer P. Early outcomes and safety of outpatient (surgery center) vs inpatient based L5-S1 anterior lumbar interbody fusion. J Clin Neurosci. 2020;73:183–6.
26. Parrish JM, Jenkins NW, Nolte MT, et al. Predictors of inpatient admission in the setting of anterior lumbar interbody fusion: a minimally invasive spine study group (MISSG) investigation. J Neurosurg Spine. 2020;1–9:S120.

# Chapter 26
# Preoperative Considerations for Anterior Lumbar Interbody Fusion Revision

**Philip C. Nelson and Stephen D. Lockey**

## Introduction

The number of spinal surgeries performed annually continues to grow [1], with anterior lumbar interbody fusion (ALIF) being one of the most utilized techniques to achieve arthrodesis [2]. There are several well-described advantages of ALIF compared to other interbody techniques. The exposure allows for excellent visualization of the anterior column, thorough disc space preparation, and a large surface area for cage placement. Other advantages include the ability to avoid extensive dissection of the back musculature and disruption of the posterior elements, superior restoration of foraminal height and local disc angle, as well as increased lumbar lordosis [3]. Open posterior approaches can also lead to epidural scarring and perineural fibrosis from nerve root retraction, making a future revision surgery more challenging if necessary [4].

Despite recent advances in implant technology and biologics to achieve fusion, some patients experience persistent or recurrent symptoms and may require a revision procedure. The reported rates of successful fusion following ALIF vary in the literature. A meta-analysis that included 55 studies reported a weighted average fusion rate of 88.2% following stand-alone ALIF [5]. Despite the advantages of ALIF, upward of 10% of patients may experience pseudarthrosis. Patients with clinically silent nonunion may not require another operation, but those with new or persistent symptoms may be considered for revision. It is critical to evaluate the individual pathology as well as optimize patients in the preoperative setting to

P. C. Nelson
Department of Orthopaedic Surgery, University of Virginia, Charlottesville, USA

S. D. Lockey (✉)
Division of Spine Surgery, Department of Orthopaedic Surgery, University of Virginia, Charlottesville, VA, USA

© The Author(s), under exclusive license to Springer Nature Switzerland AG 2023
J. R. O'Brien et al. (eds.), *Lumbar Spine Access Surgery*,
https://doi.org/10.1007/978-3-031-48034-8_26

achieve a successful result with a revision procedure. The purpose of this chapter is to review the important preoperative considerations and to discuss the options for surgical approach and technique when performing revision ALIF.

## Discussion

### *Patient Evaluation*

Proper patient evaluation with a detailed history is imperative in ascertaining whether it is appropriate to move forward with revision spine surgery. Obtaining a thorough medical and surgical history as well as reviewing prior operative reports may prove helpful in complication avoidance and appropriate patient selection. Creating a timeline of symptoms starting prior to the index procedure can help discern the source of pathology and improve clinical decision-making. For example, if the patient did not experience any relief following the initial procedure, it is important to consider an incorrect preoperative diagnosis, inadequate decompression, or even a wrong-level surgery [6, 7]. Alternatively, an early recurrence or development of new symptoms may indicate nerve root irritation or injury [8]. A gradual onset of symptoms in the intermediate to late postoperative timeframe may be from the development of scar tissue such as epidural fibrosis [9]. Adjacent segment disease and stenosis may present with new or recurrent symptoms in the late postoperative period [10]. Sudden onset pain and recurrent symptoms preceded by relative improvement can be indicative of hardware failure or a symptomatic pseudarthrosis [11]. In addition to the history, a thorough physical exam should be performed and compared to findings documented prior to the index procedure. Range of motion, gait, alignment, and sagittal balance should be assessed as well as a careful neurologic examination to elicit information about the level of pathology and any associated deficits. Examination of the hips or knees in patients with leg pain should also be performed to exclude potential sources of symptoms outside the axial skeleton [12]. The history and physical exam considered in the context of appropriate medical imaging can lead to a more accurate diagnosis and therefore appropriate targeted therapy.

It is also important to optimize modifiable risk factors like morbid obesity, which increases the risks of readmission and poor outcomes [13]. The patient's bone health must also be assessed before proceeding with revision. Osteoporosis reduces the likelihood of successful fusion, and the use of bisphosphonates or bone-forming medications like teriparatide may improve the rate of arthrodesis in patients with poor bone health [14]. Additionally, it is important to consider the role of bone quality when planning revision interbody fusion as endplate violations are more likely to occur in patients with lower bone mineral density [15]. Smoking and alcohol cessation are also modifiable risk factors to consider as each contributes to the risk of pseudarthrosis [16, 17]. Social factors like the desire to return to work after surgery predict better outcomes and patient satisfaction, which can help with appropriate patient selection [18]. Finally, some patients may also be on anticoagulation therapy for a variety of conditions. A multidisciplinary approach to determining the cessation timeline in the perioperative setting will be important in avoiding both surgical and medical complications following the operation [19].


## Diagnostic Testing

Imaging prior to revision ALIF should include radiographs with flexion/extension views, computed tomography (CT) scan, and magnetic resonance imaging (MRI). Sagittal motion on plain radiographs and the presence of broken hardware and haloed screws serve as indirect evidence of pseudarthrosis [20, 21]. Thin-cut CT provides the most detailed evaluation of fusion mass outside of surgical exploration, and MRI is useful in detailing residual stenosis or adjacent segment issues. A careful analysis of the levels included in the index surgery as well as adjacent segments can be helpful in discerning the source of pathology and should involve factors such as disc height, spondylolisthesis, sagittal alignment, and evidence of hardware loosening, malposition, and subsidence. When the source of pain remains unclear based on patient history and preoperative imaging, diagnostic injections are another important tool in the work up. Injections, particularly in the setting of equivocal examination and imaging, can further elucidate the location and level of pathology and may act to exclude or confirm a diagnosis [22]. Diagnostic injections can be performed in outpatient setting with relatively low risk and cost to the patient [23]. One caveat to be aware of is that due to the presence of fibrosis and adhesions within the soft tissue, the efficacy of injections may be impacted by the limited dispersion of medication [24].


## Preoperative Procedures

While primary ALIF provides excellent exposure of the anterior column, major structures including the great vessels, ureters, and abdominal viscera are at risk during the procedure. Injury to the iliac veins can be life-threatening, and careful preoperative planning and assessment of the vascular anatomy are essential to improve patient safety [25]. The risk to these structures is increased in the revision setting due to the presence of adhesions and extensive scar tissue which can distort the anatomy. Due to this risk, it may be necessary to perform prophylactic interventions as a means of avoiding the potentially devastating surgical complications associated with injury. For example, placement of ureteral stents is sometimes performed before open abdominal surgery and can be helpful in revision ALIF to identify and protect the structures during exposure [26]. Some authors advocate for a preoperative arteriogram and venogram to clearly define the vessels and optimize the surgical approach, which should be performed in conjunction with a vascular surgeon [27]. In the absence of preoperative stenting of the major vessels, it is essential to prep in bilateral groins to ensure hemorrhage can be controlled by a transfemoral balloon or stent if necessary [28].

### *Revision ALIF: Approach and Technique*

While a detailed discussion of the surgical techniques involved in revision anterior lumbar surgery is outside the scope of this chapter, a basic understanding of the pearls and pitfalls are essential to appropriate preoperative planning. Exposure for revision ALIF can be done by a transperitoneal or retroperitoneal approach. The retroperitoneal approach has the advantage of providing a reduced risk of postoperative complications including retrograde ejaculation and ileus [29]. Once the field is prepped and draped to include bilateral transfemoral access, the incision is centered over the appropriate level, often from the contralateral side. Most approach surgeons will opt for a left-sided approach as the arterial structures are more resilient to injury compared to the right-sided vena cava and common iliac veins. It may be beneficial to access the spine from the right side to take advantage of virginal anatomy in a revision setting. However, if the spinal pathology or adjacent structures preclude a right-sided approach, the incision of the index procedure can be utilized [27]. One study investigating the results of revision anterior lumbar surgery discussed the theoretical risk of venous congestion if bilateral segmental arteries are ligated. The authors advocate for careful review of the index surgery operative report to see which vessels were sacrificed [27]. The same study reported successful results in nine revision ALIFs performed over a 16-month period with only 22% of cases requiring a transperitoneal exposure due to extensive adhesions [27].

The transperitoneal approach is well established with reports in the literature of providing access to the anterior lumbar spine since the middle of the twentieth century [30]. The transperitoneal approach provides direct access to the L5-S1 interspace between the major vessels. There is currently limited use of the transperitoneal approach when accessing levels above the lumbosacral junction as the aorta and common iliac vessels have yet to bifurcate, thereby placing them at increased risk of injury [31]. Therefore, if a retroperitoneal exposure is unlikely to be successful, then alternative treatment strategies should be used to revise levels above L5-S1.

## Conclusion

Anterior lumbar surgery is a powerful technique to achieve anterior column arthrodesis. Access to the disc space grants the spine surgeon excellent sagittal correction power and surface area to provide for large cage placement, foraminal height restoration, and fusion biology. Revision anterior-based surgery can be safely achieved only with adequate preoperative planning. In appropriately indicated patients, a careful review of the index procedure report and analysis of advanced imaging can help create an individualized plan that improves safety and probability of a successful outcome for the patient. Close consultation with a vascular surgeon is essential to determine if anterior access is feasible or if alternative approaches should be utilized to address the relevant levels of pathology.

# References


1. Martin BI, Mirza SK, Spina N, Spiker WR, Lawrence B, Brodke DS. Trends in lumbar fusion procedure rates and associated hospital costs for degenerative spinal diseases in the United States, 2004 to 2015. Spine. 2019;44:369–76.
2. Reisener M-J, Pumberger M, Shue J, Girardi FP, Hughes AP. Trends in lumbar spinal fusion-a literature review. J Spine Surg. 2020;6:752–61.
3. Lee S-H, Choi W-G, Lim S-R, Kang H-Y, Shin S-W. Minimally invasive anterior lumbar interbody fusion followed by percutaneous pedicle screw fixation for isthmic spondylolisthesis. Spine J. 2004;4:644–9.
4. Burkus JK, Gornet MF, Dickman CA, Zdeblick TA. Anterior lumbar interbody fusion using rhBMP-2 with tapered interbody cages. J Spinal Disord Tech. 2002;15:337–49.
5. Manzur M, Virk SS, Jivanelli B, Vaishnav AS, McAnany SJ, Albert TJ, Iyer S, Gang CH, Qureshi S. The rate of fusion for stand-alone anterior lumbar interbody fusion: a systematic review. Spine J. 2019;19:1294–301.
6. Baber Z, Erdek MA. Failed back surgery syndrome: current perspectives. J Pain Res. 2016;9:979–87.
7. Palumbo MA, Bianco AJ, Esmende S, Daniels AH. Wrong-site Spine Surgery. J Am Acad Orthop Surg. 2013;21:312–20.
8. Dowlati E, Alexander H, Voyadzis J-M. Vulnerability of the L5 nerve root during anterior lumbar interbody fusion at L5-S1: case series and review of the literature. Neurosurg Focus. 2020;49:E7.
9. Bosscher HA, Heavner JE. Incidence and severity of epidural fibrosis after back surgery: an endoscopic study. Pain Pract. 2010;10:18–24.
10. Saavedra-Pozo FM, Deusdara RAM, Benzel EC. Adjacent segment disease perspective and review of the literature. Ochsner J. 2014;14:78–83.
11. Raizman NM, O'Brien JR, Poehling-Monaghan KL, Yu WD. Pseudarthrosis of the spine. J Am Acad Orthop Surg. 2009;17:494–503.
12. Mobbs RJ, Loganathan A, Yeung V, Rao PJ. Indications for anterior lumbar interbody fusion. Orthop Surg. 2013;5:153–63.
13. Phan K, Lee NJ, Kothari P, Kim JS, Cho SK. Risk factors for readmissions following anterior lumbar interbody fusion. Spine. 2018;43:364–9.
14. Govindarajan V, Diaz A, Perez-Roman RJ, Burks SS, Wang MY, Levi AD. Osteoporosis treatment in patients undergoing spinal fusion: a systematic review and meta-analysis. Neurosurg Focus. 2021;50:E9.
15. Satake K, Kanemura T, Yamaguchi H, Segi N, Ouchida J. Predisposing factors for intraoperative endplate injury of extreme lateral interbody fusion. Asian Spine J. 2016;10:907–14.
16. Berman D, Oren JH, Bendo J, Spivak J. The effect of smoking on spinal fusion. Int J Spine Surg. 2017;11:29.
17. Passias PG, Bortz C, Alas H, Segreto FA, Horn SR, Ihejirika YU, Vasquez-Montes D, Pierce KE, Brown AE, Shenoy K, et al. Alcoholism as a predictor for pseudarthrosis in primary spine fusion: an analysis of risk factors and 30-day outcomes for 52,402 patients from 2005 to 2013. J Orthop. 2019;16:36–40.
18. Guyer RD, Patterson M, Ohnmeiss DD. Failed back surgery syndrome: diagnostic evaluation. J Am Acad Orthop Surg. 2006;14:534–43.
19. Porto GBF, Jeffrey Wessell DO, Alvarado A, Arnold PM, Buchholz AL. Anticoagulation and spine surgery. Global Spine J. 2020;10:53S–64S.
20. Lee Y-P, Sclafani J, Garfin SR. Lumbar Pseudarthrosis: diagnosis and treatment. Semin Spine Surg. 2011;23:275–81.
21. Lockey S, Fakhre E, Mo AZ. Revision of lumbar pseudarthrosis after posterolateral fusion. Semin Spine Surg. 2022;34:100925.
22. Bartleson JD, Maus TP. Diagnostic and therapeutic spinal interventions: epidural injections. Neurol Clin Pract. 2014;4:347–52.

23. Kim BY, Concannon TA, Barboza LC, Khan TW. The role of diagnostic injections in spinal disorders: a narrative review. Diagnostics (Basel). 2021;11:11.
24. Urits I, Schwartz RH, Brinkman J, Foster L, Miro P, Berger AA, Kassem H, Kaye AD, Manchikanti L, Viswanath O. An evidence based review of Epidurolysis for the Management of Epidural Adhesions. Psychopharmacol Bull. 2020;50:74–90.
25. Capellades J, Pellisé F, Rovira A, Grivé E, Pedraza S, Villanueva C. Magnetic resonance anatomic study of Iliocava junction and left iliac vein positions related to L5–S1 disc. Spine. 2000;25:1695.
26. Isiklar ZU, Lindsey RW, Coburn M. Ureteral injury after anterior lumbar interbody fusion. A case report. Spine. 1996;21:2379–82.
27. Gumbs AA, Hanan S, Yue JJ, Shah RV, Sumpio B. Revision open anterior approaches for spine procedures. Spine J. 2007;7:280–5.
28. Brau S, Delamarter RB, Kropf MA, Watkins RG III, Williams LA, Schiffman ML, Bae HW. Access strategies for revision in anterior lumbar surgery. Spine. 2008;33:1662–7.
29. Mobbs RJ, Phan K, Daly D, Rao PJ, Lennox A. Approach-related complications of anterior lumbar interbody fusion: results of a combined spine and vascular surgical team. Global Spine J. 2016;6:147–54.
30. Lane JD Jr, Moore ES Jr. Transperitoneal approach to the intervertebral disc in the lumbar area. Ann Surg. 1948;127:537–51.
31. Laratta JL, Davis EG, Glassman SD, Dimar JR. The transperitoneal approach for anterior lumbar interbody fusion at L5- S1: a technical note. J Spine Surg. 2018;4:459.

# Chapter 27
# Anterior and Lateral Interbody Techniques for Revision Lumbar Fusion

Edward Fakhre, Stephen D. Lockey, Seleem Elkadi, and S. Babak Kalantar

## Introduction

Interbody fusion is a powerful tool to provide anterior column stability and indirect decompression of the neural elements. These techniques were developed to optimize fusion rates in degenerative lumbar conditions but can also be used in the revision setting for postlaminectomy instability, recurrent stenosis, or pseudarthrosis [1]. Interbody fusion is now used to manage a wide array of spinal disorders, including degenerative pathologies, neoplasias, trauma, and infection, and in the revision lumbar fusion [2].

Interbody technology is a powerful tool as it aids in proper load transmission throughout the thoracolumbar spine. In the neutral position, 80% of the spinal load is transferred across the intact intervertebral discs. Interbody fusion, therefore, provides a more stable construct to promote fusion as well as increase the surface area available for healing [3]. The purpose of this review is to discuss the utility of anterior interbody technology in the revision setting following primary lumbar fusion.

E. Fakhre · S. D. Lockey
Department of Orthopaedics, Medstar Georgetown University Hospital, Washington, DC, USA

S. Elkadi
Georgetown University School of Medicine, Washington, DC, USA
e-mail: She27@georgetown.edu

S. B. Kalantar (✉)
Department of Orthopaedic Surgery, Georgetown University School of Medicine, Medstar Orthopaedic Institute, Washington, DC, USA

© The Author(s), under exclusive license to Springer Nature Switzerland AG 2023
J. R. O'Brien et al. (eds.), *Lumbar Spine Access Surgery*,
https://doi.org/10.1007/978-3-031-48034-8_27

## Indications for Revision Lumbar Fusion

Revision of a primary fusion can be due to various conditions such as pseudarthrosis, degenerative disease progression in adjacent segments, residual stenosis, or surgical implant failure [4]. The risk of pseudarthrosis is increased if the patient has a smoking history, increased age, osteoporosis, alcoholism, or malnourishment [5, 6]. Additionally, longer fusion constructs are subject to a higher rate of pseudarthrosis due to the increased stress across the fusion mass [7]. In deformity surgery, patients with a positive sagittal imbalance $\geq$5 cm, kyphosis $\geq$20°, and unilateral sacropelvic fixation or sacropelvic fixation without anterior column support have been shown to be at an increased risk of developing pseudarthrosis [8]. Patients with pseudarthrosis may present with recurrence of symptoms after a period of relief following the index procedure [9]. Interbody technology increases the fusion surface area and in primary fusion constructs has been shown to decrease the rate of pseudarthrosis compared to isolated posterolateral arthrodesis [10]. Residual stenosis following the initial decompression is another leading cause for revision procedures with up to 20% of patients experiencing persistent symptoms [11]. In these cases, interbody devices can provide indirect decompression of the neural elements. These features make interbody technology an attractive option for the surgeon managing pseudarthrosis or residual stenosis following primary lumbar fusion [12, 13].

Proximal junctional kyphosis (PJK) refers to forward bending of the spine at the cranial end of a fusion construct. Revision for PJK often involves the extension of fusion cranially to a stable vertebral level while also correcting sagittal imbalance [14]. Interbody fusion can aid in correcting lumbar lordosis and restoring sagittal balance. Adjacent segment disease (ASD) occurs when patients experience symptomatic degeneration of the level above or below a fusion segment. This process is largely believed to be a result of increased stress and motion at the levels above or below a fusion construct, though iatrogenic damage during instrumentation and progression of preexisting disease are also thought to contribute [15, 16]. Degenerative changes seen in ASD include disc degeneration or bulging, disc herniation, facet joint arthropathy, and spondylolisthesis and instability [15, 17]. These changes can lead to stenosis at the adjacent level, resulting in radiculopathy and/or neurogenic claudication necessitating a revision procedure [17]. Interbody techniques may be useful in this setting particularly in achieving indirect foraminal decompression while avoiding the morbidity of a repeated posterior approach.

## Techniques

In performing revision surgery, multiple anterior-based approaches are available with various technical considerations either supporting or discouraging their use. The techniques discussed here are anterior lumbar interbody fusion (ALIF), oblique lumbar interbody fusion (OLIF), and lateral lumbar interbody fusion (LLIF). For all these examples, adequate intravenous access should be obtained prior to positioning in anticipation of blood loss according to the length and difficulty of the surgery. Additionally, lumbar spine imaging should be clearly displayed, and a portable C-arm machine should be available [18]. Finally, intraoperative neuromonitoring should be considered according to regional standards and surgeon discretion. The use of intraoperative monitoring must be discussed with the anesthesia team in preparation for surgery.

## *Anterior Lumbar Interbody Fusion (ALIF)*

When performing an ALIF, the patient is placed in the supine position. The patient should have arm supports and restraining devices to ensure the trunk is stabilized. Caution should be taken to ensure there is no pressure on any peripheral nerves or vessels of the arms and legs. The assistance of an access surgeon is often utilized due to the risks of mobilizing and retracting intraperitoneal and retroperitoneal structures such as the intestines, aorta, and inferior vena cava (IVC) [19]. The use of an access surgeon is associated with similar intraoperative complications, arterial injuries, and retrograde ejaculation ileus but lower prosthesis complications, reoperation rates, and postoperative complications; therefore, an access surgeon is recommended for patients with potentially difficult exposures [20].

The anterior retroperitoneal approach is classically made through a left-sided incision and approach. The vessels on the left, particularly the left common iliac vein, travel more medially over the disc space than the right-sided vessels. Exposure of the disc at L4–L5 or above requires mobilization of the left common iliac vein medially, which is facilitated by a left-sided approach. In the setting of a previously performed left-sided approach, a right-sided approach may be performed after careful review of vascular anatomy and discussion with the approach surgeon.

Once the disc space is exposed and the borders are clearly identified, the anterior longitudinal ligament (ALL) is divided into two flaps in an H-shaped configuration. Next, the disc is separated from the superior and inferior end plates with Cobb elevators and rongeurs. If the disc space is still obscured due to osteophytes, an anterior osteotomy is performed with medium-sized osteomes. If there was a previous transforaminal interbody fusion (TLIF) (Figs. 27.1 and 27.2), a disc retractor is inserted next to the spacer which is then distracted. Then, curettage is performed around the TLIF spacer to ensure separation from the end plates and the posterior longitudinal ligament (PLL). Proper care must be taken to ensure the preservation of the end plates to prevent subsidence of the new cage [19].

In revision surgery where a previously placed interbody cage is present, an osteotome can be used to create space above and below the cage along the end plate surface. In cases with excessive scar tissue, straight and curved curettes may be helpful to further loosen the cage. Once the prior device is appropriately free, a hook or pituitary with teeth can be used to extract the device [21].

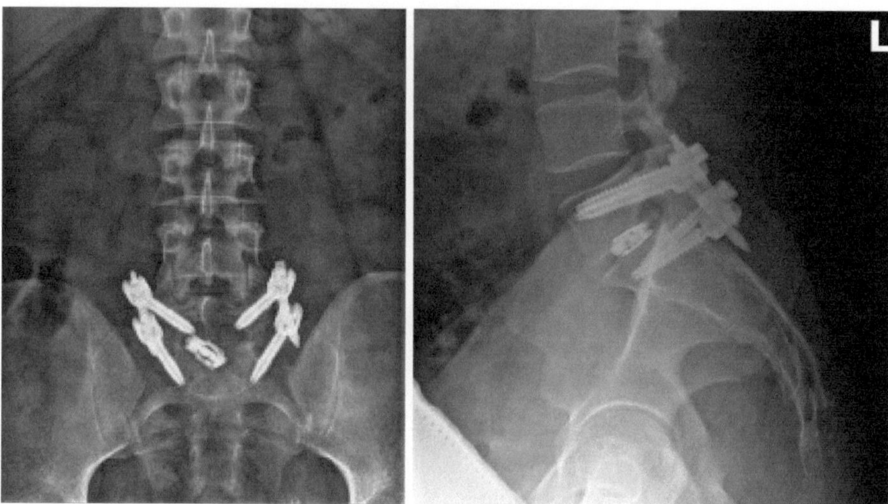

**Fig. 27.1** 35 year-old male with pseudarthrosis after L5-S1 TLIF. He presented with persistent axial back pain and radiculopathy. The existing TLIF cage required revision involving removal through an anterior approach and placement of an ALIF cage

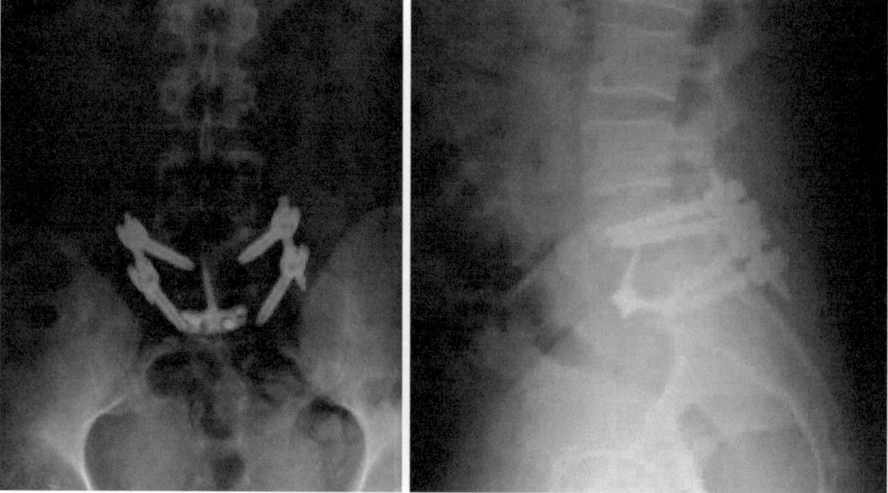

**Fig. 27.2** Patient in Fig. 27.1 after revision of pseudarthrosis with an ALIF

Once the disc space is separated, extensive exposure is performed to ensure a wide discectomy/release can be achieved. The ALL is released followed by discectomy posteriorly to the PLL. The PLL can also be released at levels not included in a prior TLIF. Next, a large paddle distractor is inserted to further pry open the disc space. To add power to the distractor, an 8-/10-mm TLIF paddle or similar instrument is inserted as far posteriorly as possible, between the blades of the distractor, and rotated approximately 90°. There is a lower probability of violating the end plate by placing the paddle as posteriorly as possible. If there is a need to address sagittal imbalance, the operating room table can be further placed in the "jackknife" position to increase the lordosis. To distract the disc further, hyperlordotic trials are inserted sequentially from smallest to largest size [19].

Finally, a hyperlordotic ALIF cage filled with the surgeon's biologic graft of choice is inserted into the disc space. Next, the cage is fixated in position using standalone screw or plate fixation to prevent extrusion. Once this step is completed, anteroposterior and lateral fluoroscopic images are obtained to ensure proper placement of the cage [19]. Most revisions through the ALIF approach attempt to correct either the L4–L5 disc space or the L5-S1 disc space; however, it is possible to address the L2–L3 and L3–L4 disc spaces through this approach [22].

Another decision that must be made when performing a revision procedure is determining the optimal cage lordotic angulation. The most common cage sizes are 6–8 degrees, 10–12 degrees, and generally up to 30 degrees. A recent study found the corrective segmental lordosis can be approximated as half the cage size. Specifically, the authors found the average change in segmental lordosis to be 6.1°, 12.5°, and 17.7° when using a 12°, 20°, and 30° cage, respectively [19]. ALIF has the powerful ability to correct mismatches in lumbar lordosis. Without proper lordosis, the issues described above such as residual stenosis, pseudoarthrosis, PJK, and ASD may arise [23].

There are several advantages to an anterior approach in the revision setting including a reduced rate of nerve damage, avoidance of paraspinal muscle trauma, and a decreased hospital stay. Furthermore, an anterior approach allows for a better disc excision and the ability to add larger interbody devices [24]. Therefore, in the revision setting, ALIF is an optimal choice in attempting aggressive correction of lordosis and restoring foraminal height, which can also lead to higher rates of fusion [25–29]. Despite these advantages, there are several complications associated with an anterior approach including retrograde ejaculation, impotence, retroperitoneal fibrosis, rectus muscle hematoma, pancreatitis, femoral nerve palsy, pseudomeningocele, and latissimus dorsi rupture [22]. Some surgeons may offer the option of preoperative sperm banking due to concerns of postoperative infertility [30]. Furthermore, a review of 1310 cases found a 0.45% incidence of left iliac artery thrombosis and a 1.4% incidence of major vein laceration [31, 32]. Many of these vascular complications can be reduced if an access surgeon is utilized for difficult approaches. Additionally, the incidence of ureteral injury has been reported in 0.3–0.5% of cases, but this complication may be reduced by preoperative placement of a ureteral stent [22, 33].

## *Oblique Lateral Interbody Fusion (OLIF)*

Patient preparation prior to OLIF is similar to ALIF as described above. For an OLIF, the patient is typically placed in the left or right lateral decubitus position. To our knowledge, there are no studies demonstrating clinical superiority of a right versus left-sided approach. However, a left-sided approach is often preferred due to the ability to avoid manipulation of the IVC. The IVC is thin walled, making it difficult to repair following injury. Despite this fact, a right-sided approach may be necessary if the patient has scoliosis, abdominal scarring, or previous lumbar surgery [34–38].

After the approach is completed and proper visualization of the disc space achieved, the discectomy can be performed using an anterolateral window that is as small as 1 cm [34, 39]. Improved visualization is then achieved through sequential dilation. While dilating, a back and forth twisting motion while going through the muscle and fascia is recommended to avoid bringing muscle into the retractor field [40]. Next, the annulus is incised to at least 18 mm, and then the discectomy is performed using pituitaries, rasps, and curettes. To release the contralateral annulus, a Cobb is placed across the disc space. This will allow for effective expansion of the disc space. The end plates can be prepared and cartilage removed using angled curettes. In revisions, where removal of previously placed interbody cages are necessary, osteotomes and straight or curved curettes can be placed to loosen the cage. Once again, it is imperative to preserve the end plates during this step. After cage removal, adequate end plate preparation is ensured, and a new cage is placed [21].

OLIF is a powerful technique as it can be used to access multiple vertebrae levels without extending the incision. By reducing incision size, the incidence of postoperative pain and potential complications such as incisional hernias may be reduced [34, 39]. Reports in the literature of OLIF to address disease from L1 to S1 make the technique an attractive option if multiple levels need to be revised [39, 41]. Studies have shown that OLIF in the revision setting has decreased operative time, intraoperative blood loss, bedridden time, and length of hospitalization when compared to posterior lumbar interbody fusion (PLIF) [42]. Another study demonstrated that patients tend to experience lower pain when compared to PLIF 1 week following surgery [41]. Similar to ALIF, one of the key advantages of OLIF for revision is that the technique provides a new surgical site following posterolateral fusion [43]. Furthermore, some of the known risks of posterior-based interbody approaches, like intraoperative durotomy, are reduced by using OLIF [44]. OLIF also allows larger cage insertion and increased disc height, allowing a similar indirect decompression and fusion surface area as ALIF [45–47]. It is worth noting, however, that indirect decompression may be limited by the presence of scar tissue and perineural adhesions from prior spine surgery [43].

## *Lateral Lumbar Interbody Fusion (LLIF)*

LLIF presents an alternative approach to the disc space that utilizes a lateral transpsoas exposure. This approach minimizes handling of the peritoneum and great vessels, decreases the risk of retrograde ejaculation, does not require the use of an approach surgeon, and allows for access to more cranial lumbar levels than anterior approaches [48].

In positioning a patient for a lateral trans-psoas approach, 90° lateral decubitus positioning ensures the most freedom of movement for the surgeon as well as the widest access to the lumbar spine. The patient is secured to the bed in this position by taping. The knees and hips are flexed, and padding is placed underneath the contralateral leg to prevent pressure on the common peroneal nerve. The arms are flexed forward to almost 90° and taped with pillows placed between them, and the ulnar nerve is padded at the elbow. An axillary roll can be considered to ensure no stretch on the brachial plexus. The patient's iliac crest is placed at the break of the bed, which can be flexed to maximize the distance between the iliac crest caudally and rib cage cranially, to allow the largest possible exposure. Additionally, a bump can be placed under the contralateral flank [48].

Factors that limit access to the lumbar spine are obstruction by the iliac crest and rib cage and the progressively anterior course of the lumbar plexus as one travels caudally in the lumbar spine [48, 49]. If necessary, LLIF can be performed in the thoracic spine through transdiaphragmatic or transthoracic approaches, but this is outside the scope of this chapter [50]. The iliac crest and vessels block access to the L5-S1 level, so L4–L5 is the most caudal level typically approached. While exposure of L4–L5 is usually possible, the exposure is made more challenging by the more anterior position of the lumbar plexus at this segment, resulting in a narrower working corridor [49]. Should neuromonitoring reveal no safe corridor, the approach should be abandoned to avoid risking devastating injury to the femoral nerve.

After sufficient exposure, discectomy and end plate decortication can be performed. Discectomy begins with an annulotomy of sufficient size to pass a cage, followed by the use of pituitary rongeurs and curettes to clear disc material [51]. In order to appropriately seat the cage, the contralateral annulus must be released by passing a Cobb elevator across the disc space and confirmed radiographically (Fig. 27.3) [51]. Biomechanical studies have shown more rigidity of the construct and less motion at the instrumented level with the use of larger cage widths (size in

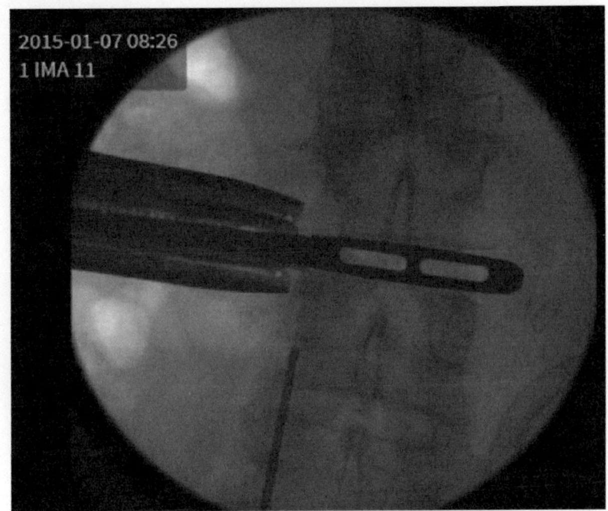


**Fig. 27.3** Intraoperative fluoroscopic image during LLIF of a trial cage crossing the contralateral annulus demonstrating the appropriate release of the contralateral annulus. A similar image with a Cobb should be obtained prior to placement of an LLIF cage

the AP dimension when referring to LLIF cages) [52]. Furthermore, the use of 22-mm cages is associated with a lower rate of subsidence relative to 18-mm implants [53]. With this in mind, insertion of larger cages should be prioritized if there is concern for poor bone quality or if the need for a highly stable construct exists in the revision setting.

LLIF is commonly described as a useful option for treating symptomatic ASD after posterolateral instrumented fusion [54, 55]. The symptoms of ASD are often a result of instability and stenosis, which can be addressed with LLIF while avoiding further destabilization of adjacent segments by leaving the ALL and PLL intact [54]. ASD commonly involves levels cranial to the instrumented levels, making the degenerated segments easily accessible through a lateral trans-psoas approach. This technique avoids the morbidity and challenge of revision posterior decompression and fusion where tissue scarring leads to a more challenging procedure and higher complication rate, which may include durotomy [56]. A further advantage over a traditional revision is the potential for correction of sagittal and coronal plane deformity. A systematic review of radiographic outcomes showed 9.1° and 7.5° of coronal and sagittal plane correction, respectively, after LLIF [57]. LLIF in this setting can be supplemented with a posterior procedure for further decompression or extension of fusion for added stability. While LLIF provides indirect decompression through disc height restoration, it may also result in indirect central and lateral recess decompression. The surgeon must carefully review preoperative imaging to assess feasibility of an indirect decompression. Generally, severe stenosis due to bony hypertrophy of the facets will require a direct posterior laminectomy [58]. LLIF can be performed with a cage as a standalone construct or supplemented with fixation, such as extension of the posterior screw-rod construct bilaterally or unilaterally (Figs. 27.4 and 27.5). Biomechanical analyses of LLIF for revision of

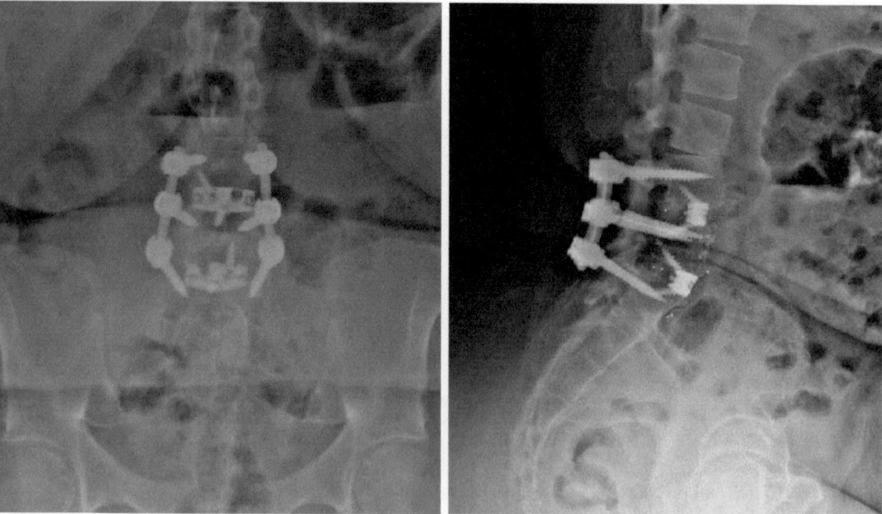

**Fig. 27.4** 51 year-old female presenting with neurogenic claudication and axial lower back pain 2 years after L4-S1 PSF and ALIF. Images demonstrate adjacent segment degeneration and kyphosis at L3–L4

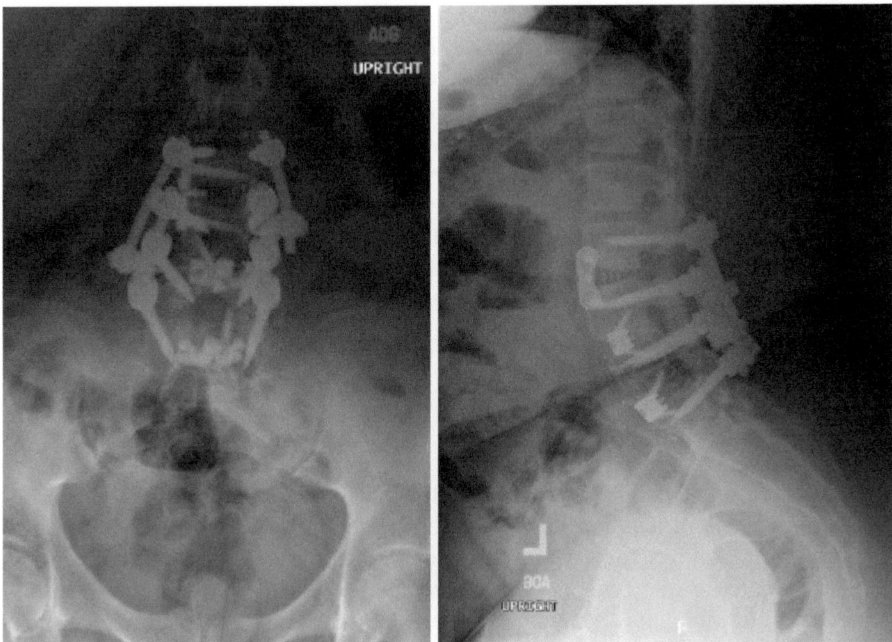


**Fig. 27.5** Patient in Fig. 27.4 after revision with LLIF at L3–L4 and laminectomy with extension of the pedicle screw construct to L3–L4

ASD showed that an interbody cage alone results in a significant increase in stiffness of the segment. The stiffness of the construct was further enhanced with supplemental fixation, including pedicle screw-rod, *in situ* screw, and lateral plate constructs [59, 60]. Standalone LLIF may therefore not be appropriate for use in cases with significant sagittal or coronal plane imbalance or with significant spondylolisthesis. These cases may benefit from either *in situ* fixation with a screw or lateral plate or extension of the posterior screw-rod construct.

While removal or revision of an existing interbody cage is usually done using an ALIF technique, LLIF has been reported for use in revising a failed TLIF [61]. In this setting, revision is likely a result of symptomatic pseudarthrosis at the level of concern. A lateral trans-psoas approach avoids the morbidity of the anterior approach and may be a safer alternative, particularly at more cranial levels in the lumbar spine. After exposure of the disc space, a cobb and osteotome can be used to create a gap between the TLIF cage and the end plate, after which a pituitary or rongeur can be used to retrieve the cage [61]. In the setting of pseudarthrosis where additional stability is needed, a large cage (22–26 mm) should be used and supplemental posterior fixation added.

Outcome data after revision LLIF are scarce and reported primarily for treatment of ASD. One study examining 100 patients treated by revision LLIF reported promising results with a mean drop of visual analogue scores from 8.6 preoperatively to 2.8 postoperatively. Additionally, the average length of hospital stay was 1.13 days, and blood loss was 1.34 g/dl [62]. Another study of 52 patients found significant improvements in pain, as well as radiographic measures, including lordosis, coronal deformity, and disc height after revision LLIF. Eleven patients (21.2%) required additional revision with 8 of 11 having received standalone LLIF. Although not statistically significant, the authors reported a trend toward higher fusion rates (87.5% vs. 53.8%) with circumferential vs. standalone fusion leading the authors to suggest that supplementation of the LLIF may be beneficial despite the added morbidity [63]. However, another study presented conflicting data demonstrating all 21 patients with ASD treated with standalone LLIF went on to solid fusion with significant improvements in leg and back pain [64]. Ultimately, existing data suggests LLIF as an effective and relatively safe treatment option for revision in ASD.

## Conclusion

Anterior interbody techniques provide a valuable alternative to traditional posterior-based approaches in revision lumbar fusion surgery. The use of a virgin surgical approach alone allows for a less complicated and morbid technique. While data comparing anterior interbody approaches to each other and to traditional posterior strategies are limited, the advantages of each approach and the clinical scenario can be used to decide on an appropriate treatment option. The corrective power in deformity surgery, as well as the ability to provide indirect decompression with enhanced stability of each technique, must be weighed against the respective complication profiles.

## References

1. Selznick LA, Shamji MF, Isaacs RE. Minimally invasive interbody fusion for revision lumbar surgery: technical feasibility and safety. J Spinal Disord Tech. 2009;22:207–13.
2. Resnick DK, Choudhri TF, Dailey AT, Groff MW, Khoo L, Matz PG, Mummaneni P, Watters WC, Wang J, Walters BC, et al. Guidelines for the performance of fusion procedures for degenerative disease of the lumbar spine. Part 7: intractable low-back pain without stenosis or spondylolisthesis. J Neurosurg Spine. 2005;2:670–2.
3. Cunningham BW, Polly DW Jr. The use of interbody cage devices for spinal deformity: a biomechanical perspective. Clin Orthop Relat Res. 2002;394:73–83.
4. Deyo RA, Martin BI, Kreuter W, Jarvik JG, Angier H, Mirza SK. Revision surgery following operations for lumbar stenosis. J Bone Joint Surg Am. 2011;93:1979–86.
5. Brown CW, Orme TJ, Richardson HD. The rate of pseudarthrosis (surgical nonunion) in patients who are smokers and patients who are nonsmokers: a comparison study. Spine. 1986;11:942–3.
6. Chun DS, Baker KC, Hsu WK. Lumbar pseudarthrosis: a review of current diagnosis and treatment. Neurosurg Focus. 2015;39:E10.
7. Cleveland M, Bosworth DM, Thompson FR. Pseudarthrosis in the lumbosacral spine. J Bone Joint Surg Am. 1948;30A:302–12.

8. Kim YJ, Bridwell KH, Lenke LG, Rhim S, Cheh G. Pseudarthrosis in long adult spinal deformity instrumentation and fusion to the sacrum: prevalence and risk factor analysis of 144 cases. Spine. 2006;31:2329–36.
9. Bederman SS, Le VH, Pahlavan S. An approach to lumbar revision spine surgery in adults. J Am Acad Orthop Surg. 2016;24:433–42.
10. Bono CM, Lee CK. Critical analysis of trends in fusion for degenerative disc disease over the past 20 years: influence of technique on fusion rate and clinical outcome. Spine. 2004;29:455–63; discussion Z5.
11. Airaksinen O, Herno A, Turunen V, Saari T, Suomlainen O. Surgical outcome of 438 patients treated surgically for lumbar spinal stenosis. Spine. 1997;22:2278–82.
12. Omidi-Kashani F, Hasankhani EG, Ashjazadeh A. Lumbar spinal stenosis: who should be fused? An updated review. Asian Spine J. 2014;8:521.
13. Hironaka Y, Morimoto T, Motoyama Y, Park Y-S, Nakase H. Surgical management of minimally invasive anterior lumbar interbody fusion with stand-alone interbody cage for L4-5 degenerative disorders: clinical and radiographic findings. Neurol Med Chir. 2013;53:861–9.
14. Lee J, Park Y-S. Proximal junctional kyphosis: diagnosis, pathogenesis, and treatment. Asian Spine J. 2016;10:593–600.
15. Park P, Garton HJ, Gala VC, Hoff JT, McGillicuddy JE. Adjacent segment disease after lumbar or lumbosacral fusion: review of the literature. Spine. 2004;29:1938–44.
16. Phillips FM, Reuben J, Wetzel FT. Intervertebral disc degeneration adjacent to a lumbar fusion. An experimental rabbit model. J Bone Joint Surg Br. 2002;84:289–94.
17. Lee CS, Hwang CJ, Lee S-W, Ahn Y-J, Kim Y-T, Lee D-H, Lee MY. Risk factors for adjacent segment disease after lumbar fusion. Eur Spine J. 2009;18:1637–43.
18. Crock HV. Anterior lumbar interbody fusion. Clin Orthop Relat Res. 1982;165:157–63.
19. Kadam A, Wigner N, Saville P, Arlet V. Overpowering posterior lumbar instrumentation and fusion with hyperlordotic anterior lumbar interbody cages followed by posterior revision: a preliminary feasibility study. J Neurosurg Spine. 2017;27:650–60.
20. Phan K, Xu J, Scherman DB, Rao PJ, Mobbs RJ. Anterior lumbar interbody fusion with and without an "Access Surgeon". Spine. 2017;42:E592–601.
21. Moisi M, Page J, Paulson D, Oskouian RJ. Technical note—lateral approach to the lumbar spine for the removal of interbody cages. Cureus. 2015;7:e268. https://doi.org/10.7759/cureus.268.
22. Gumbs AA, Hanan S, Yue JJ, Shah RV, Sumpio B. Revision open anterior approaches for spine procedures. Spine J. 2007;7:280–5.
23. Rothenfluh DA, Mueller DA, Rothenfluh E, Min K. Pelvic incidence-lumbar lordosis mismatch predisposes to adjacent segment disease after lumbar spinal fusion. Eur Spine J. 2015;24:1251–8.
24. Zdeblick TA, David SM. A prospective comparison of surgical approach for anterior L4-L5 fusion: laparoscopic versus mini anterior lumbar interbody fusion. Spine. 2000;25:2682–7.
25. Mobbs RJ, Phan K, Malham G, Seex K, Rao PJ. Lumbar interbody fusion: techniques, indications and comparison of interbody fusion options including PLIF, TLIF, MI-TLIF, OLIF/ATP, LLIF and ALIF. J Spine Surg. 2015;1:2–18.
26. Hsieh PC, Koski TR, O'Shaughnessy BA, Sugrue P, Salehi S, Ondra S, Liu JC. Anterior lumbar interbody fusion in comparison with transforaminal lumbar interbody fusion: implications for the restoration of foraminal height, local disc angle, lumbar lordosis, and sagittal balance. J Neurosurg Spine. 2007;7:379–86.
27. Phan K, Thayaparan GK, Mobbs RJ. Anterior lumbar interbody fusion versus transforaminal lumbar interbody fusion—systematic review and meta-analysis. Br J Neurosurg. 2015;29:705–11.
28. Malham GM, Parker RM, Ellis NJ, Blecher CM, Chow FY, Claydon MH. Anterior lumbar interbody fusion using recombinant human bone morphogenetic protein-2: a prospective study of complications. J Neurosurg Spine. 2014;21:851–60.

29. Rao PJ, Maharaj MM, Phan K, Abeygunasekara ML, Mobbs RJ. Indirect foraminal decompression after anterior lumbar interbody fusion: a prospective radiographic study using a new pedicle-to-pedicle technique. Spine J. 2015;15:817–24.
30. Cohn EB, Ignatoff JM, Keeler TC, Shapiro DE, Blum MD. Exposure of the anterior spine: technique and experience with 66 patients. J Urol. 2000;164:416–8. https://doi.org/10.7759/cureus.268.
31. Gumbs AA. The open anterior Paramedian retroperitoneal approach for spine procedures. Arch Surg. 2005;140:339.
32. Brau SA, Delamarter RB, Schiffman ML, Williams LA, Watkins RG. Vascular injury during anterior lumbar surgery. Spine J. 2004;4:409–12.
33. Faciszewski T, Winter RB, Lonstein JE, Denis F, Johnson L. The surgical and medical perioperative complications of anterior spinal fusion surgery in the thoracic and lumbar spine in adults. A review of 1223 procedures. Spine. 1995;20:1592–9.
34. Silvestre C, Mac-Thiong J-M, Hilmi R, Roussouly P. Complications and morbidities of mini-open anterior retroperitoneal lumbar interbody fusion: oblique lumbar interbody fusion in 179 patients. Asian Spine J. 2012;6:89.
35. Molinares DM, Davis TT, Fung DA. Retroperitoneal oblique corridor to the L2-S1 intervertebral discs: an MRI study. J Neurosurg Spine. 2016;24:248–55.
36. Molloy S, Butler JS, Benton A, Malhotra K, Selvadurai S, Agu O. A new extensile anterolateral retroperitoneal approach for lumbar interbody fusion from L1 to S1: a prospective series with clinical outcomes. Spine J. 2016;16:786–91.
37. Davis TT, Hynes RA, Fung DA, Spann SW, MacMillan M, Kwon B, Liu J, Acosta F, Drochner TE. Retroperitoneal oblique corridor to the L2-S1 intervertebral discs in the lateral position: an anatomic study. J Neurosurg Spine. 2014;21:785–93.
38. Jagannathan J, Chankaew E, Urban P, Dumont AS, Sansur CA, Kern J, Peeler B, Elias WJ, Shen F, Shaffrey ME, et al. Cosmetic and functional outcomes following paramedian and anterolateral retroperitoneal access in anterior lumbar spine surgery. J Neurosurg Spine. 2008;9:454–65.
39. Li JXJ, Phan K, Mobbs R. Oblique lumbar interbody fusion: technical aspects, operative outcomes, and complications. World Neurosurg. 2017;98:113–23.
40. Orita S, Inage K, Furuya T, Koda M, Aoki Y, Kubota G, Nakamura J, Shiga Y, Matsuura Y, Maki S, et al. Oblique Lateral Interbody Fusion (OLIF): indications and techniques. Oper Tech Orthop. 2017;27:223–30.
41. Li R, Li X, Zhou H, Jiang W. Development and application of oblique lumbar interbody fusion. Orthop Surg. 2020;12:355–65.
42. Zhu G, Hao Y, Yu L, Cai Y, Yang X. Comparing stand-alone oblique lumbar interbody fusion with posterior lumbar interbody fusion for revision of rostral adjacent segment disease: a STROBE-compliant study. Medicine. 2018;97:e12680.
43. Jung J, Lee S, Cho D-C, Han I-B, Kim CH, Lee Y-S, Kim K-T. Usefulness of oblique lumbar interbody fusion as revision surgery: comparison of clinical and radiological outcomes between primary and revision surgery. World Neurosurg. 2021;149:e1067–76.
44. Hentenaar B, Spoor AB, de Waal Malefijt J, Diekerhof CH, den Oudsten BL. Clinical and radiological outcome of minimally invasive posterior lumbar interbody fusion in primary versus revision surgery. J Orthop Surg Res. 2016;11:2.
45. Lee YS, Park SW, Kim YB. Direct lateral lumbar interbody fusion: clinical and radiological outcomes. J Korean Neurosurg Soc. 2014;55:248–54.
46. Ohtori S, Orita S, Yamauchi K, Eguchi Y, Aoki Y, Nakamura J, Miyagi M, Suzuki M, Kubota G, Inage K, et al. Change of lumbar ligamentum flavum after indirect decompression using anterior lumbar interbody fusion. Asian Spine J. 2017;11:105–12.
47. Sato J, Ohtori S, Orita S, Yamauchi K, Eguchi Y, Ochiai N, Kuniyoshi K, Aoki Y, Nakamura J, Miyagi M, et al. Radiographic evaluation of indirect decompression of mini-open anterior retroperitoneal lumbar interbody fusion: oblique lateral interbody fusion for degenerated lumbar spondylolisthesis. Eur Spine J. 2017;26:671–8.

48. Ozgur BM, Aryan HE, Pimenta L, Taylor WR. Extreme lateral interbody fusion (XLIF): a novel surgical technique for anterior lumbar interbody fusion. Spine J. 2006;6:435–43.
49. Park DK, Lee MJ, Lin EL, Singh K, An HS, Phillips FM. The relationship of Intrapsoas nerves during a Transpsoas approach to the lumbar spine. J Spinal Disord Tech. 2010;23:223–8.
50. Berjano P, Lamartina C. Far lateral approaches (XLIF) in adult scoliosis. Eur Spine J. 2013;22(Suppl 2):S242–53.
51. Billinghurst J, Akbarnia BA. Extreme lateral interbody fusion—XLIF. Curr Orthop Pract. 2009;20:238–51.
52. Pimenta L, Turner AWL, Dooley ZA, Parikh RD, Peterson MD. Biomechanics of lateral interbody spacers: going wider for going stiffer. ScientificWorldJournal. 2012;2012:381814.
53. Le TV, Baaj AA, Dakwar E, Burkett CJ, Murray G, Smith DA, Uribe JS. Subsidence of polyetheretherketone intervertebral cages in minimally invasive lateral retroperitoneal transpsoas lumbar interbody fusion. Spine. 2012;37:1268–73.
54. Palejwala SK, Sheen WA, Walter CM, Dunn JH, Baaj AA. Minimally invasive lateral transpsoas interbody fusion using a stand-alone construct for the treatment of adjacent segment disease of the lumbar spine: review of the literature and report of three cases. Clin Neurol Neurosurg. 2014;124:90–6.
55. Tobert DG, Makanji HS, Cha TD. Lumbar interbody fusion for adjacent segment disease: An illustrative case of the lateral transpsoas approach (XLIF-DLIF). Semin Spine Surg. 2018;30:258–64.
56. Khan MH, Rihn J, Steele G, Davis R, Donaldson WF, Kang JD, Lee JY. Postoperative management protocol for incidental Dural tears during degenerative lumbar spine surgery. Spine. 2006;31:2609–13.
57. Phan K, Rao PJ, Scherman DB, Dandie G, Mobbs RJ. Lateral lumbar interbody fusion for sagittal balance correction and spinal deformity. J Clin Neurosci. 2015;22:1714–21.
58. Younus A, Kelly A, Lekgwara P. Minimally invasive extreme lateral lumbar interbody fusion (XLIF) to manage adjacent level disease—a case series and literature review. Interdiscip Neurosurg. 2021;23:101014.
59. McMains MC, Jain N, Malik AT, Cerier E, Litsky AS, Yu E. A biomechanical analysis of lateral interbody construct and supplemental fixation in adjacent-segment disease of the lumbar spine. World Neurosurg. 2019;128:e694–9.
60. Liang Z, Cui J, Zhang J, He J, Tang J, Ren H, Ye L, Liang D, Jiang X. Biomechanical evaluation of strategies for adjacent segment disease after lateral lumbar interbody fusion: is the extension of pedicle screws necessary? BMC Musculoskelet Disord. 2020;21(1):117. https://doi.org/10.21203/rs.2.17339/v2.
61. Al-Rabiah AM, Alghafli ZI, Almazrua I. Using an extreme lateral interbody fusion (XLIF) in revising failed Transforaminal lumbar interbody fusion (TLIF) with exchange of cage. Cureus. 2021;13(3):e14123. https://doi.org/10.7759/cureus.14123.
62. Rodgers WB, Gerber EJ, Cox C. Minimally invasive treatment (XLIF) of adjacent segment disease after prior lumbar fusions. Internet J Minim Invasive Spinal Technol. 2009;3:3.
63. Aichmair A, Alimi M, Hughes AP, Sama AA, Du JY, Hartl R, Cammisa FP, Girardi FP. Single-level lateral lumbar interbody fusion for the treatment of adjacent segment disease: a retrospective two-center study. Spine J. 2014;14:S158–9.
64. Wang MY, Vasudevan R, Mindea SA. Minimally invasive lateral interbody fusion for the treatment of rostral adjacent-segment lumbar degenerative stenosis without supplemental pedicle screw fixation. J Neurosurg Spine. 2014;21:861–6.

# Chapter 28
# Understanding Spine Biologics for the Access Surgeon

Jay Shah, Naina Rao, and Rahul G. Samtani

## Introduction

Spine fusion continues to be one of the most common procedures utilized to treat various spinal pathologies, with the goal of achieving spinal stability through solid bony union [1]. Pseudarthrosis continues to be a common occurrence after spinal fusion procedures and has clearly been shown to negatively affect patient outcomes and represent a large economic burden to the healthcare system [2, 3].

In the last two decades, a variety of new biologics and bone graft substitutes have been introduced with the goal of augmenting local biology and achieving successful fusion.

To this effect, the growing demand has led to a bone graft market valuation of $2.78 billion dollars globally as of 2020 and is slated to grow exponentially. North America makes up 41% of the global market share in ancillary bone materials, with spine fusions accounting for 60% of that share [4].

Significant variability exists in bone graft material choice among spine surgeons [5]. This variability suggests the absence of a clear, evidence-based approach to informed decision-making. The spine surgeon's choice of bone graft substitute is often guided by limited evidence regarding clinical efficacy and outcomes in specific case scenarios. The choice of bone graft material in spine surgery is often influenced by factors other than level 1 clinical evidence, including preclinical data,

J. Shah
Department of Orthopedic Surgery, University of California San Francisco, San Francisco, CA, USA

N. Rao
Department of Orthopedic Surgery, NYU Langone, New York, NY, USA

R. G. Samtani (✉)
Southern California Orthopedic Institute, Bakersfield, CA, USA

© The Author(s), under exclusive license to Springer Nature Switzerland AG 2023
J. R. O'Brien et al. (eds.), *Lumbar Spine Access Surgery*,
https://doi.org/10.1007/978-3-031-48034-8_28

lower-level clinical trials, training, expert opinion, personal experience, and cost [6]. Therefore, it is critical that all surgeons involved in any procedure that has the goal of achieving a successful fusion understand the different types of bone graft and biologics, along with their risks, benefits, and evidence-based indications.

## Spinal Fusion Biology and Graft Properties

Successful spinal fusion inherently depends on a complex interplay between local and systemic factors and recapitulates the phases of fracture healing. On the microscopic level, healing occurs through the hemorrhagic, inflammatory, reparative, and remodeling phases. Fusion requires marrow access, vascularization, and migration of osteoprogenitor cells to the fusion mass. Additionally, a low strain and compressive mechanical environment is critical throughout the fusion process [1, 7]. Finally, different spinal regions have differing baseline fusion potentials due to unique environments and characteristics. Interbody fusion, utilized in anterior and lateral surgery, benefits from a large cancellous surface area with excellent vascular supply in a naturally compressive environment. On the other hand, posterolateral fusion at the intertransverse junction is naturally more difficult due to a smaller surface area, gapping between bony levels, and tensile or distractive forces [8].

The function of bone grafting and biologics is similar to that of native cancellous bone. The goal is to provide bone, blood cells, and proteins with a structural support matrix. For a graft to be clinically useful, it must have at least one of the three capabilities that native cancellous bone possesses—osteoconduction, osteoinduction, or osteogenesis. It is important to note that biologics can possess different combinations of these three qualities (Fig. 28.1) [9].

Osteoconductive materials provide a structural framework into which bone can grow. The role of an osteoconductive material is to act as a nonviable scaffold that supports and permits bony ingrowth, healing, and neovascularization. Purely osteoconductive materials, sometimes referred to as "passive" bone grafts, do not formally contain cells nor growth factors needed to induce bone formation and fusion. Materials with osteoconductive potential include autologous bone, allograft bone, bone matrix, collagen, and ceramics.

Osteoinductive materials contain growth factors that stimulate bone formation and proteins that induce cell differentiation toward bone. Mineralized graft has minimal osteoinductivity and is demineralized to promote osteoinductive potential. Other osteoinductive materials include bone morphogenetic proteins, several bone-promoting cytokines, and autologous/allograft bone.

Osteogenic materials directly provide any of the critical cells involved in the bone-forming and healing processes. These cells include osteoblasts, osteocytes, and mesenchymal stem cells, and for a material to be osteogenic, it must contain these cells directly. The potential to produce bone is a characteristic of autologous bone and marrow cells [1, 6, 7].

**TABLE 1. Spinal Bone Graft Properties**

| Material | Osteoconductive | Osteoinductive | Osteogenic | Comments |
|---|---|---|---|---|
| Autograft | X | X | X | ie, iliac crest bone graft (ICGB), local autograft from same incision |
| Allograft (mineralized-fresh frozen or freeze-dried) | X | Variable | Variable, but limited | Extender |
| Allograft (processed-fresh frozen or lyophilization) | X | Variable, but limited | | Osteoinductivity varies depending on mode of preparation and sterilization<br>Osteogenic capacity eliminated due to removal of osteogenic cells<br>Extender |
| Demineralized bone matrix (DBM) | X | Variable | | Contains variable amounts of osteoinductive proteins depending on manufacturer; least immunogenic of allografts<br>Extender; possible enhancer |
| Synthetic ceramics | X | | | ie, calcium salts, tri-calcium phosphate, coralline, hydroxyapatite<br>Extender |
| Composite grafts | X | Variable | | ie, hydroxyapatite/tri-calcium phosphate composite<br>May combine DBM, growth factors, or ions (eg silicate, magnesium) to enhance osteoinductivity<br>Extender; possible enhancer |
| rh-BMP-2 | X | X | | Enhancer |
| rh-BMP-7 | X | X | | Enhancer |
| Autologous mesenchymal stem cells | | X | X | ie, bone marrow aspirate (BMA) (via pedicle or iliac crest)<br>Enhancer |
| Autologous growth factor concentrate | | | X | Ultraconcentration of platelets |
| Allogenic mesenchymal stem cell products | | | X | Wide variation in regard to age at harvest, total cellular concentration, percentage of MSC, shelf life, and viability after defrosting |

**Fig. 28.1** Spinal bone graft properties. A comparison of the ostoconductive, osteoinduction, and osteogenic properties of biologics and grafts. *MSC* mesenchymal stem cells, *rh-BMP* recombinant human bone morphogenic protein

Graft materials are often described in relation to autograft as extenders, enhancers, or substitutes. Bone graft extenders are adjuvant materials that allow the use of less autologous bone graft with comparable results. Bone graft enhancers are supplemental materials combined with autograft that increase successful fusion compared to autograft alone. Bone graft substitutes are materials that can replace autologous bone in its entirety [10]. The rest of this chapter will discuss the different types of bone graft and biologics currently being considered and utilized in spine fusion.

# Autograft

Autograft is the gold standard for grafting material in spinal fusion procedures. It is the only current graft material that has osteogenic, osteoinductive, and osteoconductive properties. Moreover, it is histocompatible and poses no risk of disease transmission or immune rejection. Two major drawbacks of autograft include potential lack of volume available within the local surgical field and donor site morbidity when harvested from a separate site. In anterior or lateral surgery, local bone is usually sparsely available compared to posterior surgery and may require a separate, possibly painful, harvest site [11, 12].

Autograft can be cancellous, cortical, or corticocancellous. Cancellous bone graft provides less structural support but possesses more osteoinductive and osteogenic properties due to increased cellularity. Cortical grafts provide more structure than cancellous bone grafts and are more useful when immediate structural integrity is needed. Corticocancellous bone provides structure while maintaining its osteoinductive, osteoconductive, and osteogenic properties [13].

Iliac crest bone graft is an example of corticocancellous autograft and has well-documented high fusion rates [14]. Additionally, a large amount of graft material can be obtained from the iliac crest. However, potential complications include increased blood loss, increased surgical time, longer length of stay, chronic postoperative donor site pain, infection, hematoma, and neurovascular injury [15, 16]. While the true clinical significance and incidence of these complications are unknown, their presence has led to the development of many alternatives.

Cortical autograft can be harvested from the spinous processes, laminae, and facets during posterior spinal decompression. Cortical graft has the benefit of containing improved structural properties compared to corticocancellous or purely cancellous grafts but lacks the porosity to promote significant vascular ingrowth and progenitor cell migration. This naturally leads to poorer osteoinductive and osteogenic properties. Local autograft has the added benefit of no donor site morbidity or complications, but it is locally volume-dependent which limits its use in isolation for multilevel fusions [17].

Bone marrow aspirate (BMA) is an osteogenic and osteoinductive autologous graft commonly harvested from the iliac crest or other sites including the vertebral body. BMA possesses autologous stem cells that contain osteogenic and osteoinductive properties but no structural or osteoconductive components. As such, BMA is often combined with allograft or synthetics with structural properties. It can also be concentrated via centrifuge to achieve a higher number of cells and is then termed bone marrow concentrate [18, 19]. The ideal harvest location, preparation method, delivery mechanism, and concentration are still debated. However, studies have clearly demonstrated that combining BMA with other autografts or biologics can lead to excellent fusion rates [20].

## Allograft

Allograft is the most common bone graft alternative, and it is readily available from cadaveric bone. It comes in fresh, frozen, and freeze-dried varieties which possess differing degrees of immunogenicity and shelf-life stability. These materials are generally osteoconductive and can be weakly osteoinductive depending on processing technique but contain no osteogenic capabilities as no viable cells remain. Fresh allograft is generally not used due to immunogenicity and risk of disease transmission. On the other hand, fresh frozen allograft is significantly less immunogenic and must be stored at around −70° Celsius. Freeze-dried allograft is dehydrated during processing and subsequently sterilized. Processing results in the lowest immunogenicity but decreases mechanical strength by 50%. Freeze-dried allograft can be stored at room temperature and can be cortical, corticocancellous, or cancellous [21].

The main advantages of allograft are its availability, lack of morbidity associated with an autograft harvest site, and safety due to modern processing techniques. It has been shown to be similarly efficacious to iliac crest autograft in anterior cervical and lumbar interbody fusions, where it can be used as a stand-alone option. However, it is limited in its ability to act as an autograft substitute in posterolateral fusions, where the biological environment is naturally less amenable to fusion, and therefore should be used as an extender in these situations [22, 23].

## Demineralized Bone Matrix

Demineralized bone matrix (DBM) is an allograft produced using cortical bone acid decalcification. This process removes the mineralized portion of bone and reduces its immunogenicity. The subsequent product contains collagens, growth factors, and non-collagenous proteins. The demineralization process allows the osteoinductive growth factors to be more readily accessible while maintaining some osteoconductivity. The main drawback of DBM is the low absolute amount of available osteoinductive growth factors [24]. Therefore, DBM is often noted to have "osteoinductive potential" but usually not said to be "osteoinductive." Furthermore, the processing technique reduces its mechanical properties, limiting its ability to function as an autograft substitute. As such, it is commonly used as a bone graft extender for autografts, especially in posterolateral fusion [25].

## Bone Morphogenic Protein

In 1965, Marshall Urist identified that the bone matrix itself contains proteins capable of directly inducing bone formation. He dedicated most of his career to identifying and characterizing these proteins, which he later called bone morphogenetic protein (BMP) which are derived from the transforming growth factor family [26]. While there are 20 known types of BMPs, BMP-2 and BMP-7 have been found to be the most osteoinductive. While these proteins were initially harvested from large amounts of bone, advances in genetic technology have made it possible to synthetically engineer them, leading to more widespread use. The most studied, popular, and clinically useful of these is recombinant human bone morphogenetic protein-2 (rhBMP-2). It acts through increased expression of genes that leads to osteoprogenitor differentiation and de novo bone formation, making it powerfully osteoinductive [27]. It currently represents one of the most successful and widely used biologics in spine fusion.

While it is only US Food and Drug Association (FDA)-approved for anterior lumbar interbody fusion, the efficacy of rhBMP-2 has been extensively studied throughout the entire spectrum of spine fusion procedures and locations. Early studies demonstrated rhBMP-2 to have superior fusion rates and outcome measures regarding operative time, blood loss, length of stay, reoperation rate, and return to work when compared to autologous iliac crest bone graft in lumbar interbody fusion [28]. This was the first biologic of its kind to show superiority to autologous iliac crest graft, leading to its widespread adoption as a bone graft substitute as opposed to just an enhancer or extender. In just 10 years, the use of BMP exponentially increased from around 1000 cases to almost 80,000 in the early 2000s [29]. However, adverse effects, including radiculitis, wound complications, osteolysis, malignancy, and heterotopic ossification, were noted, especially in posterior lumbar fusions. Retrograde ejaculation, infection, urogenital events, and implant failure were associated with BMP use in anterior lumbar interbody fusions. BMP was also associated with seroma formation and subsequent life-threatening airway compromise in the cervical spine, leading to an FDA black box warning [30, 31]. These complications are attributed to the potent osteoinductive effects of rhBMP-2, which leads to significant local inflammation, activation of osteoclasts, and bone formation. Overall complication rates were noted to have an incidence of 10–50% depending on the procedure [30].

This controversy led to an independent review of the original industry-sponsored data and a push for more studies to provide evidence-based guidelines for the use of rhBMP-2 in spine fusion. The result of several recent studies and meta-analysis has had mixed results, but overall suggest that the actual complication rates are most likely significantly lower and failed to find an association with new cancer formation [31–33]. Further studies have also substantiated that rhBMP-2 is at least equivalent, if not superior, to the gold standard of autologous iliac crest graft in terms of fusion rates throughout the spine. This includes anterior lumbar interbody fusion, transforaminal lumbar interbody fusion, and posterior lumbar fusion [34–36].

Finally, patient-specific variables such as smoking, revision surgery, and poor bone quality all play a role in the risk benefit analysis of rhBMP-2 use [37]. Randomized controlled trials will play a significant role in the future of rhBMP-2 use and help clarify its true complication profile. Overall, it appears to be a powerful biologic substitute and tool in preventing pseudarthrosis of the spine but has limitations including possible adverse effects and high cost.

## Synthetic Bone Substitutes (Ceramics)

Synthetic bone substitutes are materials that mimic the inorganic phase of bone. They were originally discovered when invertebrate corals were determined to share a similar microscopic porous structure to bone, and thus they were also named ceramics. Hydroxyapatite, tricalcium phosphate, calcium sulfate, calcium carbonate, and natural coral are common ceramics. As they mimic the inorganic phase of bone, these products have no natural osteogenic or osteoinductive properties and are only used as osteoconductive agents. These products are readily available and biocompatible, create no donor site morbidity, and have virtually no risk of disease transmission. However, they are brittle and unable to withstand significant forces before fracturing and require rigid instrumentation to protect their viability. Since these products do not have osteoinductive or osteogenic properties, they best function as bone graft extenders and as carriers for other graft material [38]. They should be used like other osteoconductive bone grafts, in combination with other osteoinductive/osteogenic biologics, and placed directly on well-decorticated local host bone to maximize their osteoconductive potential [39].

## Recent Developments

Biologics and bone graft being studied include autologous and allogenic stem cells, gene therapies, and biomaterial scaffolds. With appropriate genetic engineering, mesenchymal and adipose-derived stem cells can become potently osteogenic and osteoinductive. In some ways, this is similar to BMA, but at much larger concentrations, making them potentially more effective. However, ethical and social limitations have impeded human trials. The efficacy of these stem cells in promoting spine fusion in animal models has surpassed any other potential biologic to date [40].

Allogenic cellular bone matrices are another interesting area of study. They are allogenic bone combined with allogenic stem cells, and while there are several products currently available, they have significant variability in cell concentration and shelf life. Furthermore, most studies are either animal-based or industry-sponsored, making it difficult to truly assess their viability in spine fusion [41].

Gene therapy, which uses nonviral or viral deoxyribonucleic acid to induce osteogenic differentiation and promote fusion by delivering and expressing specific genes, is also being studied. Animal models have demonstrated successful and rapid spinal fusion rates. However, concerns over systemic viral or bacterial toxicity and transmission, as well as ethical considerations, have stalled human research [42].

Finally, biomaterial scaffolds are created from ceramics and newer polypeptide-based compounds. P-15 is a polypeptide which imitates the cell-binding domain of type 1 collagen on inorganic bone [43]. These scaffolds can be engineered in different sizes and shapes. Novel studies have suggested that altering the microscopic and even nanoscopic structural, physiological, and chemical properties could potentially impart osteoinductive properties to these grafts [44]. Both ceramics and P-15 are also being studied as potential growth factor carriers. The theoretical goal is that these scaffolds will allow for time-dependent growth factor release, thereby decreasing complication rates by reducing the therapeutic dose necessary for successful fusion [45].

## Conclusion

Spinal fusion remains one of the most common techniques to treat spinal pathology, and numerous biological augmentations and grafting choices are available to improve fusion rates and prevent pseudarthrosis. Autologous graft is the gold standard as it provides excellent enhancement of the existing biological environment through its osteoconductive, osteoinductive, and osteogenic properties. However, the volume of local autograft available is not always adequate, and donor site morbidity continues to be a concerning obstacle. Allograft has the advantage of being ubiquitously available and cost-effective while avoiding a second procedure sometimes required for autograft harvest. However, it lacks the powerful osteogenic properties of other biologics and is only weakly osteoinductive. DBM is an allograft-derived tissue that is processed to have the potential to be increasingly osteoinductive, though at a variable rate. This comes at the cost of structural integrity, requiring it to be supplemented with more structural grafts and/or protected with rigid fixation. rhBMP-2 is derived from the transforming growth factor family and is both osteoinductive and osteogenic, acting through increased expression of genes that lead to osteoprogenitor differentiation. It represents one of the most successful and widely used biologics in spine fusion, although its risk profile has been a concern, especially in the cervical spine. Ceramics and newer polypeptide-based compounds are synthetic biomaterial scaffolds and utilize osteoconductive materials that offer more diverse properties and pose low to no risk of antibody formation. Finally, autologous and allogenic stem cells are pluripotent cells which can be isolated from bone marrow or adipose tissue and, with appropriate development, are osteogenic and can differentiate into osteoprogenitor cells, but limited human studies currently exist. In the future, technological advances aimed at maximizing the osteogenic properties of biologics and graft materials and minimizing their cost and risk profiles may improve spinal fusion rates and lower overall morbidity and healthcare expenditures.

## References


1. Boden SD. Overview of the biology of lumbar spine fusion and principles for selecting a bone graft substitute. Spine (Phila Pa 1976). 1976;2002(27):S26–31. [PMID: 12205416].
2. Klineberg E, Gupta M, McCarthy I, Hostin R. Detection of pseudarthrosis in adult spinal deformity: the use of health-related quality-of-life outcomes to predict pseudarthrosis. Clin Spine Surg. 2016;29(8):318–22.
3. Jain A, Yeramaneni S, Kebaish KM, Raad M, Gum JL, Klineberg EO, Hassanzadeh H, Kelly MP, Passias PG, Ames CP, Smith JS, Shaffrey CI, Bess S, Lafage V, Glassman S, Carreon LY, Hostin RA, International Spine Study Group. Cost-utility analysis of rhBMP-2 use in adult spinal deformity surgery. Spine (Phila Pa 1976). 2020;45(14):1009–15. https://doi.org/10.1097/BRS.0000000000003442. PMID: 32097274.
4. 2016. https://www.grandviewresearch.com/industry-analysis/orthopedic-implants-market. Accessed 10 Oct 2020.

5. Rihn JA, Kirkpatrick K, Albert TJ. Graft options in posterolateral and posterior interbody lumbar fusion. Spine (Phila Pa 1976). 2010;35(17):1629–39.

6. Grabowski G, Cornett CA. Bone graft and bone graft substitutes in spine surgery: current concepts and controversies. J Am Acad Orthop Surg. 2013;21(1):51–60.

7. Boden SD, Schimandle JH, Hutton WC, Chen MI. Volvo award in basic sciences. The use of an osteoinductive growth factor for lumbar spinal fusion. Part I: biology of spinal fusion. Spine. 1995;20(24):2626–32.

8. Boden SD, Sumner DR. Biologic issues in lumbar spinal fusion introduction. Spine. 1995;20(24 suppl):102S–12S.

9. Gupta A, Kukkar N, Sharif K, Main BJ, Albers CE, El-Amin Iii SF. Bone graft substitutes for spine fusion: a brief review. World J Orthop. 2015;6(6):449–56.

10. Abdullah KG, Steinmetz MP, Benzel EC, Mroz TE. The state of lumbar fusion extenders. Spine (Phila Pa 1976). 2011;36(20):E1328–34.

11. Sandhu HS, Grewal HS, Parvataneni H. Bone grafting for spinal fusion. Orthop Clin North Am. 1999;30(4):685–98.

12. Khan WS, Rayan F, Dhinsa BS, Marsh D. An osteoconductive, osteoinductive, and osteogenic tissue-engineered product for trauma and orthopaedic surgery: how far are we? Stem Cells Int. 2012;2012:236231.

13. Tarpada SP, Morris MT, Burton DA. Spinal fusion surgery: a historical perspective. J Orthop. 2017;14(1):134–6.

14. Zdeblick TA. A prospective, randomized study of lumbar fusion. Preliminary results. Spine (Phila Pa 1976). 1993;18:983–91. https://doi.org/10.1097/00007632-199306150-00006.

15. Cockin J. Autologous bone grafting: complications at the donor site. J Bone Joint Surg. 1971;53:153.

16. Dimitriou R, Mataliotakis GI, Angoules AG, Kanakaris NK, Giannoudis PV. Complications following autologous bone graft harvesting from the iliac crest and using the RIA: a systematic review. Injury. 2011;42(Suppl 2):S3–15. https://doi.org/10.1016/j.injury.2011.06.015. Epub 2011 Jun 25. PMID: 21704997.

17. Ohtori S, Koshi T, Suzuki M, et al. Uni- and bilateral instrumented posterolateral fusion of the lumbar spine with local bone grafting: a prospective study with a 2-year follow-up. Spine (Phila Pa 1976). 2011;36(26):E1744–8.

18. Hernigou P, Desroches A, Queinnec S, et al. Morbidity of graft harvesting versus bone marrow aspiration in cell regenerative therapy. Int Orthop. 2014;38(9):1855–60.

19. Salama R, Burwell RD, Dickson IR. Recombined grafts of bone and marrow. The beneficial effect upon osteogenesis of impregnating xenograft (heterograft) bone with autologous red marrow. J Bone Joint Surg Br. 1973;55(2):402–17.

20. Morris MT, Tarpada SP, Cho W. Bone graft materials for posterolateral fusion made simple: a systematic review. Eur Spine J. 2018;27:1856–67. https://doi.org/10.1007/s00586-018-5511-6.

21. Blanco JS, Sears CJ. Allograft bone use during instrumentation and fusion in the treatment of adolescent idiopathic scoliosis. Spine. 1997;22(12):1338–42.

22. Ehrler DM, Vaccaro AR. The use of allograft bone in lumbar spine surgery. Clin Orthop Relat Res. 2000;371(38–45):29.

23. Vaccaro AR, Chiba K, Heller JG, et al. Bone grafting alternatives in spinal surgery. Spine J. 2002;2(3):206–15.

24. Bae H, Zhao L, Zhu D, Kanim LE, Wang JC, Delamarter RB. Variability across ten production lots of a single demineralized bone matrix product. J Bone Joint Surg Am. 2010;92(2):427–35.

25. Buser Z, Brodke DS, Youssef JA, et al. Allograft versus demineralized bone matrix in instrumented and noninstrumented lumbar fusion: a systematic review. Global Spine J. 2018;8(4):396–412.

26. Urist MR. Bone: formation by autoinduction. Science. 1965;150:893.

27. Bragdon B, Moseychuk O, Saldanha S, King D, Julian J, Nohe A. Bone morphogenetic proteins: a critical review. Cell Signal. 2011;23:609.

28. Burkus JK, Transfeldt EE, Kitchel SH, et al. Clinical and radiographic outcomes of anterior lumbar interbody fusion using recombinant human bone morphogenetic protein-2. Spine (Phila Pa 1976). 2002;27:2396–408.
29. Cahill KS, Chi JH, Day A, Claus EB. Prevalence, complications, and hospital charges associated with use of bone-morphogenetic proteins in spinal fusion procedures. J Am Med Assoc. 2009;302(1):58–66.
30. Carragee EJ, Hurwitz EL, Weiner BK. A critical review of recombinant human bone morphogenetic protein-2 trials in spinal surgery: emerging safety concerns and lessons learned. Spine J. 2011;11(6):471–91.
31. Center for Devices and Radiological Health. Public Health Notifications (Medical Devices)—FDA Public Health Notification: Life-threatening complications associated with recombinant human bone morphogenetic protein in cervical spine fusion. 2008. Accessed 10 Oct 2022.
32. Fu R, Selph S, McDonagh M, et al. Effectiveness and harms of recombinant human bone morphogenetic protein-2 in spine fusion: a systematic review and meta-analysis. Ann Intern Med. 2013;158(12):890–902.
33. Simmonds MC, Brown JVE, Heirs MK, et al. Safety and effectiveness of recombinant human bone morphogenetic protein-2 for spinal fusion: a meta-analysis of individual-participant data. Ann Intern Med. 2013;158(12):877–89.
34. Galimberti F, Lubelski D, Healy AT, et al. A systematic review of lumbar fusion rates with and without the use of rhBMP-2. Spine. 2015;40(14):1132–9.
35. Zhang H, Wang F, Ding L, et al. A meta analysis of lumbar spinal fusion surgery using bone morphogenetic proteins and autologous iliac crest bone graft. PLoS One. 2014;9(6):e97049.
36. Crandall DG, Revella J, Patterson J, Huish E, Chang M, McLemore R. Transforaminal lumbar interbody fusion with rhBMP-2 in spinal deformity, spondylolisthesis, and degenerative disease—part 2: BMP dosage-related complications and long-term outcomes in 509 patients. Spine. 2013;38(13):1137–45.
37. Laurie AL, Chen Y, Chou R, Fu R. Meta-analysis of the impact of patient characteristics on estimates of effectiveness and harms of recombinant human bone morphogenetic protein-2 in lumbar spinal fusion. Spine (Phila Pa 1976). 2016;41(18):E1115–23.
38. Nickoli MS, Hsu WK. Ceramic-based bone grafts as a bone grafts extender for lumbar spine arthrodesis: a systematic review. Global Spine J. 2014;4(3):211–6.
39. Delécrin J, Deschamps C, Romih M, Heymann D, Passuti N. Influence of bone environment on ceramic osteointegration in spinal fusion: comparison of bone-poor and bone-rich sites. Eur Spine J. 2001;10(suppl 2):S110–3.
40. Schroeder J. Stem cells for spine surgery. World J Stem Cells. 2015;7(1):186.
41. Skovrlj B, Guzman JZ, Al Maaieh M, Cho SK, Iatridis JC, Qureshi SA. Cellular bone matrices: viable stem cell-containing bone graft substitutes. Spine J. 2014;14(11):2763–72.
42. Wegman F, Bijenhof A, Schuijff L, Oner FC, Dhert WJ, Alblas J. Osteogenic differentiation as a result of BMP-2 plasmid DNA based gene therapy in vitro and in vivo. Eur Cell Mater. 2011;21:230–42. discussion 42.
43. Jacobsen MK, Andresen AK, Jespersen AB, et al. Randomized double blind clinical trial of ABM/P-15 versus allograft in noninstrumented lumbar fusion surgery. Spine J. 2020;20(5):677–84.
44. Chai YC, Carlier A, Bolander J, et al. Current views on calcium phosphate osteogenicity and the translation into effective bone regeneration strategies. Acta Biomater. 2012;8(11):3876–87.
45. Lee SS, Hsu EL, Mendoza M, et al. Gel scaffolds of BMP-2-binding peptide amphiphile nanofibers for spinal arthrodesis. Adv Healthc Mater. 2015;4(1):131–41.

# Chapter 29
# Lumbar Access Surgery Performed by a Spine Surgeon

Jeffrey B. Weinreb and Joseph R. O'Brien

## Introduction

The anterior approach to the lumbar spine was developed in the 1930s in the treatment of Pott disease and is now a commonly utilized exposure in spine surgery, especially for anterior lumbar interbody fusion (ALIF) [1, 2]. The anterior approach to the lumbar spine is commonly organized into either an extraperitoneal or a transperitoneal approach, and the extraperitoneal approach can be subdivided into paramedian and anterolateral access [3]. Complications from the anterior approach differ from those of either a standard posterior or a lateral approach, but in general it is accepted as a safe and effective method to access the anterior lumbar spine [3]. Broadly, complications associated with the anterior approach relate either to the proximity to the anterior vasculature such as the iliac vessels or to postoperative ileus from bowel mobilization, while complications associated with the posterior approach relate to dural or neural element injury [4]. The risk of infection between the two approaches has not been well established [4]. Experience with the anterior approach during orthopedic or neurosurgical training varies widely depending on when and where training occurred [1]. In current practice, many spine surgeons elect to utilize the services of a general or vascular "access" surgeon to perform the approach [5]. The assistance of an access surgeon is utilized due to the concern that the anterior approach risks injury to intraperitoneal or retroperitoneal structures that may need to be repaired on short notice by a general, urological, or vascular surgeon [5]. There is evidence that there is an acceptable complication rate when a spine

J. B. Weinreb (✉)
Department of Orthopedic Surgery, The George Washington University, Washington, DC, USA

J. R. O'Brien
Aligned Orthopaedics, Bethesda, MD, USA
e-mail: JOBrien@alignedortho.com

© The Author(s), under exclusive license to Springer Nature Switzerland AG 2023
J. R. O'Brien et al. (eds.), *Lumbar Spine Access Surgery*,
https://doi.org/10.1007/978-3-031-48034-8_29

surgeon performs the approach alone [6]. The purpose of this chapter is to provide an overview of the anterior approach and potential complications, with specific attention paid to whether the approach is performed by a spine surgeon or access surgeon, and trends in experience with this approach during residency.


# Results


Multiple studies have evaluated complication rates between approaches performed by a spine surgeon or an access surgeon. Jarrett et al. retrospectively reviewed 296 consecutive patients who underwent an anterior approach to the lumbar spine between 2003 and 2005, with 265 patients ultimately included in the study [5]. The spine surgeon performed the approach for 24% of patients, and a vascular surgeon performed the approach in 76% of cases. A total of 8% and 12% of patients experienced at least one intraoperative complication in the spine and vascular surgeon groups, respectively. A similar rate of complications occurred when cases were stratified by a number of surgical levels. The authors attributed the overall higher rate of vascular complications in the vascular surgery cases to the increased level of complexity of cases for which an access surgeon was recruited [5].

In a retrospective study by Smith et al., 96 consecutive patients who underwent anterior lumbar spine surgery from L3 and caudal between 1995 and 2008 were reviewed [3]. The first 56 patients underwent exposure performed by a general surgeon, and the remainder underwent exposure by two fellowship-trained spine surgeons [3]. Of note, one patient from the second cohort had exposure completed by a general surgeon due to multiple previous abdominal surgeries. In this study, when the operation was performed by a spine surgeon alone, there was significantly lower estimated blood loss (EBL), operative time, and length of stay compared to when exposure was performed by an access surgeon [3]. The estimated blood loss was 204 mL, operative time was 2.8 h, and length of stay was 3.5 days, when the spine surgeon performed the exposure compared to 420 mL, 3.93 h, and 4.7 days for exposure with an access surgeon, respectively ($p < 0.01$ for all parameters) [3].

In a series of 450 patients who underwent anterior spinal fusion between T1 and S1 from 1985 to 1997 by an orthopedic spine surgeon, Holt et al. examined factors including surgical length, complications, and EBL [6]. These authors separated surgeries into anterior-only and anterior plus posterior procedures and found that the operative time for the anterior-only procedures and anterior/posterior procedures was an average of 99.3 min (range 60–370 min) and 247.5 min (range 120–240 min), respectively. Average EBL for anterior-only procedures was 385 mL (50–2700 mL), and the mean EBL for combined anterior and posterior procedures was 880.30 mL (200–3000 mL) [6]. Fifty (11.11%) patients had surgical complications, including superficial wound infection (1.5%), incisional hernia (1.5%), venous injury (1.5%), peritoneal injury (1.5%), and ileus (0.2%) [6]. Although there was no direct comparison to access surgeon results, the authors suggested their operative metrics were similar to those found in the literature and their complication rates were lower than those reported in the literature [6].

In another study that examined only cases performed by a spinal surgeon, Quraishi et al. reported a series of 304 consecutive patients who underwent anterior lumbar spine surgery between L2 and S1 from 2000 to 2010 [7]. All patients underwent a paramedian incision with retroperitoneal dissection, and these authors defined a major vascular injury as any bleeding where a suture repair or vascular reconstruction was required [7]. In this series, the authors report a 20% complication rate including a 6.2% major vascular complication rate comprised of 4.6% venous injuries and 1.6% arterial injuries. Minor complications included a 4.3% infection rate and a 1.6% venous injury rate requiring only hemostatic agents or pressure [7]. Of note, a vascular surgeon was on standby at all times in the hospital and was required for assistance with a vascular injury 3% of the time, indicating the spinal surgeon was able to manage the vascular injury in 71% of cases [7].

A large meta-analysis on ALIF with and without an access surgeon was conducted by Phan et al. in 2017 [8]. In total, 58 studies were included with a total of 8028 individual patients with 4382 utilizing an access surgeon and 3645 without an access surgeon [8]. This study demonstrated higher rates of certain complications when an access surgeon was utilized, including arterial injuries (1.16% vs. 0.44%, $p < 0.001$), retrograde ejaculation (0.96% vs. 0.41%, $p = 0.005$), and ileus (2.26% vs. 1.93%, p < 0.001), and certain complication rates were increased with no access surgeon, including total postoperative complications (5.95% vs. 4.08%, $p < 0.001$), prosthesis complications (1.59% vs. 0.89%, $p < 0.001$), reoperation rates (2.28% vs. 1.31%, $p < 0.001$), peritoneal injury (0.44% vs. 0.16%, $p = 0.034$), and neurological injury (0.99% vs. 0.11%, $p < 0.001$) [8].

## Discussion

The anterior approach to the lumbar spine is utilized to potentially reduce operative time, restore disc height for indirect decompression and sagittal deformity correction, reduce blood loss, reduce infection, and improve fusion rates [9–12]. In addition, the overall rate of the anterior approach for ALIF is increasing and was shown to increase by about 24% per year from 3650 to 6151 between 2007 and 2014 in one study utilizing the MarketScan database [13]. Though this approach may have specific benefits, it also has unique risks including large vessel injury, postoperative ileus, peritoneal injury, abdominal hernia, hypogastric sympathetic injury leading to retrograde ejaculation, or sympathectomy leading to limb thermoregulation issues or edema [12]. In the current medicolegal environment, some authors have advocated the utilization of an access surgeon to assist in all anterior lumbar surgery cases [1, 14]. Despite the common practice of utilizing an access surgeon, no reliable reduction in complications has been shown to be associated with this practice, and in many cases, a higher rate of certain complications is associated with access surgeon assistance in exposure [7, 8, 12]. Counterintuitively, multiple studies have demonstrated a higher rate of vascular complications when exposure was performed by an access surgeon [5, 7, 10, 15]. However, the significantly higher rates of certain complications with access surgeons may be related to the tendency to involve a vascular or general surgeon in more complex cases including those with prior abdominal surgery or multiple operative levels [10]. Other complex cases including those involving abnormal anatomy from a pelvic kidney, kidney transplant, or inverted vascular anatomy may also benefit from the assistance of an approach surgeon [10].

Though not well reported in the literature, the timing and geographic location of training may also affect a surgeon's ability to safely perform the anterior approach to the lumbar spine. Neurosurgical spine training in the United Kingdom has virtually no exposure to vascular surgery [1]. In the United States, orthopedic surgery training requirements have changed substantially over time [16, 17]. Prior to 1957, the American Board of Orthopaedic Surgery (ABOS) accepted preceptorship training including 1 year of internship, 1 year of surgery, and 5 years of full-time assistantship to a board-certified orthopedic surgeon and then 5 years of practice at an approved hospital [16]. Until 1958, the ABOS required a full year of general surgery training [16]. This was then updated to *recommending* a full year of general surgery training in 1964 [16]. Prior to July 1, 2013, the ABOS required 9 months of non-orthopedic training during the first postgraduate year (intern year) [17]. This was changed to 6 months after July 1, 2013 [17]. This is similar to neurosurgical training requirements, which as of July 1, 2019, required "a minimum of six months of structured education in general patient care (e.g., trauma, general surgery, neurosurgery, orthopedic surgery, otolaryngology, or plastic surgery)" [18]. Though the effects of these changes on the overall quality of spine surgery training are beyond the scope of this chapter, these changes appear to have decreased the exposure to non-orthopedic specialties during orthopedic training over time, potentially leading to a younger generation of orthopedic-trained spine surgeons with less exposure to the anterior lumbar approach than their predecessors [16, 17].

## Conclusion

Numerous studies have compared complication rates with and without assistance from an access surgeon when approaching the lumbar spine, but no dramatic differences in complications have been reliably reproduced. Some complications may even be increased with the assistance of an approach surgeon, though current studies often do not account for the increased difficulty of cases when assistance is utilized. The current literature suggests that, with proper training and comfort, a spine surgeon can safely and effectively perform the anterior approach to the lumbar spine, though current patterns in training suggest that more recently trained spine surgeons have less exposure to this approach during training than their predecessors. The decision to perform this approach must be weighed in the context of individual training, access to a vascular surgeon in the event of a serious complication out of the scope of the spine surgeon's training, and the medicolegal environment in which they practice and on a case-by-case basis, as always with a focus on achieving the safest and best results for the patient.

# References


1. Asha MJ, Choksey MS, Shad A, Roberts P, Imray C. The role of the vascular surgeon in anterior lumbar spine surgery. Br J Neurosurg. 2012;26(4):499–503.
2. Ito H, Tsuchiya J, Asami G. A new radical operation for Pott's disease. J Bone Jt Surg. 1934;16(3):499–515. https://journals.lww.com/jbjsjournal/Abstract/1934/16030/THE_TREATMENT_OF_LEGG_CALV__PERTHES_DISEASE.2.aspx. Accessed 28 July 2021.
3. Smith MW, Rahn KA, Shugart RM, Belschner CD, Stout KS, Cheng I. Comparison of perioperative parameters and complications observed in the anterior exposure of the lumbar spine by a spine surgeon with and without the assistance of an access surgeon. Spine J. 2011;11(5):389–94.
4. Scaduto AA, Gamradt SC, Yu WD, Huang J, Delamarter RB, Wang JC. Perioperative complications of threaded cylindrical lumbar interbody fusion devices: anterior versus posterior approach. J Spinal Disord Tech. 2003;16(6):502–7. https://doi.org/10.1097/00024720-200312000-00003.
5. Jarrett CD, Heller JG, Tsai L. Anterior exposure of the lumbar spine with and without an "access surgeon": morbidity analysis of 265 consecutive cases. J Spinal Disord Tech. 2009;22(8):559–64. https://doi.org/10.1097/BSD.0b013e318192e326.
6. Holt RT, Majd ME, Vadhva M, Castro FP. The efficacy of anterior spine exposure by an orthopedic surgeon. J Spinal Disord Tech. 2003;16(5):477–86. https://doi.org/10.1097/00024720-200310000-00007.
7. Quraishi NA, Konig M, Booker SJ, et al. Access related complications in anterior lumbar surgery performed by spinal surgeons. Eur Spine J. 2013;22(1):16–20.
8. Phan K, Xu J, Scherman DB, Rao PJ, Mobbs RJ. Anterior lumbar interbody fusion with and without an "access surgeon": a systematic review and meta-analysis. Spine. 2017;42(10):E592–601.
9. Manzur M, Virk SS, Jivanelli B, et al. The rate of fusion for stand-alone anterior lumbar interbody fusion: a systematic review. Spine J. 2019;19(7):1294–301.
10. Phan K, Thayaparan GK, Mobbs RJ. Anterior lumbar interbody fusion versus transforaminal lumbar interbody fusion–systematic review and meta-analysis. Br J Neurosurg. 2015;29(5):705–11.
11. Pradhan BB, Nassar JA, Delamarter RB, Wang JC. Single-level lumbar spine fusion: a comparison of anterior and posterior approaches. Clin Spine Surg. 2002;15(5):355–61.
12. Mobbs RJ, Phan K, Daly D, Rao PJ, Lennox A. Approach-related complications of anterior lumbar interbody fusion: results of a combined spine and vascular surgical team. Glob Spine J. 2016;6(2):147–54.
13. Varshneya K, Medress ZA, Jensen M, et al. Trends in anterior lumbar interbody fusion in the United States: a MarketScan study from 2007 to 2014. Clin Spine Surg. 2020;33(5):E226–30.
14. Ikard RW. Methods and complications of anterior exposure of the thoracic and lumbar spine. Arch Surg. 2006;141(10):1025–34.
15. Brau SA, Delamarter RB, Schiffman ML, Williams LA, Watkins RG. Vascular injury during anterior lumbar surgery. Spine J. 2004;4(4):409–12.
16. Kettelkamp DB. The evolving structure of orthopaedic residency education. Clin Orthop Relat Res. 2006;449:16–9.
17. Dougherty PJ, Marcus RE. ACGME and ABOS changes for the orthopaedic surgery PGY-1 (intern) year. Clin Orthop Relat Res. 2013;471(11):3412–6.
18. The American Board of Neurological Surgery. Training Requirements abnsorg Published. 2021. www.abns.org/training-requirements/.

# Chapter 30
# Prone Lateral Interbody Fusion

Leland C. McCluskey Jr and Mathew Cyriac

## Introduction

Lateral interbody fusion techniques have gained popularity since their inception, becoming more widely accepted as a safe alternative to posterior or anterior approaches [1, 2]. The advantages of the lateral interbody fusion technique are beyond the scope of this chapter and will be discussed elsewhere in the textbook. In the traditional standard lateral (SL) technique, the interbody fusion is generally supplemented with placement of pedicle screws, which requires repositioning of a patient from the lateral to the prone position, colloquially known as "flipping," which adds to operative time. Thus, there has been recent focus on "single-position surgery," in which pedicle screws are placed while the patient remains in the lateral position. Placement of pedicle screws in this position is unnatural for the surgeon, and several studies have demonstrated the challenges associated with this technique [3–5]. A novel twist on single-position lateral surgery is to perform the lateral lumbar interbody fusion with the patient in the prone position, thus providing posterior access in the more familiar prone position without repositioning. The focus of this chapter is to describe the prone lateral (PL) technique, to present the advantages and disadvantages of PL vs SL, and to review the current data on PL interbody fusion.

L. C. McCluskeyJr (✉) · M. Cyriac
Department of Orthopaedic Surgery, Tulane University School of Medicine,
New Orleans, LA, USA
e-mail: lmccluskey@tulane.edu

© The Author(s), under exclusive license to Springer Nature Switzerland AG 2023

J. R. O'Brien et al. (eds.), *Lumbar Spine Access Surgery*,
https://doi.org/10.1007/978-3-031-48034-8_30

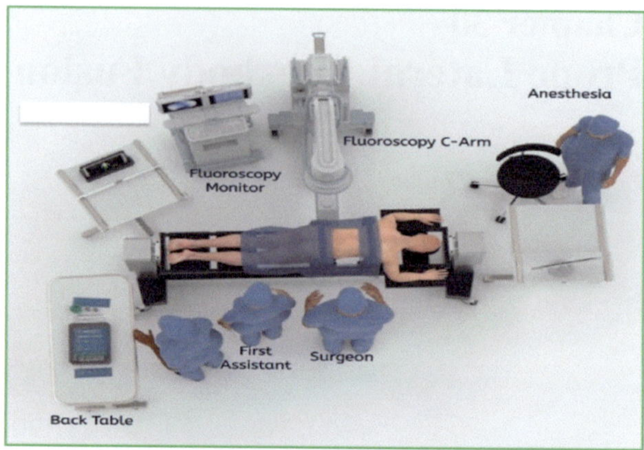

**Fig. 30.1** Room setup (image courtesy of ATEC Spine Carlsbad, CA)



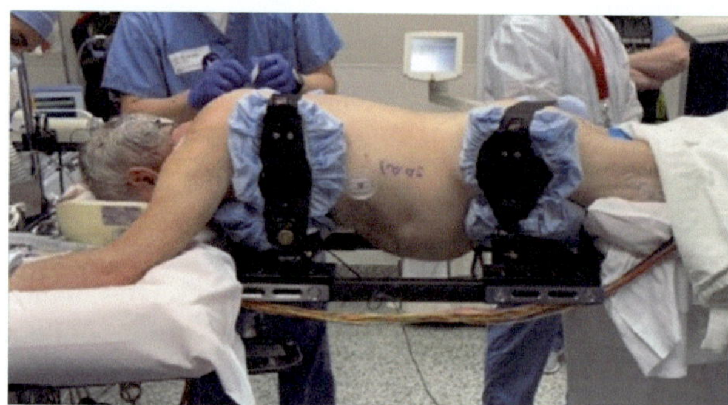

**Fig. 30.2** Patient positioning with commercially available bolsters avoids the need for taping (image courtesy of ATEC)

## *Technique*

### Positioning

Room setup is demonstrated in Fig. 30.1. The patient is positioned prone on a Jackson table or similar frame that allows the abdomen to hang freely. Ensure all bony prominences are well-padded. The chest and pelvic support pieces can be removed and exchanged for commercially available bolsters which can be adjusted to provide coronal plane "jackknife" effect to open the disc space (Fig. 30.2). Alternatively, the patient can be taped from the pelvic brim on the operative side to the contralateral corner of the bed and likewise from the ribs to the contralateral corner at the top of the bed to provide the same effect. This replaces the "jackknife" position of the bed in a standard lateral positioning and serves to tension the skin on the operative side. Neuromonitoring is utilized, including saphenous somatosensory-evoked potential monitoring when available. Positioning is verified using fluoroscopy, and the patient position is adjusted to obtain perfect anteroposterior and lateral radiographs with the C-Arm and OR table in neutral position. The laterality of the incision can be determined preoperatively based on the patient's anatomy. If anatomy is equivocal, we prefer the left-sided approach due to the location of the large vessels.

## Incision

A lateral fluoroscopic image is used to mark the appropriate location of the incision with a radio-opaque instrument. First, the appropriate disc space is identified. Next, the posterior aspect of the foramen is marked, as well as the midline of the disc space, and a line connecting these two points is used as the incision (Fig. 30.3). The incision is made slightly posterior compared to a traditional lateral to resist the effect of gravity on the retractor. We recommend extending the skin marking posteriorly to provide a visual cue to assist in obtaining the correct vector during retractor placement and instrumentation (Fig. 30.4).

## Superficial and Deep Dissection

The incision is made and external oblique fascia opened sharply. The subsequent layers, external oblique, internal oblique, and transversus abdominis muscles, are opened with digital dissection or Metzenbaum scissors. We advise to cheat slightly posterior during this portion of the approach to avoid a natural tendency to drift anterior which may result in violation of the peritoneum or inadvertently placing the dilator anteriorly. Once inside the retroperitoneal space, the retroperitoneal fat is encountered. The fat and peritoneum are swept anteriorly with a finger and the psoas is then palpated. The retroperitoneal fat and peritoneum are further released

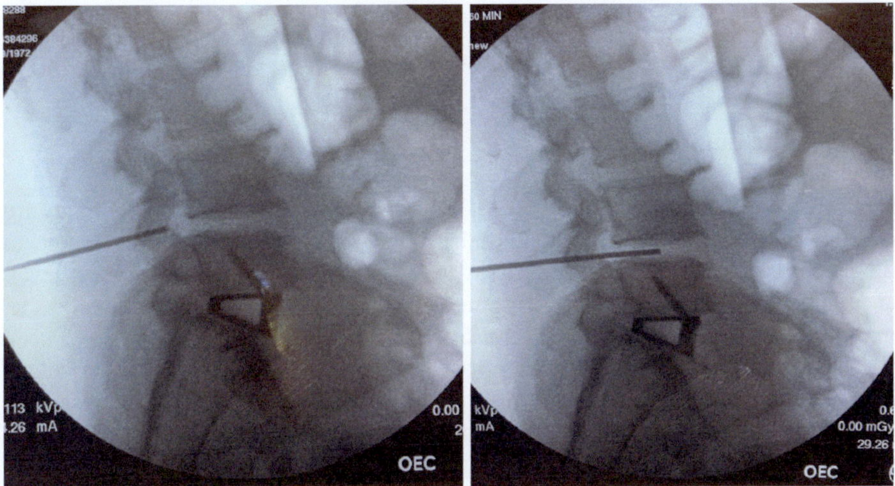

**Fig. 30.3** Marking the posterior aspect of the foramen and the 50-yd. line utilizing fluoroscopy

**Fig. 30.4** Line is extended posteriorly to visually assist with retractor placement and instrumentation vectors

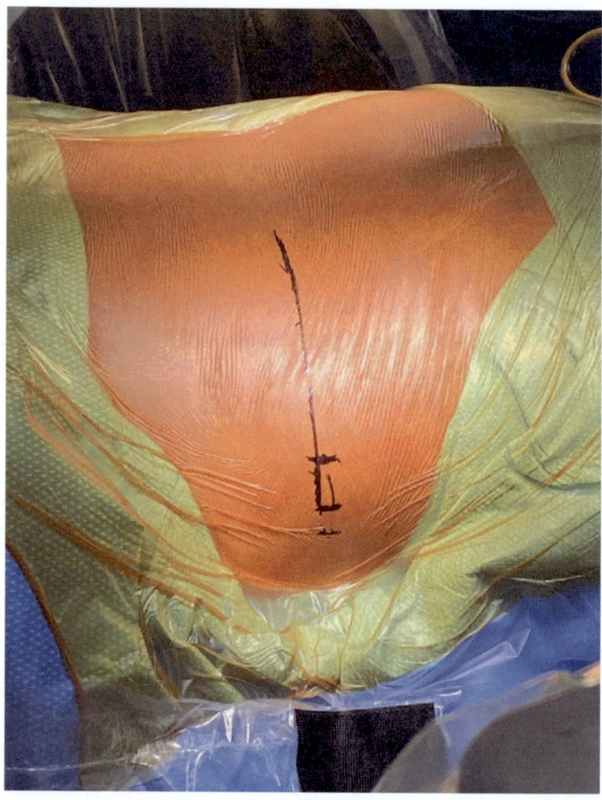

with digital dissection cranially and caudally. The initial dilator is introduced and carefully guided to the surface of the psoas with a finger to avoid peritoneal damage (Fig. 30.5). Fluoroscopy is then used to determine that the correct level is being approached.

## Avoiding the Lumbar Plexus

Next, triggered electromyography (EMG) is used to ensure the neural elements are posterior to the dilator. Once satisfied, the dilator is advanced through the psoas to the level of the disc space. Again, fluoroscopy is used to confirm the correct level, and neuromonitoring is used to ensure safe placement of the dilator. The ideal docking point is between the middle (L4–L5 level) and posterior 1/3 of the disc space (L1–L4 levels) (Fig. 30.6). Fluoroscopy is used to verify the appropriate trajectory of the initial dilator, ensuring that the corridor created through the psoas is parallel to the end plates and aiming directly across the disc space. Slight anterior to posterior angulation is permissible, but the opposite should be avoided to avoid damaging the anterior longitudinal ligament (ALL) or vascular structures [2].

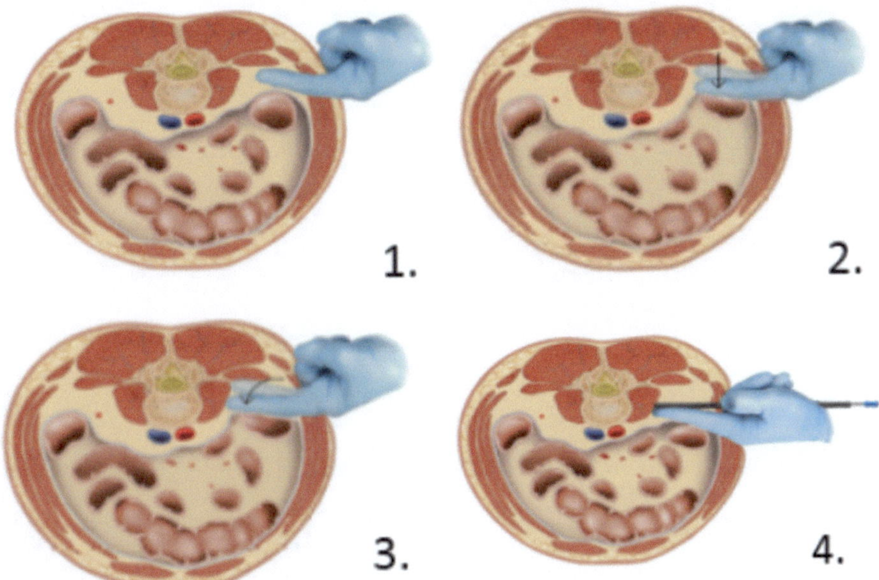


**Fig. 30.5** Illustration courtesy of a-tec spine demonstrating (1) introduction of finger into retroperitoneal space, (2) development of retroperitoneal space via blunt dissection, (3) sweeping peritoneum anterior and palpation of psoas, and (4) guiding initial dilator to the psoas with finger to protect the peritoneum

## Retractor Placement

Sequential dilation is performed to the desired diameter based on the particular system being employed. Triggered EMG measurements should be employed after each dilation to ensure safe placement anterior to the lumbar plexus. With the retractor blades closed, the retractor is placed over the dilators and docked at the appropriate level. Fluoroscopy can be used to verify location and orientation. We use a two-blade retractor. The anterior and posterior blades are opened to allow a working window for a 18-mm or 22-mm cage (Fig. 30.7). Again, triggered EMG can be used to ensure no nerves are in the working corridor once retractor deployment is complete. We typically place a shim either anteriorly or posteriorly depending on the level to decrease retractor migration.

## Disk Preparation

Next, the bed can be rotated away from the surgeon approximately 30° to provide ergonomic line of sight down the working corridor. The fluoroscopy unit should be rotated to match the patient. Another option, to avoid having the C arm in an offset direction, is to sit on a stool without rotating the table 30°. Sitting on the stool

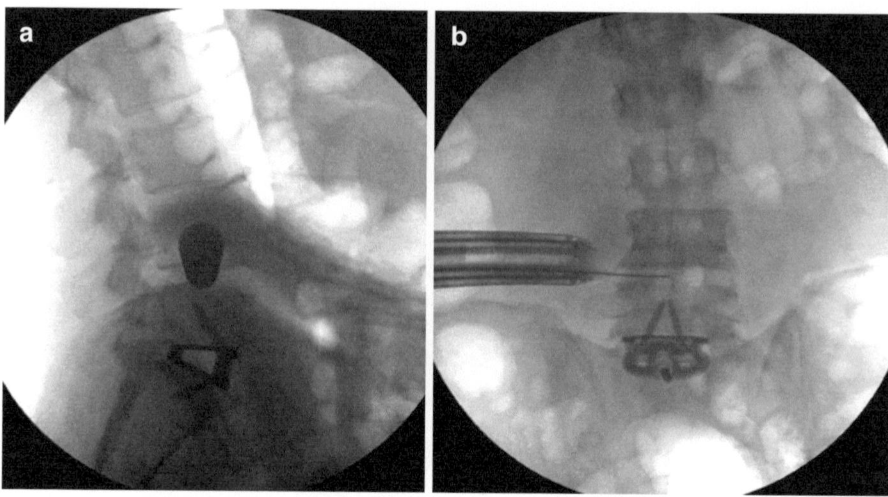

**Fig. 30.6** (**a**) Fluoro shot showing placement of initial dilator at the appropriate disk space in line with disk in the lateral view (**b**) Retractor in appropriate position with respect to disc space in AP view with stimulation probe visualized for triggered EMG monitoring to ensure safe placement prior to deployment

**Fig. 30.7** Lateral fluoroscopic image showing placement of retractor in appropriate position after deployment

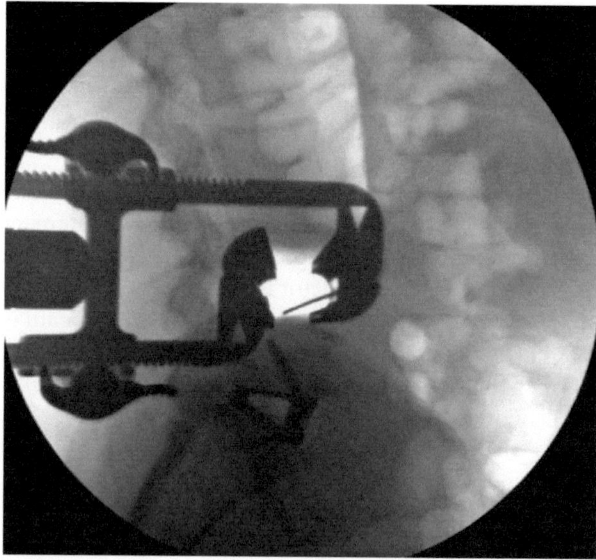

allows the surgeon to be eye level with the incision without having to raise the table too high. Next, an ipsilateral annulotomy is made, and a Cobb elevator is passed across the disc space along the superior and inferior end plates and to release the contralateral annulus. Disc material is removed using forward angle curettes and pituitary rongeurs. Fluoroscopy can be used to verify appropriate depth and orientation of the instrument. Additionally, orienting the instrument handles parallel to the retractors blades helps guide the instruments in the proper trajectory.

## Placement of Interbody Device

An interbody device and bone graft are selected from the surgeon's manufacturer of choice and are trialed and implanted (Fig. 30.8). Interbody device and size principles for a prone lateral are usually the same as for standard lateral. Compared to a

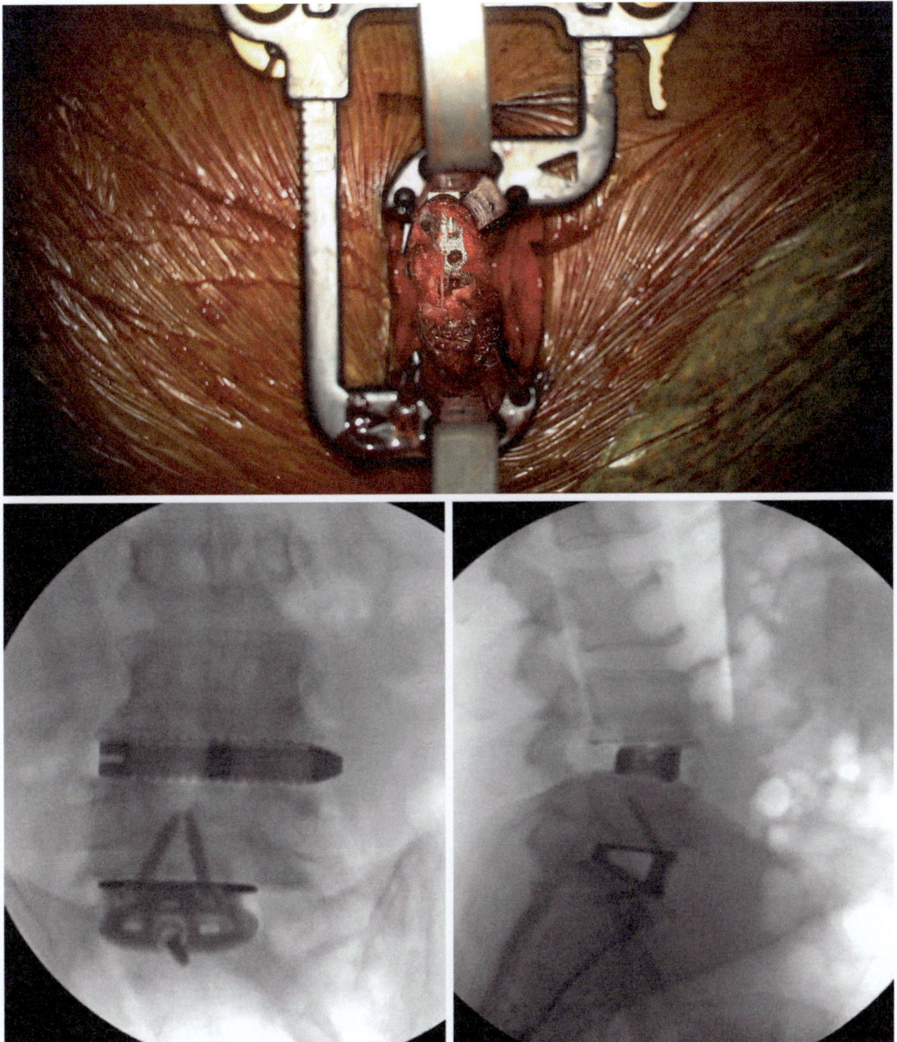

**Fig. 30.8** Photograph and fluoroscopic images of cage placement in the AP and lateral projections

standard lateral, by placing the patient prone, there is increased lordosis, making it possible to place a more lordotic cage. The interbody device height should be maximized to provide indirect decompression.

## Closure

The retractor is slowly removed under direct visualization to ensure no active bleeding is encountered. The external oblique fascial layer is closed followed by deep dermal and skin closure per the surgeon's preference.

## Posterior Instrumentation

When satisfied with the interbody device placement, the coronal bend should be released (tape or bolsters). At this time, pedicle screws can be placed along with any other posterior-based procedures indicated for the patient (Fig. 30.9). An alternative sequence is to percutaneously place pedicle screws prior to the lateral interbody portion of the procedure and then return to place rods after the interbody device has been placed. This is useful if using robotics or navigation to place the screws as it obviates the need for merging new images with the robot or navigation software after interbody device placement.

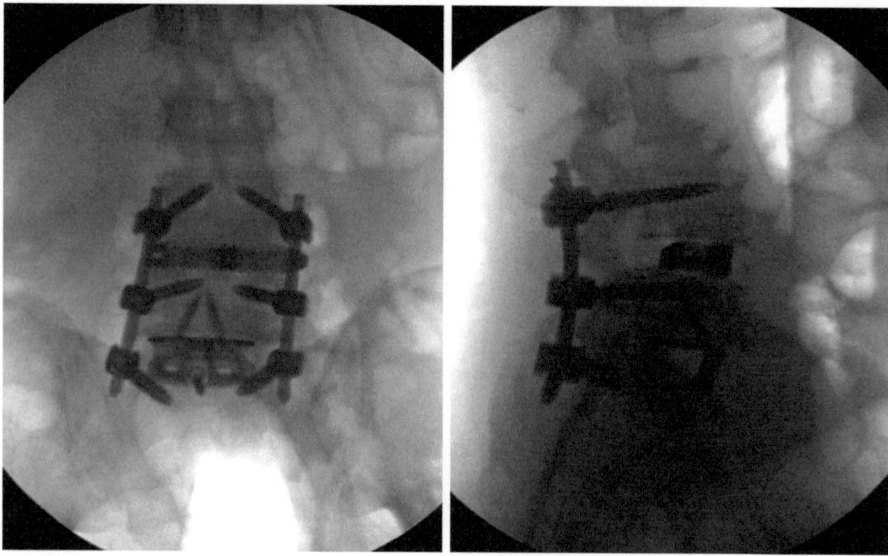

**Fig. 30.9** Final AP and lateral fluoroscopic images with cage and pedicle screws

## Advantages of Prone Technique Vs Standard Lateral Positioning

While tempting to discuss the many inherent advantages of a lateral technique, whether SL or PL, that discussion is beyond the scope of this chapter. The PL technique offers several unique advantages over the SL technique. First, the prone position offers access to the posterior spine for instrumentation and direct decompression without the need for repositioning. Additionally, placement of pedicle screws in the prone position is more familiar for the spine surgeon. Repositioning time is variable at each institution, but decreasing time in the OR and time under anesthesia is safer for the patient and financially beneficial for the institution.

Prone positioning also improves sagittal alignment and can help with reduction of spondylolisthesis. This phenomenon has been well-studied in the literature and is a major advantage of prone surgery [6, 7]. Amaral et al. compared lateral vs prone positioning with regard to lumbar lordosis. They found increased lumbar lordosis when measured from both L1-S1 ($57.6°$ vs $46.5°$, $P < 0.001$) and L4-S1 ($40.4°$ vs $36.9°$, $P < 0.01$) [8]. Sagittal balance has been shown to correlate to improved patient outcomes[23]. In our practice, for grade 2 or greater spondylolisthesis, we place the pedicle screws first, lock the caudal set screws, and then use the rod to partially reduce the spondylolisthesis. We leave the cranial set screws partially lose to allow for disc prep and placement of an adequate height lateral interbody cage. After placement of the lateral cage, we lock all the set screws.

Another advantage of prone positioning is that the psoas muscle is thought to be located more posteriorly at the level of the disc space due to hip extension. This is counterintuitive as one might expect the psoas to be more anterior with prone positioning due to the effect of gravity. Theoretically, a more posterior position of the psoas muscle results in less retraction of the psoas and therefore less risk of traction injury to the lumbar plexus to reach the ideal retractor docking position. Amaral et al. looked at psoas position based on magnetic resonance imaging in 24 healthy patients. They noted a shift of the psoas muscle posteriorly when the patient is in the prone position compared to supine and lateral positions, with no change in location of the lumbar plexus (Fig. 30.10). This is especially important at L4–L5 where the plexus is in the anterior 1/4th of the disc space in up to 83% of patients [9]. A cadaveric study by Alluri et al. demonstrated that in the prone position, extension of the hips moves the femoral nerve more posterior at L4–L5 when compared to hip flexion, such as when SL positioning is used [10]. This is a point of contention, however, as hip flexion in standard lateral positioning is thought by many to be protective of the lumbar plexus by relaxing the psoas. To our knowledge, there is no data supporting this claim. The effect of psoas position on neurologic injury requires additional investigation, but, so far, the data shows that performing a transpsoas approach and docking of a retractor in the prone position (hips extended) is at least as safe as standard lateral with hips flexed [8, 11].

Finally, some authors have also anecdotally noted that the prone position is more amenable to the use of navigation, as the patient is more secure on the table which

**Fig. 30.10** Amaral et al.
showing posterior location
of psoas with hips
extended (PL) vs
flexed (SL)

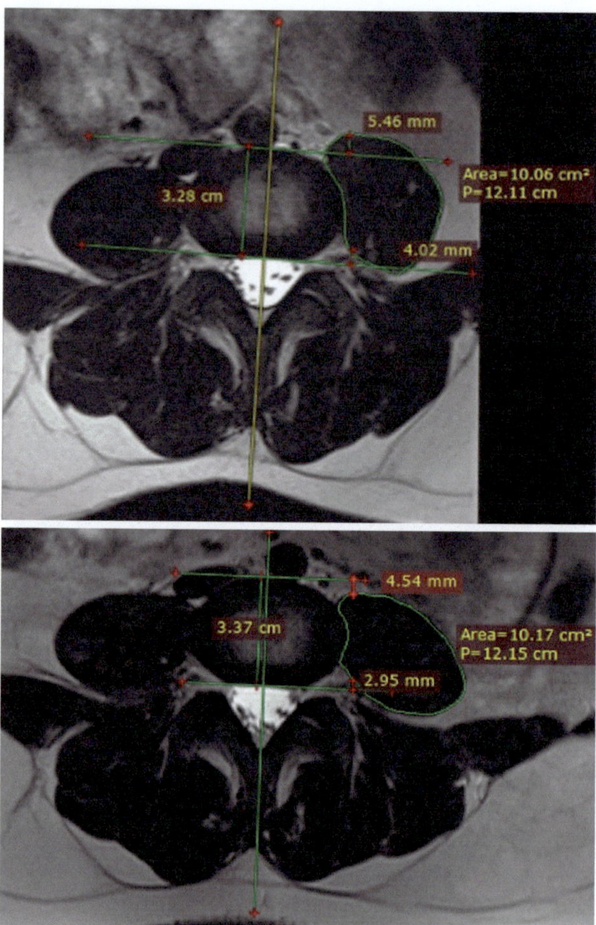

minimizes the risk of rotatory movements which can make navigation less accurate [1].

## *Limitations*

Although there are many advantages to lateral access, there are disadvantages as well. Reliance on indirect decompression is commonly cited. A full discussion of limitations of lateral surgery is beyond the scope of this chapter. The learning curve is one disadvantage of PL vs SL. Additionally, as mentioned above, while the extended position of the hips in PL has shown to move the psoas more posteriorly and thus offer safer access to the central portion of disk space by protecting the neurologic structures, it is also true that hip flexion and relaxing the psoas have been regarded as a safety measure to prevent damage to the lumbar plexus. The extended position causes the psoas to be under more tension than when hips are flexed, which could potentially lead to taut neural structures and increase the rate of neurologic injury. These observations are theoretical and limited by the lack of data in the literature.

## *Current Data*

There are limited studies on the prone lateral technique due to its recent inception, first being described in the literature by three separate publications in late 2019 and early 2020 [1, 2, 12]. At the time of publication of this chapter, only eight studies reported outcomes for the PL technique [1, 2, 11–14].

A 2021 systematic review and meta-analysis by Mills et al. reviewed available data for single-position SL and single-position PL [15]. Not surprisingly, they found that single-position surgery decreased operative times compared to flipping the patient, saving a mean of approximately 60 min of operative time. There was no difference in rates of neurologic injury, patient-reported outcome measures, or postoperative lumbar lordosis. The PL group did have a statistically significant increase in segmental lumbar lordosis compared to the single-position SL group. They also note increased rates of misplaced pedicle screws when performed in the lateral position compared to prone position [15].

Only one study to date compares PL and traditional SL. Lamartina and Berjano published their preliminary results of PL in a prospective study where they compared PL cohort to a matched SL cohort [12]. They enrolled 17 patients, 7 in the PL cohort and 10 in the SL cohort; the mean follow-up was 6 months (3–12 months). They found one instance of intraoperative cage subsidence and one ALL rupture in the PL group. Three instances of postoperative psoas weakness were identified in each group, all of which resolved by postop day four. There were four cases of thigh hypoesthesia in the PL group, one of which resolved by postoperative day 4, two more resolved by postoperative day 90, and one had not yet resolved at the 90-day postop visit. The SL group had one case of thigh hypoesthesia which resolved by postoperative day 90. Similar, significant average improvements in Oswestry Disability Index and back and leg pain by numerical rating scale were reported between the two groups, but no statistical analysis was performed due to the small sample size. The authors found longer setup times for the PL cohort as well and increased fluoroscopy exposure; however, these results are likely due to the learning curve associated with a new procedure. They conclude that the procedure is a viable alternative to SL, that there were no major complications in their limited cohort, and that they see the potential benefits of single-position surgery in the prone position once the learning curve has been taken out of the equation.

Radiographic analyses have also been performed. Pimenta et al. published radiographic outcome data from 32 patients undergoing PL surgery [16]. They reported increases in mean index-level segmental lumbar lordosis (8.7 to 14.8, $p < 0.001$) and lumbar lordosis (42.1 to 45.8, $p = 0.11$, which improved to 41.9 to 46.7, $p = 0.003$ when an outlier was excluded). Pelvic incidence-lumbar lordosis (PI-LL) mismatch of more than $10°$ was improved to less than $10°$ in 45% (10/22) patients. They concluded that the PL procedure produces improvements in sagittal alignment, but more data is needed to truly compare to SL. In 2022, Soliman et al. compared radiographic outcomes in PL vs SL [13]. In a retrospective matched cohort analysis, the PL group had better improvement in lumbar lordosis ($P < 0.05$) and PI-LL mismatch ($P = 0.05$).

# Conclusion

The PL procedure is an upgrade to the previously described SL, which we believe makes the procedure more attractive than its predecessor. Additionally, attempts to perform single-position surgery in the lateral position have proven difficult primarily due to challenges with pedicle screw placement in the lateral position. In addition to the benefits of SL over posterior approaches, the advantages of PL vs SL are improved sagittal alignment and lumbar lordosis from prone positioning, posterior access without the need to reposition, and theoretically safer access to the spine due to hip extension and thus a more posterior position of the psoas and lumbar plexus. This procedure does, however, involve a learning curve, as is true with any new procedure. Due to the novelty of the PL technique, there is inadequate data at this time to establish significant evidence as to whether the theoretical and anecdotal advantages of PL are shown in the data and are found to be widely reproducible.

# References

1. Godzik J, et al. Single-position prone lateral approach: cadaveric feasibility study and early clinical experience. Neurosurg Focus. 2020;49(3):E15.
2. Pimenta L, Taylor WR, Stone LE, Wali AR, Santiago-Dieppa DR. Prone transpsoas technique for simultaneous single-position access to the anterior and posterior lumbar spine. Oper Neurosurg (Hagerstown). 2020;20(1):E5–E12.
3. Blizzard DJ, Thomas JA. MIS single-position lateral and oblique lateral lumbar interbody fusion and bilateral pedicle screw fixation: feasibility and perioperative results. Spine. 2018;34:440–6.
4. Sellin JN, Mayer RR, Hoffman m, Ropper AE. Simultaneous lateral interbody fusion and pedicle screws (SLIPS) with CT-guided navigation. Clin Neurol Neurosurg. 2018;175:91–7.
5. Ozgur BM, et al. Extreme lateral interbody fusion (XLIF): a novel surgical technique for anterior lumbar interbody fusion. Spine J. 2006;6:435.
6. Peterson MD, Nelson LM, McManus AC, Jackson RP. The effect of operative position on lumbar lordosis: a radiographic of patients under anesthesia in the prone and 90-90 positions. Spine. 1995;20:1419–24.
7. Glassman SD, Berven S, Bridwell K, et al. Correlation of radio- graphic parameters and clinical symptoms in adult scoliosis. Spine. 2005;30:682–8.

8. Amaral R, Daher MT, Pratali R, Arnoni D, Pokorny G, Rodrigues R, Batista M, Fortuna PP, Pimenta L, Herrero CF. The effect of patient position on psoas morphology and in lumbar lordosis. World Neurosurg. 2021;153:e131–40. https://doi.org/10.1016/j.wneu.2021.06.067. Epub 2021 Jun 22.

9. Callahan RA, Brown MD. Positioning techniques in spinal surgery. Clin Orthop. 1981;154:22–6.

10. Alluri R, Clark N, Sheha E, Shafi K, Geiselmann M, Kim HJ, Qureshi S, Dowdell J. Location of the femoral nerve in the lateral decubitus versus prone position. Glob Spine J. 2021;13:1765.

11. Pimenta L, Pokorny G, Amaral R, Ditty B, Batista M, Moriguchi R, Filho FM, Taylor WR. Single-position prone transpsoas lateral interbody fusion including L4L5: early postoperative outcomes. World Neurosurg. 2021;149:e664–8. Epub 2021 Feb 4

12. Lamartina C, Berjano P. Prone single-position extreme lateral interbody fusion (pro-XLIF): preliminary results. Eur Spine J. 2020;29(Suppl 1):6–13.

13. Soliman MAR, Khan A, Pollina J. Comparison of prone transpsoas and standard lateral lumbar interbody fusion surgery for degenerative lumbar spine disease: a retrospective radiographic propensity score-matched analysis. World Neurosurg. 2021;S1878-8750(21):01274–2. https://doi.org/10.1016/j.wneu.2021.08.097.

14. Mills ES, Treloar J, Idowu O, Shelby T, Alluri RK, Hah RJ. Single position lumbar fusion: a systematic review and meta-analysis. Spine J. 2021;22:429.

15. Soliman MA, Aguirre AO, Ruggiero N, Kuo CC, Mariotti BL, Khan A, Mullin JP, Pollina J. Comparison of prone transpsoas lateral lumbar interbody fusion and transforaminal lumbar interbody fusion for degenerative lumbar spine disease: a retrospective radiographic propensity score-matched analysis. Clin Neurol Neurosurg. 2021;213:107105.

16. Pimenta L, Amaral R, Taylor W, Tohmeh A, Pokorny G, Rodrigues R, Arnoni D, Guirelli T, Batista M. The prone transpsoas technique: preliminary radiographic results of a multicenter experience. Eur Spine J. 2021;30(1):108–13. Epub 2020 May 29.

# Chapter 31
# Minimally Invasive Thoracolumbar Approaches with Diaphragm Preservation

Katriel E. Lee, Robert F. Rudy, and Juan S. Uribe

## Introduction

Despite the effectiveness of the canonical posterior and anterior approaches to the thoracolumbar spine in providing wide exposure, they also involve considerable morbidity and risk of complications [1]. The first reports of access to the ventral thoracolumbar spine appeared in the 1920s and 1930s, with access obtained via a retroperitoneal approach [2] and later with a transpleural, retroperitoneal approach [3, 4]. Soon after, Dwyer and Harrington reported instrumentation of the anterior and posterior thoracolumbar spine, which required large, open exposures [5]. For decades, the accepted approach to the thoracolumbar spine has been based on these techniques, with the approach beginning with a large incision from the lateral thoracic cage to the medial abdomen [6] for a retroperitoneal exposure of the lumbar spine and either a transpleural or a retropleural exposure of the thoracic spine [4]. Originally described by Capener in 1954 [7] and later by Larson and colleagues in 1976 [8], the lateral extracavitary approach became a workhorse corridor to the thoracolumbar spine because it enabled both ventral decompression and dorsal fixation through a single incision. However, the lateral extracavitary approach is associated with a high incidence of clinically significant morbidity, due in large part to the technical challenges and exposure of the pleura, which increases the risk of pulmonary complications [9]. Additionally, incising the diaphragm requires repair and may cause patients to develop postoperative hernias. These limitations drove the development of access strategies that decrease surgical time and reduce patient morbidity.

K. E. Lee · R. F. Rudy · J. S. Uribe (✉)
Department of Neurosurgery, Barrow Neurological Institute, St. Joseph's Hospital and Medical Center, Phoenix, AZ, USA
e-mail: Neuropub@barrowneuro.org

© The Author(s), under exclusive license to Springer Nature Switzerland AG 2023

J. R. O'Brien et al. (eds.), *Lumbar Spine Access Surgery*,
https://doi.org/10.1007/978-3-031-48034-8_31

321

With the advent of minimally invasive spine surgery, new technology and growing expertise are redefining standard approaches to the spine. This transition is particularly true for procedures in the lumbar spine, where lateral transpsoas approaches are enabling interbody fusion with large surface area cages and relatively little morbidity. However, the thoracolumbar junction poses unique anatomical challenges. The inferior rib cage and diaphragm can obstruct or complicate access. Anterior diaphragmatic attachments include the xiphoid process and the aponeurosis of the transversus abdominis muscle; lateral attachments include the medial aspects of the 7th and 8th ribs anteriorly, the 9th and 10th ribs laterally, and the 11th and 12th ribs posterolaterally; and posterior attachments include the medial and lateral arcuate ligaments and the left and right crura [10, 11]. The minimally invasive lateral extracoelomic approach was developed to address these anatomic challenges, with mobilization of the diaphragm anteriorly to facilitate access to the thoracolumbar junction.

## Minimally Invasive Lateral Approach to the Thoracolumbar Junction: Anatomical Considerations

In 1993, Moskovich et al. [12] described the extracoelomic approach to the thoracic spine, in which both the parietal pleura and the visceral pleura are reflected together from the chest wall, offering an operative corridor to the ventral spine without the risk of traversing the pleura. As surgeons have gained experience with minimally invasive spine surgery over decades of practice, this approach continued to evolve, with increasing emphasis placed on minimizing tissue trauma during access.

The contemporary version of this approach is a lateral retropleural or lateral retroperitoneal dissection through a small incision [13]. This approach is referred to as a *mini-open* technique. Mini-open approaches are promising because they provide direct visualization with minimal damage to surrounding tissue [14]. Overall, there are three lateral mini-open approaches to the thoracolumbar junction:

1. Approach via T12-L2 disc space access, with the retropleural space as the primary corridor
2. Approach via T12-L2 disc access but with significant overhang of the rib cage that requires a retroperitoneal approach and mobilization of the diaphragm
3. Approach via T11–T12 disc access achieved through retropleural dissection

Two reports of cadaveric studies of this mini-open, minimally invasive, lateral extracoelomic approach describe the technique well [10, 13]. The patient is carefully placed in the lateral decubitus position, with careful attention so that the iliac crest rests at the level of the table break (Fig. 31.1). A 6-cm oblique incision is created at the midaxillary line. Exposure requires thorough knowledge of this anatomical area. On the anterolateral surface of the abdomen, proceeding from superficial to deep, the surgeon will encounter the external oblique muscle, which originates

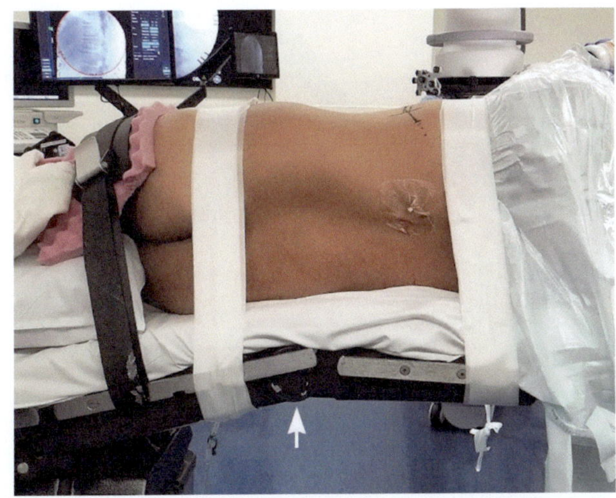

**Fig. 31.1** Patient position for the mini-open, minimally invasive, lateral extracoelomic approach. Note the lateral decubitus position, with the iliac crest position (*arrow*) at the level of the table break. (*Used with permission from J Neurosurg Spine*)

from the bottom six ribs and runs caudally and medially to terminate on the anterior iliac crest; the internal oblique muscle, which originates from the anterior iliac, iliopsoas, and thoracolumbar fasciae and runs superiorly and medially to the bottom three ribs; and the transversus abdominis muscle, which originates with the internal oblique muscle and runs anteriorly to the linea alba and the diaphragm. In this approach, the lower three ribs are encountered. On the chest wall surface, from superficial to deep, the surgeon will encounter the latissimus dorsi muscle, which originates from the spinous processes of T7-L5 and the posterior iliac crest and terminates on the medial humerus, the external oblique muscle, the external intercostal muscles (muscle fibers running inferoanteriorly), the internal intercostal muscles (muscle fibers running inferoposteriorly), and the diaphragm.

About 4–6 cm of the rib is removed at the affected level (typically, the 10th rib for T12, the 11th rib for L1, etc.). Blunt dissection of the plane between the endothoracic fascia and the parietal pleura is required at the levels of the 10th and 11th ribs. The 12th rib is more complicated because of the insertion of the diaphragm, so the pleura is bluntly mobilized anteriorly together with the diaphragm by using a finger or sponge stick until the lateral portions of the vertebral bodies and discs are visible. At the L1 level, the lumbar and posterior attachments are best transected sharply off the transverse process of L1. Cutting the arcuate ligaments can then expose the lateral vertebral body. After the diaphragm is dissected, the retropleural and retroperitoneal spaces can be connected, and the expandable tube retractor system can then be inserted. Figure 31.2 demonstrates the approaches to the different levels; Fig. 31.3 demonstrates the surgical view with the tubular retractor in place; and Fig. 31.4 shows a view of the cavities seen through this lateral approach.

There are many benefits to this surgical approach. First, because it is extracoelomic, both right-side and left-side approaches are feasible. In addition, no repair of the diaphragm is required [10, 13].

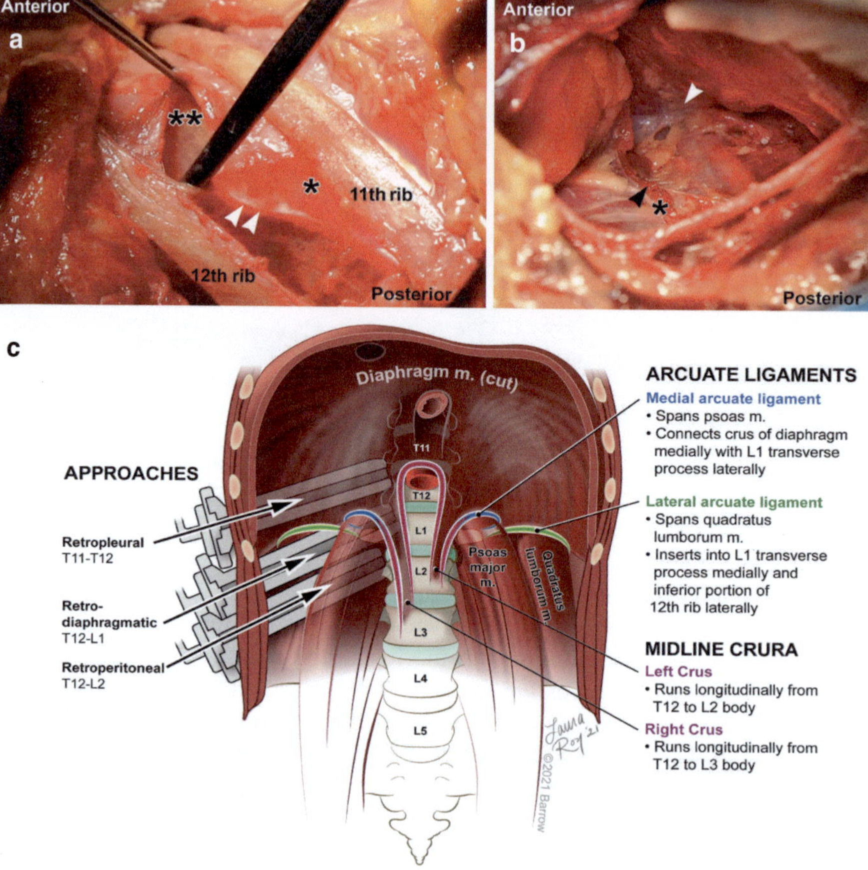



**Fig. 31.2** Relevant anatomic features of the diaphragm when approaching the thoracolumbar junction. (**a**) A photograph from a cadaveric dissection of the thoracic wall and its relevance to the lateral approach to the thoracolumbar junction. *Double arrowheads* indicate the diaphragm; *single asterisk* indicates the parietal pleura; and *double asterisks* indicate the peritoneum. (**b**) Further dissection after removal of the 11th and 12th ribs. *White arrowhead* indicates the medial attachment of the medial arcuate ligament; *black arrowhead* indicates the remaining muscle cuff of the medial lateral arcuate ligament; and *asterisk* indicates the attachment point of the medial and lateral arcuate ligament. (**c**) Illustration demonstrating the medial and lateral diaphragm attachments. *m*, muscle. (*Used with permission from Barrow Neurological Institute, Phoenix, Arizona*)

## *Surgical Considerations and Patient Selection*

Anterior approaches to the thoracolumbar spine have become increasingly preferred over posterior approaches for compressive lesions of the ventral spinal cord because of the questionable durability of kyphosis correction and overall results in patients who undergo standard posterior approaches. For patients who are candidates for the anterolateral approaches to the thoracolumbar junction, a few factors should be

**Fig. 31.3** Operative view of a cadaveric specimen with the tubular retractor in place in the mini-open, minimally invasive, lateral extracoelomic approach. (*Used with permission from J Neurosurg Spine*)

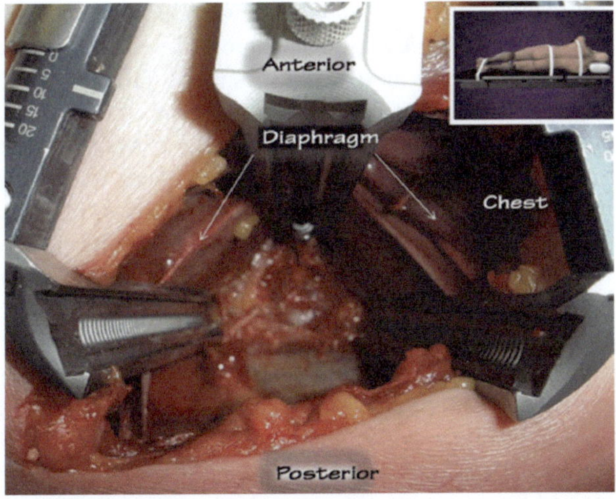


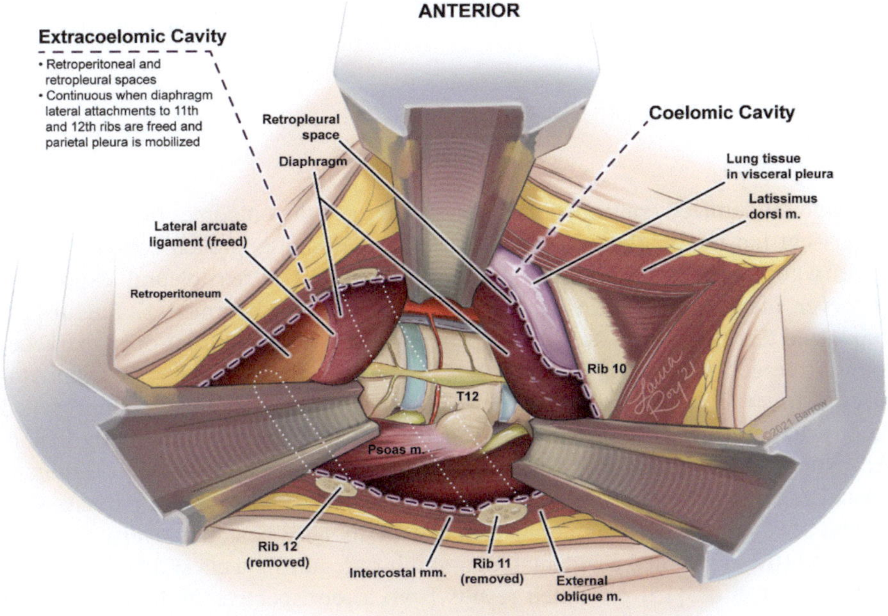


**Fig. 31.4** Artist's rendition of the anatomy as seen through the tubular retractor in the mini-open, minimally invasive, lateral extracoelomic approach. *m*, muscle. (*Used with permission from Barrow Neurological Institute, Phoenix, Arizona*)

considered. The traditional transpleural approach requires the anesthesia team to aerate only one lung during the procedure, which creates a transient but significant impairment in pulmonary function [15]. Single-lung ventilation may be of limited use in elderly patients, in patients with lung metastases, and in patients with severe pulmonary or cardiovascular comorbidities because vital capacity can be reduced up to 30% during these types of surgery [16–18]. In addition, thoracoscopic techniques can cause iatrogenic dissemination of infection or tumor cells [15].

Patients who have had previous surgery via an ipsilateral thoracotomy or a retroperitoneal approach may be poor candidates for modern mini-open extracoelomic approaches because of the possibility that significant scarring or adhesions can obscure the dissection plane. In addition, the minimally invasive approach may be less suitable for patients who require extensive repair and a wider field of exposure [19]. However, large open variations of the lateral extracoelomic approach are associated with considerable morbidity, with approximately one-third of patients experiencing clinically significant postoperative pain and one-fourth of patients reporting subsequent limitations in their activities of daily living [20].

Notably, an endoscopic approach could also be used for select patients. Trocars can be placed intrathoracically in the phrenicocostal sinus before the diaphragm is incised for exposure. However, this exposure requires diaphragm repair and carries a risk of hernia. These techniques typically have a steep learning curve, require expensive tools, and may be poorly suited for management of complications [21].

## Outcomes

No large randomized controlled trials have examined the outcomes of patients who underwent the minimally invasive lateral extracoelomic approach compared with those who underwent traditional larger transpleural or retropleural exposures. However, many smaller retrospective studies have been performed. El Saghir [19] conducted a retrospective study of 21 patients who underwent mini-open extracoelomic approaches for burst fractures ($n = 5$), degenerative discs ($n = 4$), spondylodiscitis ($n = 9$), pathologic fractures ($n = 2$), or pseudarthrosis after failed reconstruction ($n = 1$). Thirteen of the 21 patients underwent an interbody fusion. All patients had a stable reconstruction, and no patients had neurological deficits related to surgery. Anterior instrumentation failed in 2 (10%) of the 21 patients. One patient (5%) acquired pneumonia and died 3 months postoperatively, and two patients (10%) sustained accidental pleural injury requiring a chest tube [19].

Scheufler et al. [15] presented results from a retrospective study assessing 38 patients who presented with disabling back pain or progressive neurological deficits and who subsequently underwent multilevel corpectomy, spinal canal decompression, and anterior column reconstruction that used expandable vertebral body replacement and ventrolateral plate fixation via a minimally invasive retropleural or combined extracoelomic thoracoabdominal approach. Operative time, blood loss, neurological function, and clinical outcomes were favorable compared with those for traditional open and endoscopic techniques. Most (76%) of the 38 patients experienced functional improvement, deformity reduction, no pain related to the thoracotomy, and relief of radicular or back pain. Complications included the need for placement of a chest tube secondary to pleural tears (8%) and dural tear (3%) [15].

Another study analyzed prospectively maintained data for 52 patients who underwent the mini-open lateral approach primarily for traumatic burst fractures with instability and neurological deficit (94.2%) [14]. About 69% of these patients had injuries at T12 or L1. Seventy-three percent of patients were neurologically intact postoperatively or had only slight neurological deficits. Complications were dural tear ($n = 2$), intercostal neuralgia ($n = 2$), deep vein thrombosis ($n = 2$), pleural effusion ($n = 1$), and superficial posterior infection ($n = 1$).

In 2020, Christiansen et al. [22] reported a multi-institutional case series of 11 patients treated with the mini-open lateral retropleural approach or the combined retropleural-retroperitoneal approach for thoracic or thoracolumbar anterior column pathologies. In this analysis of prospectively maintained data, all 11 patients underwent successful decompression and reconstruction. The mean length of stay was 7.2 days. Axial back pain improved from a mean of 8.2 to a mean of 2.2 on the visual analog scale with a mean follow-up of 16.7 months. Complications ($n = 1$ for each) included deep vein thrombosis and pulmonary embolism, pneumonia, and cage subsidence.

Overall, the consensus in the recent literature is that the mini-open, lateral extracoelomic approach is a safe and effective treatment for patients with anterior thoracolumbar pathology and that it has an acceptable rate of pulmonary complications. The mean surgical operative time ranged from 101.2 to 181 min, the mean estimated blood loss ranged from 280 mL to 724 mL, and the mean length of stay ranged from 4 to 7.4 days [14, 15, 19, 22, 23]. However, the amount of overall evidence is limited because the published reports are only small retrospective case series.

## Conclusion

Modern mini-open extracoelomic approaches to the thoracolumbar junction are an appealing alternative to large, open surgeries because of their lung- and diaphragm-sparing capability. Patients tolerate the surgeries well, with minimal morbidity. Advances still need to be made in endoscopic, diaphragm-sparing techniques.

**Acknowledgments** We thank the staff of Neuroscience Publications at Barrow Neurological Institute for the assistance with manuscript preparation.

## References

1. McDonnell MF, Glassman SD, Dimar JR 2nd, Puno RM, Johnson JR. Perioperative complications of anterior procedures on the spine. J Bone Joint Surg Am. 1996;78(6):839–47. Epub 1996/06/01.
2. Ito H, Tsuchiya J, Asami G. A new radical operation for Pott's disease: report of ten cases. JBJS. 1934;16(3):499–515.
3. Hodgson AR, Stock FE. Anterior spinal fusion a preliminary communication on the radical treatment of Pott's disease and Pott's paraplegia. Br J Surg. 1956;44(185):266–75. Epub 1956/11/01.

4. Ikard RW. Methods and complications of anterior exposure of the thoracic and lumbar spine. Arch Surg. 2006;141(10):1025–34. Epub 2006/10/18.

5. Schafer MF. Dwyer instrumentation of the spine. Orthop Clin North Am. 1978;9(1):115–22. Epub 1978/01/01

6. Heitmiller RF. The left thoracoabdominal incision. Ann Thorac Surg. 1988;46(2):250–3. Epub 1988/08/01

7. Capener N. The evolution of lateral rhachotomy. J Bone Joint Surg Br. 1954;36-b(2):173–9. Epub 1954/05/01.

8. Larson SJ, Holst RA, Hemmy DC, Sances A Jr. Lateral extracavitary approach to traumatic lesions of the thoracic and lumbar spine. J Neurosurg. 1976;45(6):628–37. Epub 1976/12/01.

9. Resnick DK, Benzel EC. Lateral extracavitary approach for thoracic and thoracolumbar spine trauma: operative complications. Neurosurgery. 1998;43(4):796–802.

10. Dakwar E, Ahmadian A, Uribe JS. The anatomical relationship of the diaphragm to the thoracolumbar junction during the minimally invasive lateral extracoelomic (retropleural/retroperitoneal) approach. J Neurosurg Spine. 2012;16(4):359–64. Epub 2012/01/10.

11. Baaj AA, Papadimitriou K, Amin AG, Kretzer RM, Wolinsky JP, Gokaslan ZL. Surgical anatomy of the diaphragm in the anterolateral approach to the spine: a cadaveric study. J Spinal Disord Tech. 2014;27(4):220–3. Epub 2014/05/30.

12. Moskovich R, Benson D, Zhang ZH, Kabins M. Extracoelomic approach to the spine. J Bone Joint Surg Br. 1993;75(6):886–93. Epub 1993/11/01.

13. Xu DS, Walker CT, Farber SH, et al. Surgical anatomy of minimally invasive lateral approaches to the thoracolumbar junction. J Neurosurg Spine. 2021;36:1–8. Epub 2022/01/01.

14. Smith WD, Dakwar E, Le TV, Christian G, Serrano S, Uribe JS. Minimally invasive surgery for traumatic spinal pathologies: a mini-open, lateral approach in the thoracic and lumbar spine. Spine (Phila Pa 1976). 2010;35(26 Suppl):S338–46. Epub 2011/01/05.

15. Scheufler KM. Technique and clinical results of minimally invasive reconstruction and stabilization of the thoracic and thoracolumbar spine with expandable cages and ventrolateral plate fixation. Neurosurgery. 2007;61(4):798–808. discussion –9. Epub 2007/11/08.

16. Faro FD, Marks MC, Newton PO, Blanke K, Lenke LG. Perioperative changes in pulmonary function after anterior scoliosis instrumentation: thoracoscopic versus open approaches. Spine (Phila Pa 1976). 2005;30(9):1058–63. Epub 2005/05/03.

17. Graham EJ, Lenke LG, Lowe TG, et al. Prospective pulmonary function evaluation following open thoracotomy for anterior spinal fusion in adolescent idiopathic scoliosis. Spine. 2000;25(18):2319–25.

18. Vedantam R, Lenke LG, Bridwell KH, Haas J, Linville DA. A prospective evaluation of pulmonary function in patients with adolescent idiopathic scoliosis relative to the surgical approach used for spinal arthrodesis. Spine (Phila Pa 1976). 2000;25(1):82–90. Epub 2000/01/27.

19. El Saghir H. Extracoelomic mini approach for anterior reconstructive surgery of the thoracolumbar area. Neurosurgery. 2002;51(5 Suppl):S118–22. Epub 2002/09/18

20. Kim DH, Jaikumar S, Kam AC. Minimally invasive spine instrumentation. Neurosurgery. 2002;51(5 Suppl):S15–25. Epub 2002/09/18.

21. Beisse R. Endoscopic surgery on the thoracolumbar junction of the spine. Eur Spine J. 2010;19(Suppl 1(Suppl 1)):S52–65. Epub 2009/08/21

22. Christiansen PA, Huang S, Smith JS, Shaffrey ME, Uribe JS, Yen CP. Mini-open lateral retropleural/retroperitoneal approaches for thoracic and thoracolumbar junction anterior column pathologies. Neurosurg Focus. 2020;49(3):E13. Epub 2020/09/02.

23. Payer M, Sottas C. Mini-open anterior approach for corpectomy in the thoracolumbar spine. Surg Neurol. 2008;69(1):25–31. discussion 31–2. Epub 2007/12/07.

# Chapter 32
# Minimally Invasive Trauma Corpectomy of the Lumbar Spine

Hao-Hua Wu, Steven Wright, Michael Flores, Kelsey Brown, Yashar Javidan, and Alekos A. Theologis

## Introduction

Vertebral burst fractures are relatively common injuries resulting from high-energy trauma, including falls and motor vehicle accidents [1, 2]. The majority occur in the thoracolumbar region, where the rigid thoracic spine transitions to the more mobile lumbar region [3]. Overall, burst fractures account for 30–60% of thoracolumbar spinal fractures [1, 3, 4].

Despite their incidence, there remains debate with regard to the best treatment modality for these injuries [1]. For patients with burst fracture without neurologic compromise, literature has demonstrated similar functional outcomes, decreased cost, and lower complication rates for nonoperative management compared to operative management [5]. Other studies, including that by Siebenga et al., report data that suggests improved functional outcome, pain, and correction of kyphotic deformity with operative management [6]. The Thoracolumbar Injury Classification and Severity (TLICS) scoring system is commonly used to delineate which patients should be treated surgically as opposed to conservative treatment [7]. Patients are given a score based on fracture morphology, neurologic involvement, and integrity of the posterior ligamentous complex. Those with scores of 3 or less are considered appropriate for nonoperative, while those with scores of 5 or more can be deemed surgical candidates [7].

H.-H. Wu · S. Wright · M. Flores · K. Brown · A. A. Theologis (✉)
Department of Orthopaedic Surgery, University of California San Francisco (UCSF), San Francisco, CA, USA
e-mail: hao-hua.wu@ucsf.edu; steven.wright6495@cnsu.edu; michael.flores@ucsf.edu; kelsey_brown@brown.edu

Y. Javidan
Department of Orthopaedic Surgery, University of California, Davis (UCD), Davis, CA, USA
e-mail: yjavidan@ucdavis.edu

© The Author(s), under exclusive license to Springer Nature Switzerland AG 2023
J. R. O'Brien et al. (eds.), *Lumbar Spine Access Surgery*, https://doi.org/10.1007/978-3-031-48034-8_32

"""

For burst fractures that require surgical management, many options for operative intervention exist. Posterior-only instrumentation with two levels of instrumentation above and below the fracture is an attractive option given it is a single approach. An alternative is an anterior corpectomy and reconstruction with posterior instrumentation one level above and one level below the fractured level [8]. The decision to perform a corpectomy and reconstruct the anterior column can be made examining fracture involvement and pattern, as proposed by McCormack et al. [9] Their system, the load-sharing classification, can be used to predict which patients are at risk of instrumentation failure if treated by the posterior approach alone [9]. This scoring system considers a degree of comminution, apposition/displacement of fragments, and degree of kyphotic correction achieved, providing a score from 0 to 9 [9]. Patients with scores of 7 or more are at risk of instrumentation failure and, thus, likely benefit from an anterior or combined approach, while those with scores of 6 or less are felt to be adequately treated with a single posterior approach [9].

While anterior lumbar/thoracolumbar corpectomies are commonly treated by a traditional open anterolateral approach, this extensile open approach is associated with important complications, including vascular injury, pulmonary embolism, postoperative ileus, incisional hernias, and wound infections [10, 11]. Given this reportedly high morbidity, minimally invasive techniques have gained popularity as a potentially beneficial treatment strategy [10].

In this chapter, we will detail the operative technique of the mini-open lateral corpectomy of the lumbar spine for treatment of thoracolumbar burst fractures, as well as the benefits, limitations, outcomes, and complications of this approach.

## Operative Technique

Several techniques have been described in the literature with regard to minimally invasive lateral corpectomy of the lumbar spine in the setting of thoracolumbar burst fractures [10, 11]. Surgical planning depends on the level of fracture, and the approaches can be divided into T12-L1 and L2–L5 [10]. A preoperative MRI can be used to determine laterality based on location of the aorta and major vessels, position of the iliac crest, and location of the lumbar plexus [12, 13]. Patients are placed in a lateral decubitus position as has been previously described, and a multimodal neuromonitoring approach (free-running EMG, triggered EMG, motor-evoked potentials, somatosensory-evoked potentials) is utilized [14].

### *T12-L1 Incision and Exposure*

For burst fractures at the level of T12 and L1, the diaphragm and lung need to be considered during this approach. Intraoperative fluoroscopy is used to identify the level of the fracture. A 5–7-cm incision can be made in line with the corresponding

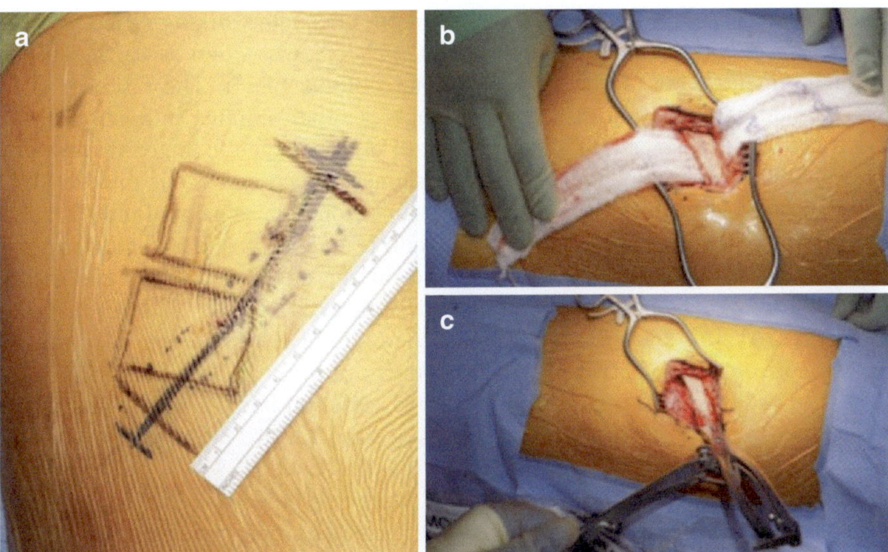

**Fig. 32.1** Intraoperative images of (**a**) skin marking of borders of vertebral bodies, overlying rib, and placement of incision. Photos of the minimally invasive retropleural approach with subperiosteal dissection of the rib (**b**) and rib cutter (**c**). (*Javidan Y and Hurley Jr. MRK. Minimally Invasive Lateral Approach to Thoracic and Lumbar Spine: For Discectomy and Corpectomy for Trauma, Tumor, Infection, and Deformity. Oper Tech Orthop 00:100721 © 2019 Published by Elsevier Inc.*)

rib from the anterior to the posterior surface of the vertebral body (Fig. 32.1) [10]. The periosteum over the rib is incised, and either a rib resection or dissection just superior to the rib can be undertaken to gain access to the retropleural space [15]. To avoid injury, a retropleural approach is utilized between the parietal pleura and the inner surface of the rib inferior to the access incision [10, 11]. The diaphragm and pleura are retracted and dissected anteriorly [10]. Once the psoas is identified, sequential tube dilation is undertaken with positioning just ventral to the posterior aspect of the vertebral body (adjacent intact vertebral body can be used as reference) [16]. Neuromonitoring is used to ensure safe retractor placement and avoidance of the lumbar plexus and genitofemoral nerve [14, 16]. The standard lateral retractor is then placed with view of the fracture as well as superior and inferior intervertebral discs [16].

## *L2–L5 Incision and Exposure*

For burst fractures of the L2–L5 vertebral bodies, a standard transpsoas retroperitoneal approach can be utilized with three modifications: (1) minimizing the break of the table to avoid disrupting the fracture, (2) using a single incision, and (3) making the incision 1–2 cm longer to allow for adequate working space for corpectomy [10, 11]. After making the skin incision, dissection is carried down through subcutaneous tissue to the external oblique fascia. The fascia is then incised, and careful blunt dissection through external oblique, internal oblique, and transversus muscles/fascia is carried out [14, 16]. A gentle finger sweep technique is then used to localize the retroperitoneal space and psoas muscle [16]. After confirming the dissection is in the retroperitoneum, sequential tube dilation is undertaken, the depth of the retractor length is measured, and a standard lateral retractor is placed to visualize fracture and intervertebral disc above and below [10, 11, 14, 16]. The position of the plexus is checked with the neuromonitoring probe [15]. The more caudal the fracture, the more likely the lumbar plexus is to have a more anterior position in relation to the posterior wall of the vertebral body [17]. The psoas muscle overlying the injured vertebral body is released, and the segmental artery is ligated, thereby exposing the fracture and discs above and below [15].

The mini-open exposure to lumbar burst fractures should be reserved for levels at L3 or above. Performing corpectomies via the mini transpsoas approach at L4 and L5 is not safe given the vascular and neural anatomy. Specifically, the increased retractor time needed to perform a corpectomy, including removal of the L4–L5 disc, precludes it from being a reproducibly safe operation for L4 fractures. At L5, the location of the major vessels and their branches as well as a high iliac crest prevent adequate exposure required to complete the required corpectomy safely via a mini-open lateral approach [17].

## *Anterior Column Reconstruction*

With the retractor in place, corpectomy and disc prep is the next step in the operation [10]. First, discectomies are performed cranial and caudal to the level of the burst fracture [10, 18]. The lateral annulus is incised in a rectangular fashion with a No. 15 blade [18]. A box osteotome, pituitary rongeur, cobb, and different angled curettes are then used to remove the intervening disc [15, 18]. While it is important to clear disc, it is also important to avoid disruption of the endplate to prevent future subsidence of the cage [11, 15]. Osteotomes are then used to remove the central vertebral body, leaving the anterior wall intact [11, 15, 18]. The posterior wall is left intact if there is no concern for neurological compromise; however, the posterior wall and the retropulsed fragments are removed if there are preoperative neurological deficits (Fig. 32.2) [11, 15].

The size of the vertebra and the degree of correction are then used to determine the size of the corresponding cage [15]. Options for reconstruction of the corpectomy defect include structural osseous graft and static versus expandable cages (titanium or PEEK) with circular or rectangular endplates [19, 20]. Expandable cages have gained popularity and are most commonly used now, as they allow one

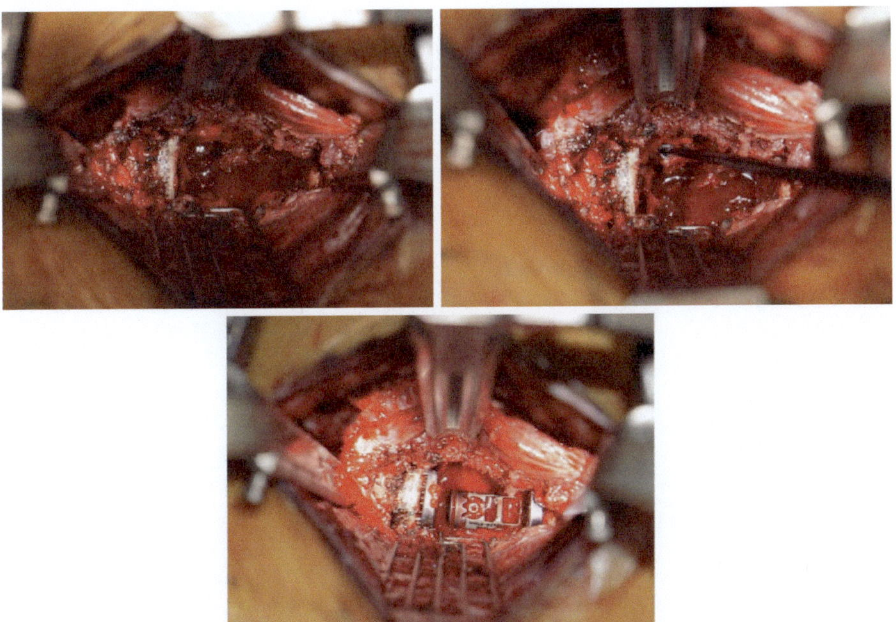

**Fig. 32.2** Intraoperative photos of (**a**) corpectomy completion with posterior wall and posterior longitudinal ligament (PLL) intact, (**b**) removal of PLL with curette, and (**c**) final anterior column reconstruction with expandable titanium cage

to fill the corpectomy defect and restore height and lordosis more adequately [21, 22]. However, expandable cages are potentially at higher rates of subsidence and catastrophic failure, especially when there is edge loading of a hyperlordotic cage [21, 23]. With respect to endplate shape, rectangular endplates have been found to provide more resistance to subsidence by creating more contact with the apophyseal ring compared to circular endplates [24–26]. After the cage or graft is placed, a plate can be placed on the lateral aspect of the vertebral body to create a more stable construct, or posterior percutaneous screws and rods can be placed to restore the posterior tension band (Fig. 32.3) [10, 12].

## Clinical Outcomes

The literature is rich with comparisons of outcomes of minimally invasive corpectomies with traditional open approaches. For example, Podet et al. compared 65 minimally invasive lateral corpectomies with 16 open lateral corpectomies and found that mini-open corpectomies had significantly shorter operative time (difference of 27 min) and a trend toward decreased estimated blood loss (EBL), although not statistically significant [11]. Similarly, in a comparison of 23

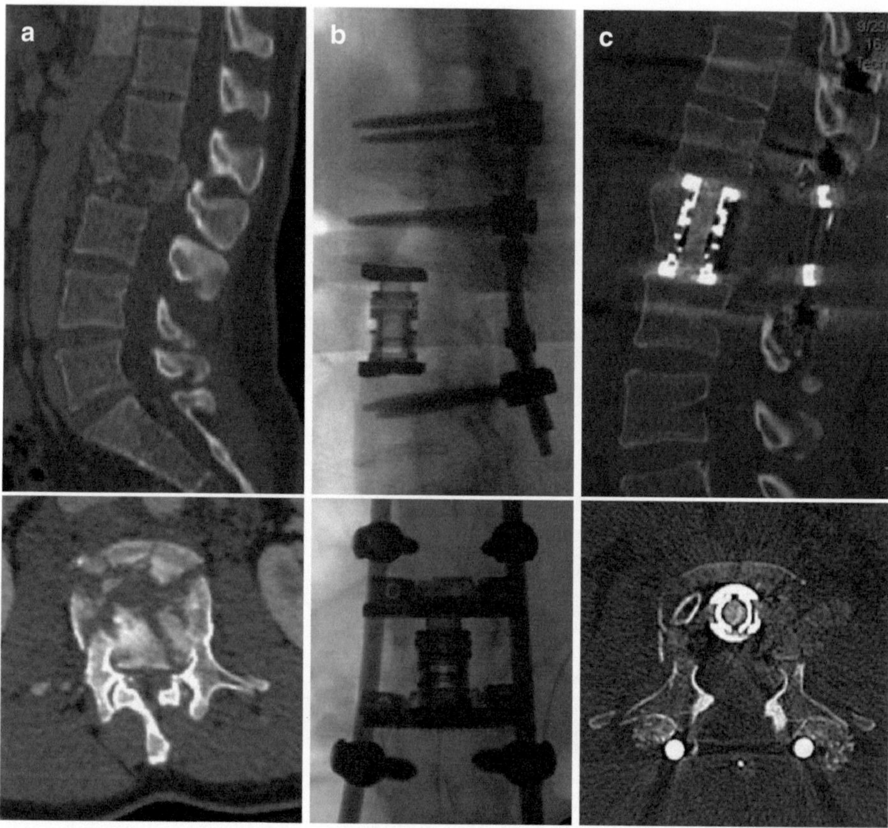

**Fig. 32.3** Preoperative CT scan of a L2 burst fracture (**a**) reconstructed with an expandable titanium cage with rectangular endplates via a mini-open lateral corpectomy as well as an open short-segment posterior fixation (**b**). Postoperative CT scan demonstrates restoration of lumbar lordosis as well as adequate neural decompression anteriorly and posteriorly (**c**)

mini-open lateral corpectomies and 43 open corpectomies, Sulaiman et al. found mini-open operations had 745 mL less EBL and shorter operative times (average 81 min) compared to open corpectomies, both of which were statistically significant [27].

With respect to length of stay, patients who undergo the mini-open approach have also been found to have decreased time spent in the hospital. One comparative study found the average length of stay for mini-open corpectomies to be 5 days shorter than patients who had undergone open lumbar corpectomies [27].

Mini-open lateral corpectomy has also been found to improve pain scores and physical and mental health outcomes. In a case series of 12 patients, Theologis et al. found that patients were satisfied with their outcomes, reporting an average Oswestry Disability Index (ODI) of 20, which was equivalent to minimal/moderate disability [15]. Additionally, these patients had improved physical component

(41.7% ± 10.4%) and mental health component (50.2% ± 11.6%) 12-item Short Form health Survey (SF-12) scores after surgery [15].

Patients with neurological compromise also have been found to improve significantly [10]. In a study of 52 patients undergoing mini-open lateral corpectomies, Smith et al. found that the American Spinal Injury Association (ASIA) Impairment Scale improved significantly at all time points postoperatively [10]. Another study examining outcomes of 16 patients who underwent acute or hyperacute lateral corpectomies for burst fractures found that 73% of patients achieved one ASIA grade improvement and 20% achieved 2 or more grade improvements [28].

Lastly, mortality associated with lateral corpectomies is reported as low in available literature [29, 30]. In a 20-patient case series of patients who underwent minimally invasive thoracolumbar corpectomy and spinal reconstruction, Le et al. reported three postoperative complications, including 1 (5%) mortality for urosepsis [30]. In a series of 25 patients, Khan et al. reported two mortalities (8%) for metastatic progression after lateral corpectomies [29].

In summary, while the reported total number of mini-open lateral corpectomies for thoracolumbar burst fractures is relatively low, the available data suggest that mini-open corpectomies for this indication lead to reduced blood loss, reduced length of stay, and improvements in ASIA grade and SF-12 physical and mental component self-reported outcome scores.

## Complications

The traditional open lateral corpectomy approach has been associated with a number of major complications, including vascular injury, peritoneal and/or bowel injury, postoperative ileus, superior hypogastric plexus disruption, retrograde ejaculation, ureter injury, and postoperative hernias [31]. Overall, it has been shown that the MIS lateral approach has significantly fewer of these specific complications and others compared to the traditional open approach [32]. Reported complication rates for the mini-open lateral approach range from 13.5% to 41% [11, 32–34].

### *Pleural Tears*

During the lateral approach, violation of the parietal lung pleura is sometimes necessary. In these cases, a chest tube is not needed, but a flat drain (Jackson-Pratt 7 mm) or red rubber catheter should be tunneled into the lateral aspect of the corpectomy cage for suction [10, 11]. If the visceral pleura is injured, a formal chest tube should be placed intraoperatively to avoid pneumothorax [11]. Although there is limited data available on rates of pneumothorax following the MIS lateral corpectomy approach, one study listed a complication rate for pneumothorax as 6.8% [11]. Additionally, hemothorax has been reported with a complication rate of 1.3% [32].

Pleural tears during MIS lateral corpectomy also led to sepsis and death after chest tube placement in one case study [30]. After all cases where the retropleural approach is utilized, serial chest radiographs and oxygen saturations should be followed to assess pulmonary function and detect any life-threatening situations (i.e., tension pneumothorax) [11].

## Dural Tear

One common complication of the MIS lateral corpectomy approach is a dural tear [35]. These most often arise iatrogenically but may also occur from the trauma itself in the case of a burst fracture [36]. In one study, it was cited as the most common complication, with a rate of 2.5% [32]. A tear in the dura of the spinal cord can cause CSF leakage, leading to further complications such as back pain, delayed healing, nerve injury, infection, and/or intracranial hypotension [37].

Dural tears are best managed with dural sutures, often using the running, locked technique [36, 38]. However, some locations, such as a ventral dural tear, can be difficult or impossible to manage with sutures due to their inaccessibility. When sutures are not an option, dural tears can be managed through grafting, including artificial dural grafts, autologous fat grafts, and fascia grafts [36, 38]. Additionally, a fibrin patch, intramural with epidural patch, fibrin glue, polyethylene glycol hydrogel sealant, or Gelfoam are sometimes used alone or in conjunction with other closure methods [36, 37].

## Neurological Complications

Neurological complications stem from trauma, infection, or iatrogenic causes. The most common postoperative neurological complications cited in literature are femoral and intercostal neuropathy [11, 15, 32, 34]. Neuralgia and numbness can resolve over time, but some patients suffer from lasting morbidity [34]. One study cited the complicate rate for intercostal neuropathy as 2.5% [32], while another study had a femoral neuropathy rate of 3.4% [11]. However, little research has focused on the complication rates for neurological complications, and many studies report no neurological complications [15, 33].

## Infection

Infection is a complication that can occur during trauma or iatrogenically. These can include infections originating from the posterior wound, chest, or paraspinal abscesses through iatrogenic contamination [11, 32]. Failure to appropriately identify or manage infection can lead to further complications such as delayed wound healing, sepsis, and death. Elderly and immunocompromised patients are especially at risk. One study identified the complication rate for infection after the MIS lateral approach as 1.3% [4].

## *Instrumentation*

Cited instrumentation complications for the MIS lateral corpectomy include cage subsidence and failure of fixation [11, 15, 34]. One study noted radiographic evidence of some cage subsidence in 13.5% of patients [15]; however, another study identified the complication rate for hardware failure as 1.3% [32].

## *Other Complications*

Other complications of the MIS lateral corpectomy approach include splenic hemorrhage, deep venous thrombosis, pulmonary embolism, pleural effusion, and inadequate decompression [11, 15].

## Conclusion

For thoracolumbar burst fractures that require anterior corpectomy to obtain stability and correction of deformity, a lateral approach is necessary to gain access to the zone of injury. Given this high morbidity associated with the traditional open lateral approach, mini-open lateral corpectomy may be utilized to minimize blood loss, case length, and length of stay and improve overall patient-reported outcomes.

## References


1. Scheer JK, Bakhsheshian J, Fakurnejad S, Oh T, Dahdaleh NS, Smith ZA. Evidence-based medicine of traumatic thoracolumbar burst fractures: a systematic review of operative management across 20 years. Glob Spine J. 2015;5(1):73–82. https://doi.org/10.1055/s-0034-1396047.
2. DeWald RL. Burst fractures of the thoracic and lumbar spine. Clin Orthop. 1984;189:150–61.
3. Gertzbein SD. Scoliosis Research Society: multicenter spine fracture study. Spine. 1992;17(5):528–40.
4. Magerl F, Aebi M, Gertzbein SD, Harms J, Nazarian S. A comprehensive classification of thoracic and lumbar injuries. Eur Spine J. 1994;3(4):184–201.
5. Gnanenthiran SR, Adie S, Harris IA. Nonoperative versus operative treatment for thoracolumbar burst fractures without neurologic deficit: a meta-analysis. Clin Orthop. 2012;470(2):567–77.

6. Siebenga J, Leferink VJM, Segers MJM, et al. Treatment of traumatic thoracolumbar spine fractures: a multicenter prospective randomized study of operative versus nonsurgical treatment. Spine. 2006;31(25):2881–90.

7. Rihn JA, Anderson DT, Harris E, et al. A review of the TLICS system: a novel, user-friendly thoracolumbar trauma classification system. Acta Orthop. 2008;79(4):461–6.

8. Dai L-Y, Jiang S-D, Wang X-Y, Jiang L-S. A review of the management of thoracolumbar burst fractures. Surg Neurol. 2007;67(3):221–31. discussion 231.

9. McCormack T, Karaikovic E, Gaines RW. The load sharing classification of spine fractures. Spine. 1994;19(15):1741–4.

10. Smith WD, Dakwar E, Le TV, Christian G, Serrano S, Uribe JS. Minimally invasive surgery for traumatic spinal pathologies: a mini-open, lateral approach in the thoracic and lumbar spine. Spine. 2010;35(26 Suppl):S338–46.

11. Podet AG, Morrow KD, Robichaux JM, Shields JA, DiGiorgio AM, Tender GC. Minimally invasive lateral corpectomy for thoracolumbar traumatic burst fractures. Neurosurg Focus. 2020;49(3):E12.

12. Hlubek RJ, Eastlack RK, Mundis GM. Transpsoas approach nuances. Neurosurg Clin N Am. 2018;29(3):407–17.

13. Kepler CK, Bogner EA, Herzog RJ, Huang RC. Anatomy of the psoas muscle and lumbar plexus with respect to the surgical approach for lateral transpsoas interbody fusion. Eur Spine J. 2011;20(4):550–6.

14. Ozgur BM, Aryan HE, Pimenta L, Taylor WR. Extreme lateral interbody fusion (XLIF): a novel surgical technique for anterior lumbar interbody fusion. Spine J. 2006;6(4):435–43. https://doi.org/10.1016/j.spinee.2005.08.012.

15. Theologis AA, Tabaraee E, Toogood P, et al. Anterior corpectomy via the mini-open, extreme lateral, transpsoas approach combined with short-segment posterior fixation for single-level traumatic lumbar burst fractures: analysis of health-related quality of life outcomes and patient satisfaction. J Neurosurg Spine. 2016;24(1):60–8.

16. Michael KW, Yoon TS. Operative techniques in spine surgery, vol. 4. 2nd ed. Philadelphia, PA: Lippincott Williams & Wilkins; 2016.

17. O'Brien J, Haines C, Dooley ZA, AWL T, Jackson D. Femoral nerve strain at L4-L5 is minimized by hip flexion and increased by table break when performing lateral interbody fusion. Spine. 2014;39(1):33–8.

18. Wiesel SW. Operative techniques in orthopaedic surgery, vol. 4. 2nd ed. Philadelphia, PA: Lippincott Williams & Wilkins; 2016.

19. Adkins DE, Sandhu FA, Voyadzis J-M. Minimally invasive lateral approach to the thoracolumbar junction for corpectomy. J Clin Neurosci. 2013;20(9):1289–94.

20. Walker CT, Xu DS, Godzik J, Turner JD, Uribe JS, Smith WD. Minimally invasive surgery for thoracolumbar spinal trauma. Ann Transl Med. 2018;6(6):102.

21. Pekmezci M, Tang JA, Cheng L, et al. Comparison of expandable and fixed interbody cages in a human cadaver Corpectomy model: fatigue characteristics. Clin Spine Surg. 2016;29(9):387–93.

22. Cappelletto B, Giorgiutti F, Balsano M. Evaluation of the effectiveness of expandable cages for reconstruction of the anterior column of the spine. J Orthop Surg. 2020;28(1):2309499019900472.

23. Pekmezci M, Tang JA, Cheng L, et al. Comparison of expandable and fixed interbody cages in a human cadaver corpectomy model, part I: endplate force characteristics: laboratory investigation. J Neurosurg Spine. 2012;17(4):321–6.

24. Mundis GM, Eastlack RK, Moazzaz P, Turner AWL, Cornwall GB. Contribution of round vs. rectangular expandable cage endcaps to spinal stability in a cadaveric Corpectomy model. Int J Spine Surg. 2015;9:53.

25. Deukmedjian AR, Manwaring J, Le TV, Turner AWL, Uribe JS. Corpectomy cage subsidence with rectangular versus round endcaps. J Clin Neurosci. 2014;21(9):1632–6.

26. Pekmezci M, McDonald E, Kennedy A, et al. Can a novel rectangular footplate provide higher resistance to subsidence than circular footplates? An ex vivo biomechanical study. Spine. 2012;37(19):E1177–81.
27. Sulaiman OAR, Garces J, Mathkour M, et al. Mini-open thoracolumbar Corpectomy: perioperative outcomes and hospital cost analysis compared with open Corpectomy. World Neurosurg. 2017;99:295–301.
28. Smith WD, Ghazarian N, Christian G. Acute and hyper-acute thoracolumbar Corpectomy for traumatic burst fractures using a mini-open lateral approach. Spine. 2018;43(2):E118–24.
29. Khan SN, Cha T, Hoskins JA, Pelton M, Singh K. Minimally invasive thoracolumbar corpectomy and reconstruction. Orthopedics. 2012;35(1):e74–9. https://doi.org/10.3928/01477447-20111122-04.
30. Le H, Barber J, Phan E, Hurley RK, Javidan Y. Minimally invasive lateral corpectomy of the thoracolumbar spine: a case series of 20 patients. Glob Spine J. 2020;12:29.
31. Hundal RS, Brooks NP, Williams SK. Lateral corpectomy and reconstruction for thoracolumbar burst fractures with neurological injury. Semin Spine Surg. 2021;33(1):100849. https://doi.org/10.1016/j.semss.2021.100849.
32. Baaj AA, Dakwar E, Le TV, et al. Complications of the mini-open anterolateral approach to the thoracolumbar spine. J Clin Neurosci. 2012;19(9):1265–7. https://doi.org/10.1016/j.jocn.2012.01.026.
33. Gandhoke GS, Tempel ZJ, Bonfield CM, Madhok R, Okonkwo DO, Kanter AS. Technical nuances of the minimally invasive extreme lateral approach to treat thoracolumbar burst fractures. Eur Spine J. 2015;24(Suppl 3):353–60. https://doi.org/10.1007/s00586-015-3880-7.
34. Yu JYH, Fridley J, Gokaslan Z, Telfeian A, Oyelese AA. Minimally invasive thoracolumbar Corpectomy and stabilization for unstable burst fractures using intraoperative computed tomography and computer-assisted spinal navigation. World Neurosurg. 2019;122:e1266–74. https://doi.org/10.1016/j.wneu.2018.11.027.
35. Nakashima H, Kanemura T, Satake K, et al. Lateral approach corpectomy and reconstruction after anterior longitudinal ligament release in cases with fixed kyphosis: a technical note and a preliminary case series. J Clin Neurosci. 2020;78:164–9. https://doi.org/10.1016/j.jocn.2020.04.084.
36. Bosacco SJ, Gardner MJ, Guille JT. Evaluation and treatment of dural tears in lumbar spine surgery: a review. Clin Orthop. 2001;389:238–47. https://doi.org/10.1097/00003086-200108000-00033.
37. Lee D-H, Kim K-T, Park J-I, Park K-S, Cho D-C, Sung J-K. Repair of inaccessible ventral Dural defect in thoracic spine: double layered Duraplasty. Korean J Spine. 2016;13(2):87–90. https://doi.org/10.14245/kjs.2016.13.2.87.
38. Cammisa FP, Girardi FP, Sangani PK, Parvataneni HK, Cadag S, Sandhu HS. Incidental durotomy in spine surgery. Spine. 2000;25(20):2663–7. https://doi.org/10.1097/00007632-200010150-00019.

# Chapter 33
# Access to L1–L2 and L2–L3

Karim A. Shafi, Junho Song, Brooks Martino, and Sheeraz A. Qureshi

## Introduction

Minimally invasive surgical (MIS) access to the upper lumbar segments (L1–L2, L2–L3) is largely limited to oblique (prepsoas) and lateral (transpsoas) approaches due to the presence of the great vessels anteriorly. Unlike the most caudal lumbar segments, in which mini-open anterior approaches are feasible, the L1–L2 and L2–L3 levels are more safely and effectively accessed via a lateral approach. Advantages of a minimally invasive lateral lumbar transpsoas approach include the ability to place large interbody grafts, preservation of the facet joints and posterior tension band, and approach execution without an access surgeon. Awareness of the position of the lumbar plexus at each segment is key to safe execution of this technique, and much prior research has been performed to establish safe working zones based on anatomic level. Similarly, patient positioning is critical to allow for optimal radiographic images intraoperatively and to minimize technical challenges with instrumentation.

K. A. Shafi · J. Song
Weill Cornell Medical College, New York, NY, USA

B. Martino
Department of Orthopaedic Surgery, Hospital for Special Surgery, New York, NY, USA

S. A. Qureshi (✉)
Weill Cornell Medical College, New York, NY, USA

Department of Orthopaedic Surgery, Hospital for Special Surgery, New York, NY, USA

© The Author(s), under exclusive license to Springer Nature
Switzerland AG 2023
J. R. O'Brien et al. (eds.), *Lumbar Spine Access Surgery*,
https://doi.org/10.1007/978-3-031-48034-8_33

# Anatomic Considerations of L1–L2 and L2–L3

A comprehensive and detailed understanding of the anatomy and biomechanics of the lumbar spine is crucial to treating its pathology in a safe and efficient manner.

## *Osseous Anatomy*

The upper lumbar vertebrae have several distinguishing features: the vertebral bodies are relatively large, and the width and anteroposterior diameter of the vertebral bodies progressively increase from L1 to L5. The lumbar spinous processes are relatively short and thick, and the laminae of the upper lumbar vertebrae are notable for their short and narrow morphology. The superior articular processes in the lumbar vertebrae are marked by the presence of mammillary processes on the posterior aspects. The zygapophyseal joints exhibit a parasagittal orientation in the upper lumbar segments and become more coronal toward the inferior lumbar segments.

The intervertebral discs are comprised of nucleus pulposus, annulus fibrosus, and cartilaginous end plates. The biomechanically important constituents of the discs include collagen fibers, elastin fibers, and aggrecan. The peripherally located annulus fibrosus receives innervation from the sinuvertebral nerve, a recurrent nerve originating from the ventral ramus. In the lumbar spine, the anterior disc height at a given level is normally greater than the posterior disc height, which is critical for the formation of lumbar lordosis. The anterior-posterior height difference is greatest between L4 and S1, which contributes 67% of the total lordosis. In contrast, the proximal lumbar segments contribute approximately 10% of overall lordosis each [1, 2].

## *Soft Tissue Anatomy*

The largest muscle in cross-sectional evaluation of the lumbar spine is the psoas major, a long fusiform muscle and key landmark in minimally invasive surgery (MIS) approaches to the lumbar spine. A thorough gross and radiographic understanding of this muscle is crucial in obtaining safe surgical access. This muscle has fibrous attachments to the transverse processes of T12-L4 and the lateral aspects of the interposed intervertebral discs. The fascicles of the psoas major are oriented inferolaterally and coalesce with the iliacus to form the iliopsoas tendon, which inserts on the lesser trochanter of the femur. From cranial to caudal, the diameter of the muscle increases linearly [3]. There can be variants of the iliopsoas tendon, with single, double, or triple tendon bundles. The psoas major is innervated by the ventral rami of L1–L4 and small branches from the femoral nerve. It has a complex arterial supply from collateral rami of lumbar arteries, the iliolumbar arteries, the circumflex iliac artery, the obturator artery, and the common femoral artery.

The diaphragm is a critical soft tissue structure to consider when approaching the thoracolumbar junction laterally. The diaphragm is a dome-shaped musculoaponeurotic structure with multiple fascial attachments: anterior/sternal, lateral/costal, and posterior/lumbar. The left and right crura of the diaphragm arise from the anterolateral surfaces of the upper lumbar vertebrae, L1–L3 on the right and L1–L2 on the left, overlapping the psoas major. The costal part of the diaphragm originates from the inner surface and upper margins of the 7th through 12th ribs. During quiet breathing, the diaphragm has approximately 2 cm of vertical motion, and it can descend up to nearly 10 cm with deep breathing [4]. Mobilization of the diaphragm is necessary for anterolateral access to the thoracolumbar junction. In the minimally invasive lateral approach, the diaphragm may be reflected anteriorly once the costal and lumbar attachments have been mobilized. To avoid iatrogenic injury to the diaphragm and pleura during the lateral approach to the upper lumbar vertebrae, spinal surgeons must consider the variations of diaphragm attachments at the midaxillary line and vertebral bodies [5].

The anterior longitudinal ligament (ALL) is a component of the anterior column of the spine which traverses the anterior aspect of all vertebral bodies and intervertebral discs. It is thicker and narrower over the vertebral bodies and thinner and wider over the intervertebral discs. The ALL reinforces the intervertebral discs and limits spine extension. In lateral access surgery, the ALL can be released in order to improve mobility of the lumbar segments, allowing for restoration of lordosis. ALL release must be performed carefully with awareness of the close proximity to the great vessels and sympathetic plexus, found intimately along its anterior aspect [6].

## Neurovascular Anatomy

The surgical corridor of the lateral transpsoas approach risks injury to the lumbar plexus which is embedded within the psoas major (Fig. 33.1). The lumbar plexus is located anteriorly to the transverse processes and is formed by the ventral rami of L1–L4 and contributions of the subcostal nerve (T12). Nerves arising from the lumbar plexus, from superior to inferior, include iliohypogastric (T12, L1), ilioinguinal (L1), genitofemoral (L1, L2), lateral femoral cutaneous (L2, L3), femoral (L2, L3, L4), and obturator nerves (L2, L3, L4) [7] (Table 33.1). Injury to the lumbar plexus can occur in the lateral transpsoas approach secondary to mechanical compression, laceration, stretch, or indirect ischemia [8, 9].

The subcostal nerve originates from the T12 root and accompanies the subcostal vessels along the inferior border of the 12th rib. The iliohypogastric nerve arises from T12-L1 nerve roots, while the ilioinguinal nerve arises from the L1 root. The subcostal, iliohypogastric, and ilioinguinal nerves innervate the anterior abdominal wall musculature while traversing between the transversus abdominis and internal oblique before terminating as anterior cutaneous sensory branches. The genitofemoral nerve originates from the L1–L2 roots, traverses obliquely through the psoas major, and courses superficially over the muscle. The nerve then reaches the

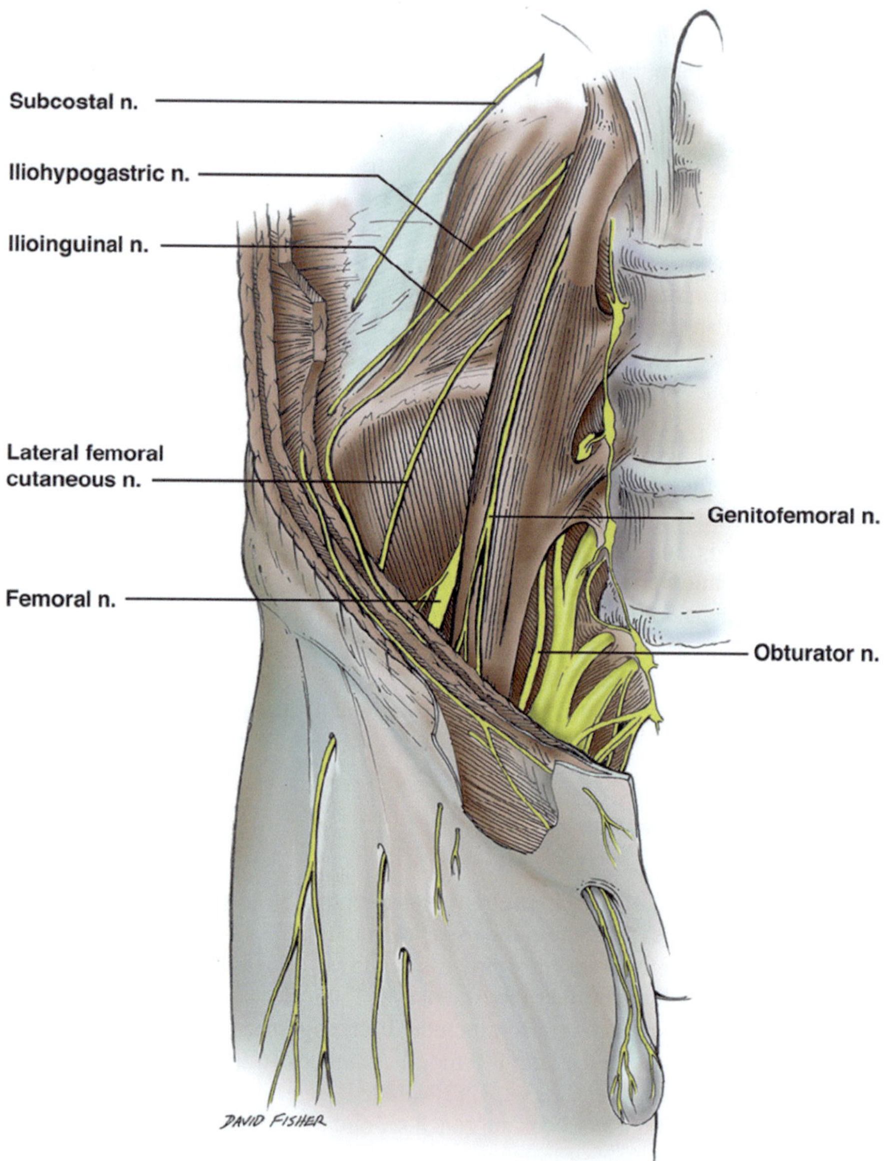


**Fig. 33.1** Schematic drawing of the anterior view of the lumbar plexus in relation to the psoas major muscle. (Tubbs RI, Gabel B, Jeyamohan S, Moisi M, Chapman JR, Hanscom RD, Loukas M, Oskouian RJ, Tubbs RS. Relationship of the lumbar plexus branches to the lumbar spine: anatomical study with application to lateral approaches. Spine J. 2017 Jul;17 (7):1012–1016. doi: 10.1016/j.spinee.2017.03.011. Epub 2017 Mar 30. PMID: 28365495)

**Table 33.1** Nerves of the lumbar plexus. Uribe JS, Arredondo N, Dakwar E, Vale FL. Defining the safe working zones using the minimally invasive lateral retroperitoneal transpsoas approach: an anatomical study. J Neurosurg Spine. 2010 Aug;13(2):260-6. doi: 10.3171/2010.3.SPINE09766. PMID: 20672964

| Nerve | Segment | Innervated Muscles | Cutaneous Branches |
| --- | --- | --- | --- |
| iliohypogastric | T12–L1 | • transversus abdominus<br>• abdominal internal oblique | • anterior cutaneous<br>• lateral cutaneous |
| ilioinguinal | L-1 | | • anterior scrotal nerves in males<br>• anterior labial nerves in females |
| genitofemoral | L1–2 | • cremaster in males | • femoral ramus<br>• genital ramus |
| lateral femoral cutaneous | L2–3 | | • lateral femoral cutaneous |
| obturator | L2–4 | • obturator externus<br>• adductor longus<br>• gracilis<br>• pectineus<br>• adductor magnus | • cutaneous ramus |
| femoral | L2–4 | • iliopsoas<br>• pectineus<br>• sartorius<br>• quadriceps femoris | • anterior cutaneous branches<br>• saphenous |
| short, direct muscular branches | T12–L4 | • psoas major<br>• quadratus lumborum<br>• iliacus<br>• lumbar intertransverse | |

transversalis fascia to enter the abdominal wall around the inguinal ring. The genitofemoral nerve can be injured during sequential dilation with a transpsoas approach, especially in the upper lumbar segments (Fig. 33.2). Given that this is a primary sensory nerve, it will not be detected via intraoperative electromyography unless the cremasteric muscle in males is also monitored [10]. The lateral femoral cutaneous nerve usually arises from the posterior divisions of L2 and L3 and emerges from the lateral border of the psoas major. It crosses the iliacus toward the anterior superior iliac spine to innervate the skin of the lateral thigh. The femoral nerve is the largest branch of the lumbar plexus and is derived from the L2–L4 spinal nerves. It passes through the psoas major and travels laterally before coursing deep to the inguinal ligament. The obturator nerve arises from L2–L4 ventral rami, descends through the psoas major, and emerges from its medial border at the pelvic brim to exit via the obturator foramen to innervate the medial compartment of the thigh [11].

The aorta descends along the left anterior aspect of the lumbar vertebrae. The paravertebral sympathetic chain is also found along the aorta and lies anterior to the vertebral bodies and extends inferiorly beyond the aortic bifurcation to form the superior hypogastric plexus. The inferior vena cava (IVC) descends along the right anterior aspect of lumbar vertebrae. The aorta and IVC are positioned more posteriorly on the lateral disc space as they progress inferiorly toward their bifurcation into the iliac vessels at L4–L5 levels. The IVC is situated more posteriorly compared to the aorta and has been suggested to be at higher risk of injury during the lateral

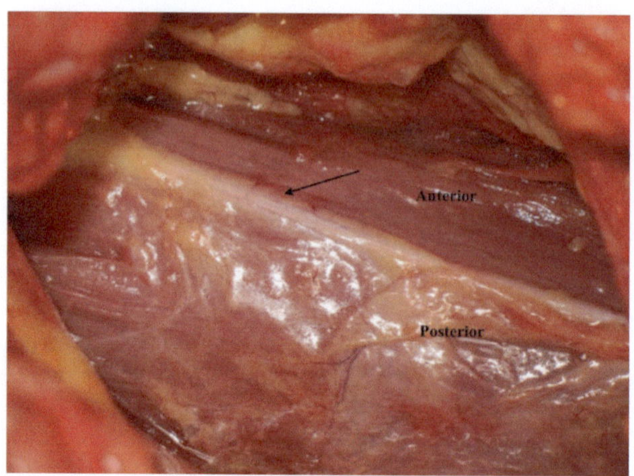


**Fig. 33.2** Genitofemoral nerve identified overlying the anterior third of the psoas musculature. *Arrow*, genitofemoral nerve. (Banagan K, Gelb D, Poelstra K, Ludwig S. Anatomic mapping of lumbar nerve roots during a direct lateral transpsoas approach to the spine: a cadaveric study. Spine (Phila Pa 1976). 2011 May 15;36 (11):E687–91. doi: 10.1097/BRS.0b013e3181ec5911. PMID: 21217450)

transpsoas approach [12]. At L1–L2 and L2–L3 segments, most individuals have a retroperitoneal fat plane providing padding to the IVC, which may reduce the risk of injury to the vessel when performing ALL release [13]. In addition to the great vessels, lumbar segmental arteries at each level arise directly from the aorta and run posterolaterally on the vertebral bodies, passing under the sympathetic trunks into the spaces between transverse processes. Anatomical variations in the lumbar arteries and veins must be considered to prevent iatrogenic vascular injury, and preoperative evaluation of the location of the major vessels is critical for operative success [14].

## *Urological Anatomy*

The kidneys are located lateral to the psoas major, with their superior border typically located at the level of the T12 vertebra and inferior border near the L3–L4 disc space. In the retroperitoneal space, the ureters are located lateral to the psoas major and anterior to the quadratus lumborum muscle and are therefore vulnerable to injury during the transpsoas approach. Although rare, the risk of injury to the kidney or ureter during the lateral transpsoas approach is greatest at the upper lumbar levels, where the distance between the kidney and the intervertebral disc space is shortest. The risk can also be heightened in the presence of anatomic variants or pathology involving the kidney or ureter [15, 16].

## *Other Anatomical Considerations*

The presence of degenerative or idiopathic scoliosis must be identified and assessed when performing MIS approaches. Scoliosis has been shown to be associated with a significantly higher incidence of vascular variants in the lumbar region [13, 17]. Axial rotation of the spine may shift the great vessels more posteriorly on the concave side of the deformity, increasing the risk of injury to the great vessels. In addition, patients with intersegmental Cobb angles greater than 14.5° have been shown to be at an increased risk of injury to the lumbar segmental artery on the concave side during the transpsoas approach [18]. Scoliosis has also been shown to be associated with a significantly higher incidence of vascular variants in the lumbar region, almost always occurring ipsilaterally to the convexity of the spine [13, 17].

Another important anatomical consideration in lateral access surgery is the presence of retroperitoneal scarring, which may be idiopathic or secondary to surgery, medication, malignancy, or infection. Fibro-inflammatory tissue in the retroperitoneum can surround the vasculature and envelop the neighboring structures, disrupting the normal anatomy. Therefore, bilateral retroperitoneal scarring may be considered a relative contraindication to the lateral approach to the spine.

## Lateral/Transpsoas Approach to L1–L2 and L2–L3

Since the 1990s, the lateral approach has gained increasing popularity as a means of obtaining extraperitoneal/retroperitoneal access to the lumbar spine. Surgeons have been drawn to the advantages of this MIS approach, including preservation of the posterior tension band and the ability to restore/increase physiologic lordosis and perform indirect decompression of the neural elements via placement of larger interbody devices. Patients have similarly benefitted from the decreased postoperative pain scores, shorter hospital stays, and favorable clinical outcomes associated with this approach when compared to traditional, open posterior procedures [3, 10, 19–21].

Initially performed using transperitoneal laparoscopy requiring insufflation and retraction of the peritoneum and abdominal contents, the lateral approach has since evolved into a mini-open/open retroperitoneal, transpsoas approach secondary to advances in neuromonitoring and instrumentation [19, 22]. In 2006, Ogzur et al. described the modern minimally invasive lateral interbody fusion (LLIF), though the nomenclature of this technique varies secondary to proprietary rights with placement of commercially available interbody devices [19]. This procedure provides lateral access to single or multiple levels from L1 to L4, limited cranially by the presence of the pleural cavity and caudally by the iliac crest. Indications for LLIF are extensive, including degenerative disc disease, adjacent segment disease in the setting of prior surgery, degenerative spondylolisthesis, and complex degenerative coronal plane deformities.

The modern lateral approach utilizes a retroperitoneal corridor through a muscle-splitting technique of the psoas major, providing direct access to the lateral spine (Fig. 33.3). Following superficial dissection through the internal oblique, external oblique, and transversus abdominus, the retroperitoneal space is entered, and the abdominal contents are retracted anteriorly. Blunt digital dissection is then performed until the quadratus lumborum is encountered, and the transverse process can be palpated anteriorly. The psoas is then palpated medially to the transverse process. Special consideration must be made when performing a lateral approach to the L1–L2 segment, given the anatomy of the pleural cavity and diaphragm. Preoperative imaging must be studied to evaluate the relationship of thoracic contents to the L1–L2 disc space. At this level, a lateral approach may require maneuvering around or partial resection of the 12th rib. This should be performed along the posterior aspect of the rib in order to preserve anterior intercostal and soft tissue attachments.

Successful completion of this approach hinges on blunt dissection through the iliopsoas with identification and posterior retraction of the lumbar plexus. Advances in neuromonitoring probes and expandable tubular retractors, in conjunction with

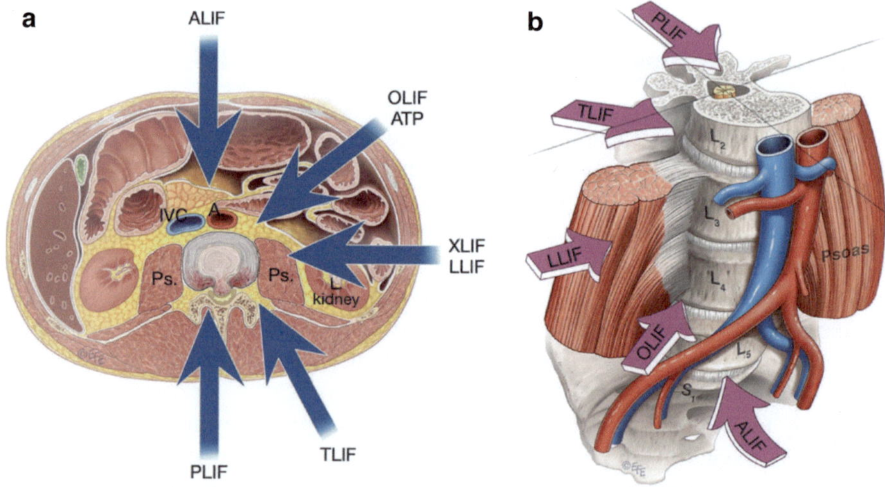


**Fig. 33.3** (**a**) Five primary approaches to the lumbar spine for interbody fusion techniques: anterior (ALIF), lateral or extreme lateral interbody fusion (LLIF or XLIF), oblique lumbar interbody fusion/anterior to psoas (OLIF/ATP), transforaminal (TLIF or MI-TLIF), and posterior (PLIF). (**b**) Surgical approaches to the lumbar spine for interbody fusion techniques: anatomy of the psoas and anterior vasculature determines approach at various levels. (Mobbs RJ, Phan K, Malham G, Seex K, Rao PJ. Lumbar interbody fusion: techniques, indications and comparison of interbody fusion options including PLIF, TLIF, MI-TLIF, OLIF/ATP, LLIF and ALIF. J Spine Surg. 2015 Dec;1 (1):2–18. doi: 10.3978/j.issn.2414-469X.2015.10.05. PMID: 27683674; PMCID: PMC5039869)

further studies of the anatomy of the lumbar plexus, have spurred utilization of this approach over the past two decades. A landmark paper by Uribe et al. defined safe working corridors when utilizing this approach. The authors performed anatomic and radiographic analysis of five cadaveric specimens (20 lumbar segments) and identified 4 working zones within the lumbar vertebral bodies (VB): Zone I (anterior quarter), Zone II (middle anterior quarter), Zone III (posterior middle quarter), and Zone IV (posterior quarter) [10] (Fig. 33.4). Based on their analysis, the safe anatomic corridor at L1–L2, L2–L3, and L3–L4 is the midpoint of Zone II (middle posterior quarter of the VB). Of note, the genitofemoral nerve, which traverses the anterior aspect of the psoas muscle, is at risk for direct injury in Zone II (middle anterior quarter) with placement of sequential dilators (Fig. 33.2).

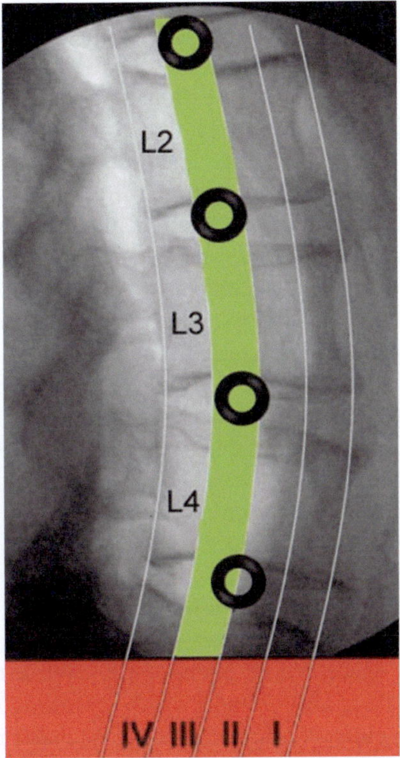


**Fig. 33.4** Lateral radiograph of the lumbar spine demonstrating the division of the vertebral bodies into four zones (Zones I–IV) from anterior to posterior. The relative "safe zone" (Zone III) depicted in green. The recommended safe working zones to prevent direct nerve injury are indicated with black circles at each level. (Uribe JS, Arredondo N, Dakwar E, Vale FL. Defining the safe working zones using the minimally invasive lateral retroperitoneal transpsoas approach: an anatomical study. J Neurosurg Spine. 2010 Aug;13 (2):260–6. doi: 10.3171/2010.3.SPINE09766. PMID: 20672964)

## *Patient Positioning: Prone Versus Lateral Decubitus*

Traditionally, the patient is placed in a 90° lateral decubitus position on a radiolucent operating table, with the iliac crest in line with the table break. The axillary neurovascular structures are protected with an axillary roll, and padding is placed between the arms and legs and the table to prevent peripheral nerve compression. The hip is flexed slightly, thereby relaxing the psoas muscle and the femoral nerve within the muscle belly. The patient is then secured to the operating room table, and slight flexion is applied through the table break, thereby opening the space between the iliac crest and the lowest rib, as well as the disc space, on the operative side. Lateral fluoroscopy is then used to confirm appropriate imaging. It is crucial that both the patient and C-arm remain in their respective orientations throughout the duration of the procedure to ensure precise working corridors when exposing and accessing the disc space.

One of the more notable limitations with LLIF is the need for intraoperative repositioning from the lateral to prone position when performing same surgery adjunct posterior decompression and instrumentation. Prior studies have demonstrated an increase of 30–200 min of additional operative time with repositioning, subsequently resulting in increased time under anesthesia and healthcare resource utilization [23–25]. The use of single-position lateral surgery, performing both LLIF and posterior open versus percutaneous fixation and/or decompression in the lateral decubitus position, was introduced as a means of performing LLIF via a more streamlined workflow. However, placement of "downsided" pedicle screws in the lateral position and accurate fluoroscopic image interpretation provide novel technical challenges with single-position lateral decubitus surgery.

More recently, single-position prone lateral (PL) or prone transpsoas (PTP) surgery has been introduced to mitigate these limitations. While similarly avoiding the need for intraoperative repositioning, this technique has several additional potential advantages. Proponents of the PTP technique have suggested both improved operative workflow and increased disc space lordosis with traditional prone positioning [26]. Additionally, the lateral working corridor is thought to be increased in the prone position, as hip extension and subsequent psoas major extension should pull the lumbar plexus more posteriorly [27]. In support of this hypothesis, a cadaveric study by Alluri et al. demonstrated consistent posterior translation of the femoral nerve at the L4–L5 disc space and L5 endplate [25]. While the working corridor is considered most favorable at L1–L2 and L2–L3, a working knowledge of the position of the plexus with either the hips flexed or extended is essential in order to perform a safe transpsoas approach. Please see Chapter 30 for additional information.

## **Anterior Approach to L1–L2 and L2–L3**

The utility of an open, direct anterior approach to L1–L2 and L2–L3 is limited by the proximity of the abdominal aorta and inferior vena cava as noted above. However, anterior retroperitoneal access to the upper lumbar segments is feasible via an oblique or pre-transpsoas approach (i.e., oblique lateral interbody fusion (OLIF)). This approach utilizes the natural corridor between the abdominal aorta and psoas muscle on the left or the IVC and psoas muscle on the right. Proponents of this approach note that blunt dissection through the psoas and subsequent risk of lumbar plexus injury are avoided, though the risk of major vascular injury is increased [28–30].

The ability to perform a prepsoas approach is dependent on each patient's unique anatomy, though prior gross specimen and magnetic resonance imaging (MRI) analysis have demonstrated this corridor to be present in 90–100% of individuals (Fig. 33.5) [29, 31]. Molinares et al. demonstrated a mean distance of 16.04 ± 5.83 mm from the lateral border of the aorta to the anterior border of the psoas muscle at the

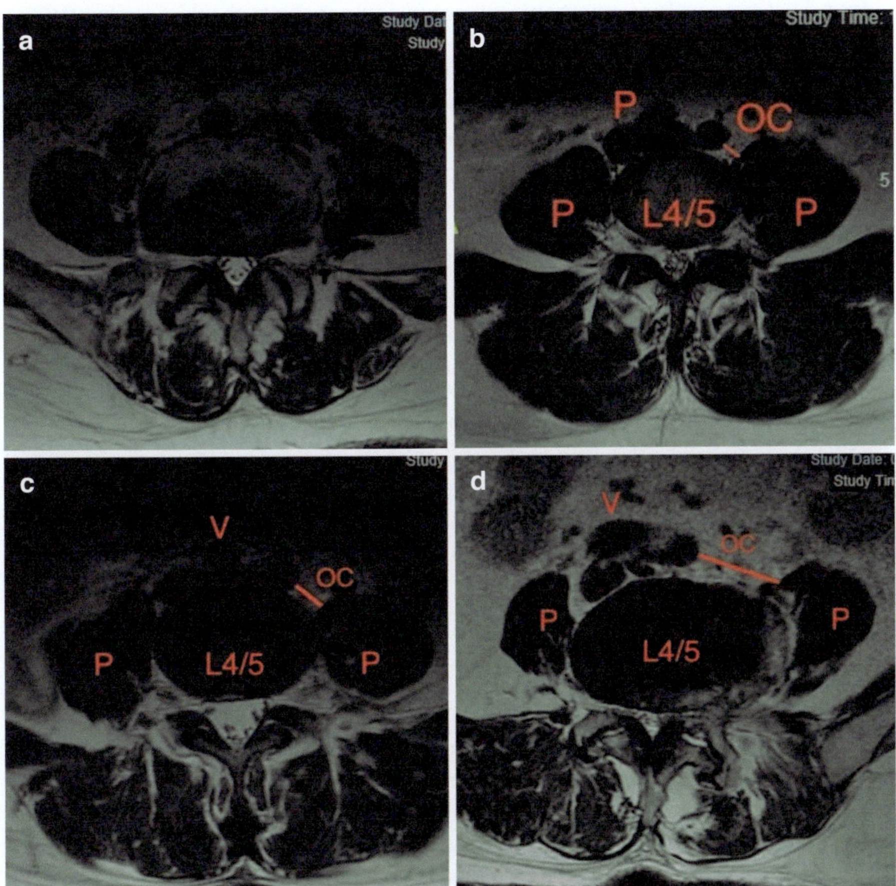

**Fig. 33.5** Axial magnetic resonance images of the L4–L5 disc level showing (**a**) OC grade 0, that is, no measurable corridor, (**b**) OC grade 1, (**c**) OC grade 2, and (**d**) OC grade 3; *V* vessel, *P* psoas, *L4/L5* L4/L5 disc. OC indicates oblique corridor. (Ng JP, Kaliya-Perumal AK, Tandon AA, Oh JY. The Oblique Corridor at L4-L5: A Radiographic-Anatomical Study Into the Feasibility for Lateral Interbody Fusion. Spine (Phila Pa 1976). 2020 May 15;45 (10):E552-E559. doi: 10.1097/BRS.0000000000003346. Erratum in: Spine (Phila Pa 1976). 2020 Aug 1;45 (15):E977. PMID: 31770312)

L2–L3 disc space based on MRI analysis. Similarly, Zhang et al. noted a mean distance of 15.53 ± 2.87 mm at L1–L2 and 13.49 ± 3.52 mm at L2–L3 in the supine position [32]. Of note, the authors demonstrated a reduction in the size of the corridor when analyzed in the right lateral decubitus position from 11.95 ± 3.41 mm to 9.56 ± 3.13 mm. Similarly, several studies have demonstrated the corridor to be largest at the most proximal lumbar segments and decreasing progressively at each lower level [29, 31–33]. However, the presence of the kidney, the renal vasculature, or the liver (if a right-sided approach is selected) may preclude this approach. Similarly, large proximal psoas muscle bulk abutting the aorta may limit this approach. As such, preoperative MRI analysis of each patient's individual soft tissue, vascular, and visceral anatomy is essential.

Typically, a left-sided approach is preferred as the tunica media of the aorta provides robust support for retractor placement in comparison to the thin-walled IVC. A right-sided approach may be used if a prior left-sided approach has been utilized or if significant coronal plane deformity precludes a traditional approach. The patient is positioned in either the supine or lateral decubitus position with the table break and kidney bolster placed directly below the level of interest to allow lateral extension of the given disc space, although this is dependent on surgeon preference. Access to L2–L3 typically requires more trunk rotation, with the patient positioned nearly perpendicular to the table. The superficial dissection is similar to the transpsoas approach, requiring identification of the abdominal wall musculature and transversalis fascia via an oblique lateral incision. Once inside the retroperitoneal cavity, blunt finger dissection is carried out along the internal aspect of the posterior abdominal wall down to the palpable bulk of the psoas muscle. The peritoneum is then swept ventrally off the psoas. The abdominal aorta is then palpated anteriorly, and retractor is slid posterior to the surgeon's finger and anterior to the psoas. A Kittner or peanut-tip dissector may be used to further develop this corridor. Of note, both the ureter and sympathetic chain are in proximity of this corridor and should be retracted anteriorly with the aorta. Commercially available self-retaining retractors and sequential dilators may then be placed per surgeon preference to help complete exposure.

## Complications

The transpsoas approach to the upper lumbar segments carries the risk of direct or traction-related trauma to the psoas major muscle and, more significantly, the lumbar plexus within (genitofemoral, femoral obturator, and lateral femoral cutaneous nerves). Prolonged retraction of these structures eventually leads to axonotmesis or neurotmesis. This may manifest as transient or lasting muscle soreness, dysesthesia/paresthesia, sensory changes, or hip flexor weakness. Rates as high as 75% of postoperative sensory changes have been reported. Prior studies have suggested that LLIF at the L2–L3 level was associated with a high incidence of postoperative anterior thigh paresthesia, thought to be secondary to the close proximity of the genitofemoral and lateral femoral cutaneous nerves at this level [34]. Injury to the femoral nerve is perhaps the most feared complication, resulting in lasting quadriceps weakness and atrophy. The exact rate of femoral nerve injury remains unknown, though rates of 3.4–23.7% of motor nerve injuries have been reported [35–37]. Although the risk of femoral nerve injury is thought to be low at L1–L2 and L2–L3 given its posterior location at these segments, surgeons must remain vigilant with regard to the direction and time of their retraction [30, 38]. While advances in neuromonitoring have helped mitigate risk, patients should be counseled extensively about the possibility of these adverse effects.

One of the most life-threatening complications in anterior or lateral approaches to the spine is major vascular injury. The incidence of major vascular injury is low, reportedly ranging from 0.1 to 0.4% [30, 39]. Injury to these vessels is less of a concern with the transpsoas approach. In theory, a left-sided transpsoas approach to the proximal lumbar segments may be safest as the vena cava is typically positioned more posteriorly relative to the aorta. There is a markedly elevated risk of vascular injury in the transpsoas approach when an anterior column release is performed, which adds to the overall technical difficulty of the procedure. Another risk factor for major vascular injury is degenerative scoliosis, in which the axial rotation of the spine can shift the aorta and vena cava more posteriorly on the concave aspect of the deformity [40].

Injury to the kidney or ureter is another rare but possible complication with anterior or lateral approaches to the upper lumbar spine. Several case reports and series have described the possibility of urological injury with an oblique approach [41, 42]. The incidence with a transpsoas approach has been described to be between 0.0 and 0.9% [43]. The kidney is in closest proximity to the operative field at the L1–L2 level. The risk of injury to the ureter is greatest at the L2–L3 level. At the upper lumbar segments, tubular retractors can overlap the ureter, predisposing injury [31]. Ureteral injury must be considered when a patient perioperatively experiences hematuria or nonspecific signs and symptoms, such as distention, pain, fever emesis, or ileus. Although not widely utilized, preoperative dual-phase contrast-enhanced computed tomography is a precautionary measure that may help avoid this complication and may be indicated in patients at elevated risk of urologic injury, such as those with known anatomical variants, which are often associated with aberrant renal vasculature. As such, preoperative imaging must be scrutinized for any low-lying renal substance or vasculature that may impede either a prepsoas or a transpsoas approach at the upper lumbar levels.

Bowel injury is another severe complication possible with lateral or anterior approaches to the spine. With oblique or lateral approaches to the spine, the peritoneum and bowel contents are mobilized anteriorly. Peritoneal laceration can occur with excessive retraction during disc space exposure. Bowel perforation is also a risk with these approaches, although its exact incidence is unknown. The risk of injury to the colon with a transpsoas approach is described to be the highest at the L2–L3 and L3–L4 levels. During removal of the retractor, the surgical area must be meticulously inspected to ensure that no injury to the bowel or peritoneum has occurred. Early recognition of acute abdominal symptoms is critical for avoiding potentially fatal outcomes of bowel perforation. Delayed presentation of visceral injury can occur, especially in the setting of a retroperitoneal leak with contained abscess formation. In addition to direct peritoneal or bowel injury, patients can also experience postoperative ileus secondary to prolonged retraction of the peritoneal contents to access the retroperitoneal space.

Lastly, abdominal pseudohernia may occur secondary to injury to the iliohypogastric, ilioinguinal, or genitofemoral nerves, which causes local ipsilateral paresis of the abdominal wall musculature. This complication is thought to occur secondarily to errant superficial dissection through the abdominal musculature, though its exact incidence is unknown [17, 30, 44]. Patients typically present with an abdominal "bulge" as well as pain, paresthesia, or other sensory changes. The differential diagnosis includes an incisional hernia, thought to occur at a rate of approximately 1%.

## Conclusion

Access to L1–L2 and L2–L3 may be performed safely via a transpsoas or prepsoas approach, with each offering unique advantages and risks. While the transpsoas approach offers an orthogonal trajectory to the vertebral body and avoids critical anterior vascular and visceral structures, retraction of the lumbar plexus poses a significant risk for postoperative transient or lasting sensory and/or motor changes. In contrast, the prepsoas approach avoids risk lumbar plexus via an anatomic corridor between the aorta/IVC and psoas, though major vascular injury risk is increased. In sum, approach selection depends both on patients' unique anatomy and surgeon preference, though a working knowledge of both approaches should be within a spine surgeon's armamentarium.

## References


1. Saadeh YS, Joseph JR, Smith BW, Kirsch MJ, Sabbagh AM, Park P. Comparison of segmental lordosis and global spinopelvic alignment after single-level lateral lumbar interbody fusion or Transforaminal lumbar interbody fusion. World Neurosurg. 2019;126:e1374–8. https://doi.org/10.1016/j.wneu.2019.03.106.
2. Roussouly P, Gollogly S, Berthonnaud E, Dimnet J. Classification of the normal variation in the sagittal alignment of the human lumbar spine and pelvis in the standing position. Spine (Phila Pa 1976). 2005;30(3):346–53. https://doi.org/10.1097/01.brs.0000152379.54463.65.
3. Verma R, Virk S, Qureshi S. Interbody fusions in the lumbar spine: a review. HSS J. 2020;16(2):162–7. https://doi.org/10.1007/s11420-019-09737-4.
4. Boussuges A, Gole Y, Blanc P. Diaphragmatic motion studied by m-mode ultrasonography: methods, reproducibility, and normal values. Chest. 2009;135(2):391–400. https://doi.org/10.1378/chest.08-1541.
5. Baaj AA, Papadimitriou K, Amin AG, Kretzer RM, Wolinsky J-P, Gokaslan ZL. Surgical anatomy of the diaphragm in the anterolateral approach to the spine: a cadaveric study. J Spinal Disord Tech. 2014;27(4):220–3. https://doi.org/10.1097/BSD.0b013e3182a18125.
6. Beckman JM, Marengo N, Murray G, Bach K, Uribe JS. Anterior longitudinal ligament release from the minimally invasive lateral retroperitoneal Transpsoas approach: techni-

cal note. Oper Neurosurg (Hagerstown). 2016;12(3):214–21. https://doi.org/10.1227/NEU.0000000000001203.

7. Abel NA, Januszewski J, Vivas AC, Uribe JS. Femoral nerve and lumbar plexus injury after minimally invasive lateral retroperitoneal transpsoas approach: electrodiagnostic prognostic indicators and a roadmap to recovery. Neurosurg Rev. 2018;41(2):457–64. https://doi.org/10.1007/s10143-017-0863-7.

8. Regev GJ, Kim CW. Safety and the anatomy of the retroperitoneal lateral corridor with respect to the minimally invasive lateral lumbar intervertebral fusion approach. Neurosurg Clin N Am. 2014;25(2):211–8. https://doi.org/10.1016/j.nec.2013.12.001.

9. Pumberger M, Hughes AP, Huang RR, Sama AA, Cammisa FP, Girardi FP. Neurologic deficit following lateral lumbar interbody fusion. Eur spine J. 2012;21(6):1192–9. https://doi.org/10.1007/s00586-011-2087-9.

10. Uribe JS, Arredondo N, Dakwar E, Vale FL. Defining the safe working zones using the minimally invasive lateral retroperitoneal transpsoas approach: an anatomical study. J Neurosurg Spine. 2010;13(2):260–6. https://doi.org/10.3171/2010.3.SPINE09766.

11. Tubbs RI, Gabel B, Jeyamohan S, et al. Relationship of the lumbar plexus branches to the lumbar spine: anatomical study with application to lateral approaches. Spine J. 2017;17(7):1012–6. https://doi.org/10.1016/j.spinee.2017.03.011.

12. Kepler CK, Bogner EA, Herzog RJ, Huang RC. Anatomy of the psoas muscle and lumbar plexus with respect to the surgical approach for lateral transpsoas interbody fusion. Eur Spine J. 2011;20(4):550–6. https://doi.org/10.1007/s00586-010-1593-5.

13. Mai HT, Schneider AD, Alvarez AP, et al. Anatomic considerations in the lateral Transpsoas interbody fusion: the impact of age, sex, BMI, and scoliosis. Clin Spine Surg. 2019;32(5):215–21. https://doi.org/10.1097/BSD.0000000000000760.

14. Alkadhim M, Zoccali C, Abbasifard S, et al. The surgical vascular anatomy of the minimally invasive lateral lumbar interbody approach: a cadaveric and radiographic analysis. Eur spine J. 2015;24(Suppl 7):906–11. https://doi.org/10.1007/s00586-015-4267-5.

15. Voin V, Kirkpatrick C, Alonso F, et al. Lateral Transpsoas approach to the lumbar spine and relationship of the ureter: anatomic study with application to minimizing complications. World Neurosurg. 2017;104:674–8. https://doi.org/10.1016/j.wneu.2017.05.062.

16. Anand N, Baron EM. Urological injury as a complication of the transpsoas approach for discectomy and interbody fusion. J Neurosurg Spine. 2013;18(1):18–23. https://doi.org/10.3171/2012.9.SPINE12659.

17. Dakwar E, Cardona RF, Smith DA, Uribe JS. Early outcomes and safety of the minimally invasive, lateral retroperitoneal transpsoas approach for adult degenerative scoliosis. Neurosurg Focus. 2010;28(3):E8. https://doi.org/10.3171/2010.1.FOCUS09282.

18. Takata Y, Sakai T, Tezuka F, et al. Risk assessment of lumbar segmental artery injury during lateral Transpsoas approach in the patients with lumbar scoliosis. Spine (Phila Pa 1976). 2016;41(10):880–4. https://doi.org/10.1097/BRS.0000000000001362.

19. Ozgur BM, Aryan HE, Pimenta L, Taylor WR. Extreme lateral interbody fusion (XLIF): a novel surgical technique for anterior lumbar interbody fusion. Spine J. 2006;6(4):435–43. https://doi.org/10.1016/j.spinee.2005.08.012.

20. Mobbs RJ, Phan K, Malham G, Seex K, Rao PJ. Lumbar interbody fusion: techniques, indications and comparison of interbody fusion options including PLIF, TLIF, MI-TLIF, OLIF/ATP, LLIF and ALIF. J spine Surg (Hong Kong). 2015;1(1):2–18. https://doi.org/10.3978/j.issn.2414-469X.2015.10.05.

21. Manzur MK, Samuel AM, Morse KW, et al. Indirect lumbar decompression combined with or without additional direct posterior decompression: a systematic review. Glob Spine J. 2021;12:21925682211013012. https://doi.org/10.1177/21925682211013011.

22. McAfee PC, Regan JJ, Peter Geis W, Fedder IL. Minimally invasive anterior retroperitoneal approach to the lumbar spine. Emphasis on the lateral BAK. Spine (Phila Pa 1976). 1998;23(13):1476–84. https://doi.org/10.1097/00007632-199807010-00009.

23. Buckland AJ, Ashayeri K, Leon C, et al. Single position circumferential fusion improves operative efficiency, reduces complications and length of stay compared with traditional circumferential fusion. Spine J. 2021;21(5):810–20. https://doi.org/10.1016/j.spinee.2020.11.002.
24. Avrumova F, Sivaganesan A, Alluri RK, Vaishnav A, Qureshi S, Lebl DR. Workflow and efficiency of robotic-assisted navigation in spine surgery. HSS J. 2021;17:15563316211026658. https://doi.org/10.1177/15563316211026658.
25. Alluri RK, Clark N, Sheha ED, et al. Location of the femoral nerve in the lateral decubitus versus prone position. Global Spine J. 2023;13(7):1765–70.
26. Godzik J, Ohiorhenuan IE, Xu DS, et al. Single-position prone lateral approach: cadaveric feasibility study and early clinical experience. Neurosurg Focus. 2020;49(3):E15. https://doi.org/10.3171/2020.6.FOCUS20359.
27. Pimenta L, Taylor WR, Stone LE, Wali AR, Santiago-Dieppa DR. Prone Transpsoas technique for simultaneous single-position access to the anterior and posterior lumbar spine. Oper Neurosurg (Hagerstown, Md). 2020;20(1):E5–E12. https://doi.org/10.1093/ons/opaa328.
28. Li JXJ, Phan K, Mobbs R. Oblique lumbar interbody fusion: technical aspects, operative outcomes, and complications. World Neurosurg. 2017;98:113–23. https://doi.org/10.1016/j.wneu.2016.10.074.
29. Molinares DM, Davis TT, Fung DA. Retroperitoneal oblique corridor to the L2-S1 intervertebral discs: an MRI study. J Neurosurg Spine. 2016;24(2):248–55. https://doi.org/10.3171/2015.3.SPINE13976.
30. Walker CT, Harrison Farber S, Cole TS, et al. Complications for minimally invasive lateral interbody arthrodesis: a systematic review and meta-analysis comparing prepsoas and transpsoas approaches. J Neurosurg Spine. 2019;30(4):446–60. https://doi.org/10.3171/2018.9.SPINE18800.
31. Davis TT, Hynes RA, Fung DA, et al. Retroperitoneal oblique corridor to the L2-S1 intervertebral discs in the lateral position: an anatomic study. J Neurosurg Spine. 2014;21(5):785–93. https://doi.org/10.3171/2014.7.SPINE13564.
32. Zhang F, Xu H, Yin B, et al. Does right lateral decubitus position change retroperitoneal oblique corridor? A radiographic evaluation from L1 to L5. Eur Spine J. 2017;26(3):646–50. https://doi.org/10.1007/s00586-016-4645-7.
33. Julian Li JX, Mobbs RJ, Phan K. Morphometric MRI imaging study of the corridor for the oblique lumbar interbody fusion technique at L1-L5. World Neurosurg. 2018;111:e678–85. https://doi.org/10.1016/j.wneu.2017.12.136.
34. Shirahata T, Okano I, Salzmann SN, et al. Association between surgical level and early postoperative thigh symptoms among patients undergoing standalone lateral lumbar interbody fusion. World Neurosurg. 2020;134:e885–91. https://doi.org/10.1016/j.wneu.2019.11.025.
35. Cummock MD, Vanni S, Levi AD, Yu Y, Wang MY. An analysis of postoperative thigh symptoms after minimally invasive transpsoas lumbar interbody fusion. J Neurosurg Spine. 2011;15(1):11–8. https://doi.org/10.3171/2011.2.SPINE10374.
36. Knight RQ, Schwaegler P, Hanscom D, Roh J. Direct lateral lumbar interbody fusion for degenerative conditions: early complication profile. J Spinal Disord Tech. 2009;22(1):34–7. https://doi.org/10.1097/BSD.0b013e3181679b8a.
37. Bergey DL, Villavicencio AT, Goldstein T, Regan JJ. Endoscopic lateral transpsoas approach to the lumbar spine. Spine (Phila Pa 1976). 2004;29(15):1681–8. https://doi.org/10.1097/01.brs.0000133643.75795.ef.
38. Cahill KS, Martinez JL, Wang MY, Vanni S, Levi AD. Motor nerve injuries following the minimally invasive lateral transpsoas approach: clinical article. J Neurosurg Spine. 2012;17(3):227–31. https://doi.org/10.3171/2012.5.SPINE1288.
39. Woods KRM, Billys JB, Hynes RA. Technical description of oblique lateral interbody fusion at L1-L5 (OLIF25) and at L5-S1 (OLIF51) and evaluation of complication and fusion rates. Spine J. 2017;17(4):545–53. https://doi.org/10.1016/j.spinee.2016.10.026.

40. Regev GJ, Haloman S, Chen L, et al. Incidence and prevention of intervertebral cage overhang with minimally invasive lateral approach fusions. Spine (Phila Pa 1976). 2010;35(14):1406–11. https://doi.org/10.1097/BRS.0b013e3181c20fb5.
41. Kubota G, Orita S, Umimura T, Takahashi K, Ohtori S. Insidious intraoperative ureteral injury as a complication in oblique lumbar interbody fusion surgery: a case report. BMC Res Notes. 2017;10(1):1–4. https://doi.org/10.1186/s13104-017-2509-9.
42. Lee H-J, Kim J-S, Ryu K-S, Park CK. Ureter injury as a complication of oblique lumbar interbody fusion. World Neurosurg. 2017;102:693.e7–693.e14. https://doi.org/10.1016/j.wneu.2017.04.038.
43. Iwanaga J, Yilmaz E, Tawfik T, et al. Anatomical study of the extreme lateral Transpsoas lumbar interbody fusion with application to minimizing injury to the kidney. Cureus. 2018;10(1):e2123. https://doi.org/10.7759/cureus.2123.
44. Wu A, March L, Zheng X, et al. Abdominal wall paresis as a complication of minimally invasive lateral transpsoas interbody fusion. Nature. 2020;388:1–14.

# Chapter 34
# Anterior Approaches to the Cervical Spine

Michael Hammer, Claire van Ekdom, Brian Panish, and Eric Feuchtbaum

## Introduction

This textbook primarily concerns the anterior and lateral approaches to the lumbar spine. However, the anterior approach to the cervical spine remains one of the most important and commonly utilized surgical techniques in spine surgery. For this reason, it is detailed here. The anterolateral approach to the cervical spine, also known as the Smith-Robinson approach, generally gives surgical access to the anterior region of the third to the seventh cervical vertebrae and, depending on patient specific anatomy, to the second cervical and first thoracic vertebrae as well [1]. It is often the approach of choice for anterior cervical discectomy and fusion (ACDF), corpectomy, and cervical disc arthroplasty.

## Anterolateral Approach

### Positioning

The patient is positioned supine on the operating table with head and neck in a neutral to slightly extended alignment [2]. The surgeon may place a rolled towel transversely between the shoulder blades to assist with shoulder retraction and neck

M. Hammer
Georgetown University School-Medicine, Washington, DC, USA

C. van Ekdom · E. Feuchtbaum (✉)
Ortho Bethesda, Bethesda, MD, USA
e-mail: efeuchtbaum@bcc-ortho.com

B. Panish
Harbor-UCLA Medical Center, Torrance, CA, USA

© The Author(s), under exclusive license to Springer Nature Switzerland AG 2023
J. R. O'Brien et al. (eds.), *Lumbar Spine Access Surgery*,
https://doi.org/10.1007/978-3-031-48034-8_34

extension [3]. Advantages to neck extension include increased surface area of the anterior aspect of the neck and increased height of the anterior portion of the inter-vertebral discs, and sufficient extension can help prevent postoperative kyphosis. However, cervical hyperextension can increase canal stenosis and result in neuro-logical injury. In some cases where the patient has critical canal stenosis, any exten-sion should be avoided, and the patient's head and neck should remain in neutral alignment.

Approach from the left or right depends on surgeon preference and training. Right-handed surgeons may find approaching from the right side easier, while left-handed surgeons may prefer the opposite [4]. If a patient has a possible laryngeal nerve palsy on one side of their neck from a prior surgery, consultation with otolar-yngology for video laryngoscopy and vocal cord analysis should be performed, and in the case of a palsy, the surgeon should choose to perform their approach on ipsi-lateral side to avoid bilateral laryngeal nerve palsy.

The surgeon verifies that there is proper padding of all bony prominences, that the eyes are protected, and that the patient has been prepped and draped in the usual sterile fashion. Intraoperative traction is achieved using halter traction, Gardner-Wells tongs, Mayfield clamp, or headrest [2]. Then, the typical time-out is performed.

## *Incision*

The surgeon locates the index level by identifying visible surface landmarks. The mandibular angle approximates the C2–C3 disc space [5]. The hyoid bone approxi-mates the C3–C4 disc space. The thyroid cartilage approximates the C4–C5 disc space, and the cricoid cartilage and the carotid tubercle approximate the sixth cervi-cal vertebrae. The surgeon may use a radiopaque marker and fluoroscopy to identify where they intend to make their incision.

A single transverse incision generally allows access to two to three levels, but by extending the incision and performing a larger fascial dissection, more levels may be accessed [4]. The surgeon begins the transverse incision about a centimeter con-tralateral to the midline, crosses the midline, and terminates the incision shortly after crossing the border of the ipsilateral sternocleidomastoid (SCM). The surgeon may opt to perform a longitudinal incision when the surgery is more than three levels [6]. The surgeon begins a longitudinal incision at the uppermost surgical level just medial to the border of the edge of the SCM and extends the incision parallel to the border of the SCM muscle to the lowermost level of surgery. Advantages to the transverse incision over a longitudinal incision are that the post-operative scar is more discrete as it tends to blend in with the natural lines of the neck [6]. However, a transverse incision may provide less exposure compared to a longitudinal incision.

## *Dissection*

After incising the skin, the dissection is carried to the level of the platysma muscle [4]. The surgeon incises the investing layer of deep cervical fascia, retracts the medial border of the SCM laterally, and skeletonizes the omohyoid muscle. The trachea and esophagus are retracted medially.

Next, the surgeon feels for the carotid pulse, thereby locating the carotid sheath. The surgeon incises the pretracheal fascia where it meets the medial side of the carotid sheath so as to separate the pretracheal fascia from the carotid sheath. The carotid sheath is moved laterally with gentle retraction. Blunt dissection is used to create an opening down to the prevertebral fascia, often with Kittner dissectors. A longitudinal incision is made to open the prevertebral fascia. The surgeon then mobilizes the longus colli muscles with bipolar electrocautery and places retractors underneath the longus colli. Caspar pins are localized with C-arm fluoroscopy to confirm the correct level before proceeding with discectomy.

It is important to note that inserting pins into the disc has been shown to contribute to disc degeneration. A less experienced surgeon and a single-level procedure are two factors that increase the likelihood of inserting a pin into a disc that was not intended for surgery. In these cases, the surgeon should consider confirming the level with other methods. One example is putting a radio-opaque marker on the anterior longitudinal ligament (ALL) in the area overlying the level being confirmed [6]. The surgeon will employ cautery to control bleeding. There is generally not much bleeding incurred with this approach, and most is typically due to the epidural venous plexus.

## The Anterior Approach to the Upper Cervical Spine/Craniovertebral Junction

The transoral approach is indicated for pathologies located at the anterior cervical spine from the lower clivus to C2, such as pannus of rheumatoid arthritis, basilar invagination, and fractures requiring stabilization [2]. The transpalatal, transmandibular, and retropharyngeal approaches are other anterior upper cervical spine access techniques.

The transoral-transpharyngeal approach is the conventional approach used to expose the lower clivus, anterior arch of C1, odontoid process of C2, and anterior C2 vertebrae [7]. The transoral-transpharyngeal approach creates a smaller surgical window than other more extensive variations of the transoral approach. Therefore, it is indicated for pathologies that can be treated with smaller surgical fields, including degeneration that can be treated with decompression in a piecemeal fashion and small tumors that do not require vascular control.

## Transoral-Transpharyngeal Approach

### *Position*

The patient is positioned supine on the operating table, and the neck is put into slight extension [8]. The head may be fixed into position by Mayfield clamps or placed on a horseshoe support [9].

### *Preparation*

Orotracheal intubation, nasotracheal intubation, and tracheostomy are the three main methods of intubation for this approach [4]. Patients with possible compression at the cervico-medullary junction or cervical instability require fiber-optic orotracheal intubation. Gauze throat packs are positioned, and the oral cavity is disinfected using a solution such as Betadine or chlorhexidine gluconate oral solution [7, 9]. Broad-spectrum antibiotics are administered intravenously. A drape is positioned over the patient's face in a manner such that the mouth and nose areas are left open. The surgeon positions a self-retaining retractor over the teeth to keep the mouth expanded [7]. An additional self-retraining retractor is placed to depress the tongue. Every 30 minutes throughout the entire operation, the tongue retraction should be released and reapplied.

### *Incision and Discectomy*

The surgeon uses their fingers to palpate the posterior oropharynx to locate the underlying anterior arch of C1 and anterior vertebral body of C2 [10]. The anterior tubercle marks midline unless there is C1–C2 rotatory subluxation or atlantoaxial dislocation. Fluoroscopic images are taken to check the alignment of the palate, head, and neck to determine the surgical trajectory.

The surgeon makes a midline longitudinal incision at the posterior oropharynx from the inferior clivus down to the superior edge of C3 [10]. Using monopolar cautery or sharp dissection depending on preference, an incision is made through the posterior pharyngeal wall mucosa, pharyngeal muscles, and the ALL to bone. Care should be taken to keep the pharyngeal mucosa and fascia intact as a single layer for proper closure [11]. Subperiosteal dissection proceeds laterally on both sides freeing the anterior clivus, the body of C1, and the body of C2 from the overlying ALL and pharyngeal musculature. Self-retaining retractors are placed to retract the pharyngeal flaps laterally.

## Complications

Given the complex anatomy of the anterior cervical region, structures such as the esophagus, trachea, vasculature, and neural elements are at risk during anterior cervical spine surgery. Complications include dural tear and cerebrospinal fluid leak (CSF), esophageal injury, vascular injury and stroke, airway obstruction, dysphagia, and adjacent segment disease (ASD).

## Dural Tear and Cerebrospinal Fluid Leak

Yee et al. found that the incidence of CSF leak was 0.5% ($n = 32,229$) across 30 retrospective and 2 prospective studies [12]. A CSF collection can present as a neck mass with dysphagia and can lead to infection [13]. This is important because a neck mass from a CSF leak should undergo computed tomography (CT) scan prior to any treatment such as surgical repair, sterile fine needle aspiration, or incision and drainage [13]. The recommended treatment for a CSF leak after a cervical spine surgery is surgical repair if possible and lumbar drain placement in irreparable tears [14]. When a dural injury occurs intraoperatively and is identified, it can be treated intraoperatively to prevent a postoperative CSF leak [15]. Direct suture repair of the dural defect can be challenging in the anterior cervical spine and may necessitate a wider exposure or corpectomy for a direct repair. Multiple treatment modalities including collagen matrix, fibrin sealant, fat/muscle patching, or synthetic patching have been described, and many surgeons opt to combine multiple treatment modalities to achieve dural closure [16].

## Esophageal Injury

Yee et al. found esophageal perforation to have an incidence of 0.2% ($n = 12,842$) across 11 retrospective studies [12]. Postoperatively, esophageal injury typically presents with dysphagia, odynophagia, or an expanding fluctuant neck mass [12]. If an esophageal injury is suspected postoperatively, a mix of diagnostic modalities including contrast CT/magnetic resonance imaging (MRI) and contrast esophagography should be used prior to attempting surgical repair [17]. If an esophageal perforation is suspected clinically, it is important to surgically explore early and proceed with aggressive management with otolaryngology consultation [12]. Primary repair and reinforcement with a flap are effective treatment options for esophageal injuries [18–20]. Perforations that have been detected and treated within 24 hours have a high mortality rate as high as 20%; however, delays in treatment have seen mortality rates as high as 50% [12]. The removal of anterior hardware is essential to the treatment of esophageal perforations [18].

## Vascular Injury and Stroke

Yee et al. determined the incidence of vertebral artery injury to be 0.4% ($n = 3884$) across 11 studies [12]. Injury to the vertebral artery is a rare but a potentially life-threatening complication during cervical spine surgery. Tortuosity of the vertebral artery and asymmetric excessive far lateral bone removal are the two main scenarios that account for iatrogenic vertebral artery injury [21]. MRI and CT studies can be used preoperatively to avoid dilated or tortuous vertebral artery anatomy intraoperatively [21]. Damage to the vertebral artery during far lateral bone removal usually occurs when a decompression is taken too far laterally and there is overly aggressive drilling [21]. Maintaining midline orientation is key to preventing vertebral artery injury. When laceration of the vertebral artery does occur, initial treatment is tamponade, followed by microvascular repair or ligation [21]. If direct repair has failed, ligation of the vertebral artery should be the next option, but ligation carries the risk of cerebellar/brain stem infarction and has been reported to have a mortality rate of 12% [22]. Carotid artery injury by anterior cervical spine surgery is fairly rare; however, retraction of the carotid artery causes a reduction in blood flow, and prolonged retraction can induce a stroke [23–25].

## Airway Obstruction

Obstruction of the airway after anterior cervical spine surgery is typically caused by soft tissue edema or retropharyngeal hematoma and has been reported to have an incidence as high as 6% [26]. Symptoms typically develop 36 h postoperatively, and maximum swelling is observed on days two to four [27–29]. Risk factors for airway obstruction after anterior cervical spine surgery include exposing more than three vertebral levels, more than 300 mL of blood loss, operative time more than 5 h, and exposures involving C2, C3, and C4 [29, 30]. Lee et al. found that retropharyngeal local steroid significantly reduced prevertebral soft tissue swelling within 2 weeks of anterior cervical spine operations compared to no treatment [27].

## Dysphagia

Yee et al. found the incidence of dysphagia to be 5.3% at any time after surgery ($n = 737,041$) [12]. However, dysphagia is commonly reported initially after anterior cervical spine operations with a rate around 50% [31]. Female sex, revision surgery, multilevel surgery, and prolonged operative time have all been identified as risk factors for dysphagia [12, 31–34]. Studies have suggested prevertebral swelling, retraction, and cervical plate prominence as possible causes for dysphagia following anterior cervical spine operations [35]. Removal of anterior plating has been found to improve symptoms in up to 87% of patients with persistent severe dysphagia [33]. Dysphagia also improves over time after surgery [31]. Several preventative measures have been identified to reduce the risk of postoperative dysphagia including decreased operative time, using smaller cervical plates, application of steroid before wound closure, and decreasing tracheal cuff pressure during medial retraction [32].

## *Adjacent Segment Disease*

Adjacent segment disease (ASD) refers to degeneration of levels above or below a fusion construct, and it has been debated whether this phenomenon is a surgical complication or simply the progression of the natural history of cervical spondylosis. The classic study by Hilibrand et al. described a relatively constant 2.9% per year rate of symptomatic ASD following ACDF over 10 years [36]. This study also determined that patients who had more levels fused had lower rates of ASD, which is attributed to the progression of the natural history of cervical spondylosis [36]. Carrier et al. found patients to have symptomatic ASD with an incidence of 11.99% and patients with asymptomatic segment degeneration with an incidence of 47.33% [37]. Yee et al. found a pooled incidence related to ASD disease to be 4.5% ($n = 2600$) with a mean time to reoperation between 2.5 years and 3.1 years [12]. Currently, there is no statistically significant evidence that surgical procedure type affects the rate of reoperation due to ASD. Verma et al. compared rates of reoperation between ACDF and total disc arthroplasty patients and did not find a significant difference in reoperation rates ($n = 1586, p = 0.44$) [38].

## Clinical Guidelines

### *Diagnostics*

The neck disability index, short form-36, short form-12, and visual analog scale have been recommended by the North American Spine Society for assessing treatment of cervical radiculopathy from degenerative disorders [39, 40]. The common presenting symptoms of cervical radiculopathy are arm pain, neck pain, scapular pain, paresthesias, numbness, sensory changes, weakness, or abnormal deep tendon reflexes [40]. The more atypical presenting symptoms of cervical radiculopathy are deltoid weakness, scapular winging, weakness of the intrinsic muscles of the hand, chest pain, and headaches [40]. Physical examination including shoulder abduction and Spurling's tests may be considered in patients with symptoms consistent with cervical radiculopathy [40]. When a presenting patient has a high likelihood of cervical radiculopathy, MRI, CT, or CT myelography should be considered. MRI is suggested for the confirmation of a compressive lesion in patients who have failed a course of conservative therapy and who may be a candidate for surgical treatment [40]. CT myelography is suggested for patients who have a contraindication to MRI or signs that are discordant with MRI findings [40]. Selective nerve root block can be useful in the evaluation of patients with multilevel degenerative lesions identified on MRI or CT to determine the symptomatic level [41].

## Nonsurgical Treatment

Cervical traction, physical therapy, medications, and injections have been associated with improvements in patient-reported pain [40]. Cervical traction alone has been determined to be no better than placebo alone; however, while paired with physical therapy, cervical traction has been found to be superior than just physical therapy at 6 and 12 months [42]. Physical therapy has been found to give patients significant improvement during the first 6 weeks of cervical radiculopathy [42]. A short course of oral corticosteroids has been found to reduce radiculopathy-related pain in the short term [42]. Transforaminal epidural steroid injection may provide relief for 60% of patients, and about 25% of patients may achieve relief to negate the need for surgery [40]. Despite the relief provided for patients, transforaminal epidural steroid injection carry the risk of spinal cord injury and even possibly death. Roughly 88% of patients will improve within 4 weeks of nonoperative management of their symptoms [42].

## Surgical Treatment and Outcomes

ACDF provides more rapid relief over a 4-month period with continued gains over a 12-month period compared to physical therapy or cervical immobilization [43]. In the treatment of single-level disease, anterior plating may reduce the risk of pseudoarthrosis and graft problems [44]. An interbody graft is also useful for improving sagittal alignment [44]. Jacobs et al. examined 2267 patients in 33 studies and demonstrated that there was no significant difference in pain relief with one- and two-level ACDF that utilized autograft, allograft, or synthetic [45]. They found moderate-quality evidence that bone graft produced more effective fusion than discectomy alone [45]. ACDF and total disc arthroplasty result in similarly successful outcomes for single-level degenerative cervical radiculopathy [40]. Boselie et al. reviewed 9 studies including 2400 patients and found high-quality evidence that segmental mobility was statistically significantly higher with arthroplasty at 1 to 2 years when comparing to cervical fusion [46].

# Conclusion

The anterior approaches to the cervical spine are versatile and, with proper execution, safe and effective. Any surgeon who operates in the area should be familiar with their implementation and aware of the possible risks to best help patients undergo informed consent, as well as identify and manage complications in the perioperative and postoperative settings. Complications such as dysphagia, spinal fluid leak, esophageal injury, vascular injury, airway obstruction, and adjacent segment disease can range from minor to life-threatening, and early identification and treatment can mean the difference between life and death in some instances.

# References


1. Arumalla K, Bansal H, Jadeja J, et al. Anterior approach to the cervical spine: elegance lies in its simplicity. Asian. J Neurosurg. 2021;16(4):669–84. Published 2021 Dec 18. https://doi.org/10.4103/ajns.AJNS_313_20.
2. Tandon M, Saigal D. Essentials of neuroanethesia: spinal surgery. Cambridge, MA: Academic; 2017. p. 399–439. https://doi.org/10.1016/B978-0-12-805299-0.00024-5.
3. Vigo V, Pastor-Escartín F, Doniz-Gonzalez A, et al. The smith-Robinson approach to the subaxial cervical spine: a stepwise microsurgical technique using volumetric models from anatomic dissections. Oper Neurosurg (Hagerstown). 2020;20(1):83–90. https://doi.org/10.1093/ons/opaa265.
4. Cheung KM, Mak KC, Luk KD. Anterior approach to cervical spine. Spine (Phila Pa 1976). 2012;37(5):E297–302. https://doi.org/10.1097/BRS.0b013e318239ccd8.
5. Siribumrungwong K, Sinchai C, Tangtrakulwanich B, Chaiyamongkol W. Reliability and accuracy of palpable anterior neck landmarks for the identification of cervical spinal levels. Asian Spine J. 2018;12(1):80–4. https://doi.org/10.4184/asj.2018.12.1.80.
6. Razi A, Saleh H, DeLacure MD, Kim Y. Anterior approach to the subaxial cervical spine: pearls and pitfalls. J Am Acad Orthop Surg. 2021;29(5):189–95. https://doi.org/10.5435/JAAOS-D-17-00891.
7. Hsu W, Wolinsky JP, Gokaslan ZL, Sciubba DM. Transoral approaches to the cervical spine. Neurosurgery. 2010;66(3 Suppl):119–25. https://doi.org/10.1227/01.NEU.0000365748.00721.0B.
8. Watkins RG. Transoral approach to C1–C2. In: Watkins III R, Watkins IV R, editors. Surgical approaches to the spine. New York, NY: Springer; 2015. https://doi.org/10.1007/978-1-4939-2465-3_2.
9. Li W, Wang B, Feng X, Hua W, Yang C. Preoperative management and postoperative complications associated with transoral decompression for the upper cervical spine. BMC Musculoskelet Disord. 2022;23(1):128. https://doi.org/10.1186/s12891-022-05081-7.
10. Crockard HA. Transoral surgery: some lessons learned. Br J Neurosurg. 1995;9(3):283–93. https://doi.org/10.1080/02688699550041304.
11. Apostolides P, Vishteh A, Galler R, Sonntag V. Technique of transoral odontoidectomy. In: Mayer HM, editor. Minimally invasive spine surgery. Berlin: Springer; 2006. https://doi.org/10.1007/3-540-29490-2_7.
12. Yee TJ, Swong K, Park P. Complications of anterior cervical spine surgery: a systematic review of the literature. J Spine Surg. 2020;6(1):302–22. https://doi.org/10.21037/jss.2020.01.14.

13. Schaberg MR, Altman JI, Shapshay SM, Woo P. Cerebrospinal fluid leak after anterior cervical disc fusion: an unusual cause of dysphagia and neck mass. Laryngoscope. 2007;117(11):1899–901. https://doi.org/10.1097/mlg.0b013e31812eee01.

14. Fountas KN, Kapsalaki EZ, Johnston KW. Cerebrospinal fluid fistula secondary to dural tear in anterior cervical discectomy and fusion. Spine. 2005;30(10):E277–80. https://doi.org/10.1097/01.brs.0000162399.93992.5c.

15. Sugawara T, Itoh Y, Hirano Y, Higashiyama N, Shimada Y, Kinouchi H, et al. Novel dural closure technique using polyglactin acid sheet prevents cerebrospinal fluid leakage after spinal surgery. Neurosurgery. 2005;57(suppl_4):ONS-290-ONS-294. https://doi.org/10.1227/01.neu.0000176410.65750.c0.

16. Fang Z, Tian R, Jia Y-T, Xu T-T, Liu Y. Treatment of cerebrospinal fluid leak after spine surgery. Chin J Traumatol. 2017;20(2):81–3. https://doi.org/10.1016/j.cjtee.2016.12.002.

17. Lee TS, Appelbaum EN, Sheen D, Han R, Wie B. Esophageal perforation due to anterior cervical spine hardware placement: case series. Int J Otolaryngol. 2019;2019:1–9. https://doi.org/10.1155/2019/7682654.

18. Dakwar E, Uribe JS, Padhya TA, Vale FL. Management of delayed esophageal perforations after anterior cervical spinal surgery. SPI. 2009;11(3):320–5. https://doi.org/10.3171/2009.3.spine08522.

19. Dantas FLR, Dantas F, Mendes PD, Sandes BL, Fonseca FG. Primary repair of esophageal perforation following anterior cervical fusion. Cureus. 2020;12(11):e11590. https://doi.org/10.7759/cureus.11590.

20. Kang MS, Kim KH, Park JY, Kuh SU, Chin DK, Jin BH, et al. Management of Esophageal and Pharyngeal Perforation as complications of anterior cervical spine surgery. World Neurosurg. 2017;102:275–83. https://doi.org/10.1016/j.wneu.2017.02.130.

21. Burke JP, Gerszten PC, Welch WC. Iatrogenic vertebral artery injury during anterior cervical spine surgery. Spine J. 2005;5(5):508–14. https://doi.org/10.1016/j.spinee.2004.11.015.

22. Hershman SH, Kunkle WA, Kelly MP, Buchowski JM, Ray WZ, Bumpass DB, et al. Esophageal perforation following anterior cervical spine surgery: case report and review of the literature. Glob Spine J. 2017;7(1_suppl):28S–36S. https://doi.org/10.1177/2192568216687535.

23. Inamasu J, Guiot BH. Iatrogenic carotid artery injury in neurosurgery. Neurosurg Rev. 2005;28(4):239–47. https://doi.org/10.1007/s10143-005-0412-7.

24. Pollard ME, Little PW. Changes in carotid artery blood flow during anterior cervical spine surgery. Spine. 2002;27(2):152–5. https://doi.org/10.1097/00007632-200201150-00006.

25. Yeh Y-C, Sun W-Z, Lin C-P, Hui C-K, Huang I-R, Lee T-S. Prolonged retraction on the Normal common carotid artery induced lethal stroke after cervical spine surgery. Spine. 2004;29(19):E431–4. https://doi.org/10.1097/01.brs.0000141177.95850.b1.

26. Sagi HC, Beutler W, Carroll E, Connolly PJ. Airway complications associated with surgery on the anterior cervical spine. Spine. 2002;27(9):949–53. https://doi.org/10.1097/00007632-200205010-00013.

27. Shintani A, Zervas NT. Consequence of ligation of the vertebral artery. J Neurosurg. 1972;36(4):447–50. https://doi.org/10.3171/jns.1972.36.4.0447.

28. Lee S-H, Kim K-T, Suk K-S, Park K-J, Oh K-I. Effect of retropharyngeal steroid on prevertebral soft tissue swelling following anterior cervical discectomy and fusion. Spine. 2011;36(26):2286–92. https://doi.org/10.1097/brs.0b013e318237e5d0.

29. Suk K-S, Kim K-T, Lee S-H, Park S-W. Prevertebral soft tissue swelling after anterior cervical discectomy and fusion with plate fixation. Int Orthop. 2006;30:290. https://doi.org/10.1007/s00264-005-0072-9.

30. Kwon B, Yoo JU, Furey CG, Rowbottom J, Emery SE. Risk factors for delayed Extubation after single-stage, multi-level anterior cervical decompression and posterior fusion. J Spinal Disord Techn. 2006;19(6):389–93. https://doi.org/10.1097/00024720-200608000-00002.

31. Bazaz R, Lee MJ, Yoo JU. Incidence of dysphagia after anterior cervical spine surgery. Spine. 2002;27(22):2453–8. https://doi.org/10.1097/00007632-200211150-00007.

32. Lee MJ, Bazaz R, Furey CG, Yoo J. Risk factors for dysphagia after anterior cervical spine surgery: a two-year prospective cohort study. Spine J. 2007;7(2):141–7. https://doi.org/10.1016/j.spinee.2006.02.024.

33. Joaquim AF, Murar J, Savage JW, Patel AA. Dysphagia after anterior cervical spine surgery: a systematic review of potential preventative measures. Spine J. 2014;14(9):2246–60. https://doi.org/10.1016/j.spinee.2014.03.030.

34. Cho SK, Lu Y, Lee D-H. Dysphagia following anterior cervical spinal surgery. Bone Joint J. 2013;95-B(7):868–73. https://doi.org/10.1302/0301-620X.95B7.31029.

35. Fogel GR, McDonnell MF. Surgical treatment of dysphagia after anterior cervical interbody fusion. Spine J. 2005;5(2):140–4. https://doi.org/10.1016/j.spinee.2004.06.022.

36. Hilibrand AS, Carlson GD, Palumbo MA, Jones PK, Bohlman HH. Radiculopathy and myelopathy at segments adjacent to the site of a previous anterior cervical arthrodesis. JBJS. 1999;81(4):519–28.

37. Carrier CS, Bono CM, Lebl DR. Evidence-based analysis of adjacent segment degeneration and disease after ACDF: a systematic review. Spine J. 2013;13(10):1370–8.

38. Verma K, Gandhi SD, Maltenfort M, Albert TJ, Hilibrand AS, Vaccaro AR, Radcliff KE. Rate of adjacent segment disease in cervical disc arthroplasty versus single-level fusion: meta-analysis of prospective studies. Spine. 2013;38(26):2253–7.

39. Mummaneni PV, Kaiser MG, Matz PG, Anderson PA, Groff MW, Heary RF, et al. Cervical surgical techniques for the treatment of cervical spondylotic myelopathy. SPI. 2009;11(2):130–41. https://doi.org/10.3171/2009.3.SPINE08728.

40. Bono CM, Ghiselli G, Gilbert TJ, Kreiner DS, Reitman C, Summers JT, et al. An evidence-based clinical guideline for the diagnosis and treatment of cervical radiculopathy from degenerative disorders. Spine J. 2011;11(1):64–72. https://doi.org/10.1016/j.spinee.2010.10.023.

41. Anderberg L, Annertz M, Rydholm U, Brandt L, Säveland H. Selective diagnostic nerve root block for the evaluation of radicular pain in the multilevel degenerated cervical spine. Eur Spine J. 2006;15(6):794–801. https://doi.org/10.1007/s00586-005-0931-5.

42. Childress MA, Becker BA. Nonoperative management of cervical radiculopathy. Am Fam Physician. 2016;93(9):746–54.

43. Matz PG, Holly LT, Groff MW, Vresilovic EJ, Anderson PA, Heary RF, et al. Indications for anterior cervical decompression for the treatment of cervical degenerative radiculopathy. SPI. 2009;11(2):174–82. https://doi.org/10.3171/2009.3.SPINE08720.

44. Matz PG, Ryken TC, Groff MW, Vresilovic EJ, Anderson PA, Heary RF, et al. Techniques for anterior cervical decompression for radiculopathy. SPI. 2009;11(2):183–97. https://doi.org/10.3171/2009.2.SPINE08721.

45. Jacobs W, Willems PC, van Limbeek J, Bartels R, Pavlov P, Anderson PG, et al. Single or double-level anterior interbody fusion techniques for cervical degenerative disc disease. Cochrane Database Syst Rev. 2011;1:CD004958. https://doi.org/10.1002/14651858.CD004958.pub2.

46. Boselie TF, Willems PC, van Mameren H, de Bie R, Benzel EC, van Santbrink H. Arthroplasty versus fusion in single-level cervical degenerative disc disease. Cochrane Database Syst Rev. 2012;9:CD009173. https://doi.org/10.1002/14651858.CD009173.pub2.

# Index



© The Editor(s) (if applicable) and The Author(s), under exclusive license to
Springer Nature Switzerland AG 2023
J. R. O'Brien et al. (eds.), *Lumbar Spine Access Surgery*,
https://doi.org/10.1007/978-3-031-48034-8

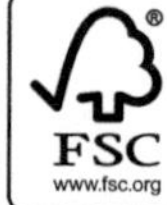

**MIX**
Papier aus verantwortungsvollen Quellen
Paper from responsible sources
FSC® C105338

If you have any concerns about our products,
you can contact us on
ProductSafety@springernature.com

In case Publisher is established outside the EU,
the EU authorized representative is:
**Springer Nature Customer Service Center GmbH
Europaplatz 3, 69115 Heidelberg, Germany**

Printed by Libri Plureos GmbH
in Hamburg, Germany